# The Best Hospitals
## in America

# THE BEST
# HOSPITALS
## IN AMERICA
—

by Linda Sunshine and John W. Wright

HENRY HOLT AND COMPANY
NEW YORK

Dedicated to the memory of both
Dr. Harold K. Sunshine and
Louis P. Forster

Library of Congress Cataloging-in-Publication Data
Sunshine, Linda.
The best hospitals in America.
Includes index.
1. Hospitals—United States—Directories.
2. Medicine—Specialties and specialists—United States—Directories.
3. Consumer education.   I. Wright, John W., 1941–    .   II. Title.
[DNLM: 1. Hospitals—United States—popular works. WX 27 AA1 S89b]
RA981.A2S86   1987      362.1′1′02573      87-7535
ISBN 0-8050-0583-8

First Edition

Designer: Ann Gold
Printed in the United States of America
1   3   5   7   9   10   8   6   4   2

ISBN 0-8050-0583-8

# Contents

# An Important Note to Our Readers

Because the practice of medicine and the administration of hospital care is conducted by fallible human beings, we cannot and do not in any way guarantee that you will receive flawless medical treatment at the hospitals, clinics, and medical centers described in this book. While this book describes some of the finest medical institutions in the world, errors in judgment can happen even at the best hospitals. We cannot, therefore, be held responsible for any medical mishap or malpractice that might occur if you choose one of these institutions as a result of reading this book.

Please note, too, that all of the facts and figures in the book have been reviewed by representatives of the hospitals we've included and are based on material gathered through January 1987. Some of the information will no doubt change—doctors can and often do switch their affiliations, and room charges usually go up each year—so we recommend that you call the hospital directly if you have any questions. This is especially true regarding admissions policies and financial requirements, which, in today's volatile hospital environment, could change suddenly at some institutions.

# Acknowledgments

Over the last decade or so several magazines have regularly run lists of "best hospitals," but as far as we know this is the first book of its kind ever published. Although our Introduction makes it clear that the results are based on extensive research, we do not claim to be professionals in the health-care field. We are writers—journalists, if you prefer—who have searched for reliable information on behalf of prospective patients, who in today's dramatically changing hospital world need all the help and advice they can get. We, of course, had a great deal of assistance.

From inception, this book has had the solid underpinning of continuous consultation with physicians in various regions of the country; we need to offer a special word of thanks to the many physicians who helped us, some of them at every stage of the book's development. At the very beginning of our research our discussions with Drs. Frank Harford and Robert Leupold helped us to develop our first set of criteria and to compile our initial list of hospitals. Over the next few months we consulted further with physicians around the country both about our criteria (which some of them helped us to refine) for determining excellence in hospital care and about specific hospitals in their regions and specialties. They included: Drs. Najib Bouz, Melvin Britton, Peter Buckley, Thomas Bunch, Harris Burstin, William Conway, Roger Enlow, John Ervin, Thomas Ferguson, Irving Fox, Charles Goldberg, Francis Goldstein, Stewart Greisman, George Griffin, James Halper, John Hurley, David Martin, Ellen Millis, Desmond O'Duffy, Martin Oster, Marc Rubinstein, Irwin Steiger, Steven Tay, Robert Treat, and Michael Wise. A number of other physicians spoke to us—and quite candidly, too—but only on the condition that they remain anonymous. As our list of hospitals continued to take shape, we went back to several of these doctors for further advice. Of course not all of them would comment on every hospital and not every hospital they recommended was included, although we frequently mention those institutions in the introductory remarks to hospitals in the same area. In the end, the final choices were ours.

We also learned a great deal from the published articles and books about hospitals written by physicians, including Arnold Relman, the editor of the prestigious *New England Journal of Medicine*, Joyce Craddick, Herbert Dietrich, Steven Jones, William Schwartz, and John Wennberg, although we wish to make clear that none of these doctors specifically recommended hospitals to us.

Throughout the project we had help and advice from numerous other sources. We would like to thank the people at the Health Care Financing Administration, especially Phillip Cotterill and Karen Beebe, for their patience and cooperation in obtaining and explaining the complexity of care lists compiled for Medicare purposes. We also wish to acknowledge the public affairs staff at the Joint Commission on Accreditation of Hospitals for their help in explaining the procedures for hospital evaluation, and numerous people in various parts of the NIH who gave us information on a continuing basis, always courteously and efficiently.

In addition, we sought and received information from a large number of organizations, including the American Academy of Nursing, the American College of Cardiology, the Arthritis Foundation, Council of Teaching Hospitals, the Cystic Fibrosis Foundation, the MS Foundation, and the Trauma Foundation.

A special word of thanks must also be given to the more than 150 people in public affairs and communications departments at all of the hospitals we contacted. Their patience in dealing with our questions and their cooperation in trying to obtain detailed facts and figures from doctors and administrators—even when they met strong resistance—have made this a much better book.

Finally, we would like to offer our gratitude to Connie Clausen for her support of this project at the very beginning; to Donald Lorimer and Jerry Kappes for their help during our initial stages of research; to the copy editor, Susan Brown; and to the extraordinary people at Henry Holt and Company—especially Pat Breinin, Rachel Christmas, and Channa Taub for their faith, trust, and patience.

# The Best Hospitals
## in America

# Introduction

When you or someone you love is ill and needs special medical attention, how do you go about finding the best possible hospital to treat that illness? Unless you need immediate emergency room services—when the closest place may be the best place—you probably select a hospital because of its location or, more likely still, on the recommendation of a single doctor. Yet hospital care can vary greatly from one institution to another, and such an uninformed decision may not serve you well. In a medical crisis you want to find the best hospital, one capable of delivering the most advanced care. This book can help.

*The Best Hospitals in America* is the first comprehensive guide to the services offered at the most prestigious medical institutions in the nation and, consequently, in the world. Based on the recommendations of physicians from around the country and supported by information from government sources, professional and popular publications, and interviews with more than 150 hospitals, this book provides the kind of authoritative background patients and their families need to choose the right hospital. For while our research has convinced us that there are hundreds of first-rate hospitals in this country, we also discovered that it is often difficult for the general public to distinguish the first-rate hospitals from those that are mediocre or even less than adequate. Our intention is to help remedy that situation by identifying hospitals and medical centers whose special qualities have earned them the highest standing in American medicine.

At these institutions can be found many of the world's leading physicians, the most up-to-date, state-of-the-art medical technology, and, in almost every instance, the most prestigious medical research programs. Most important, these hospitals are known within the medical community for their ability to treat the most complicated types of illness in a wide range of specialties or, for a few of the hospitals included, in specific areas, such as cancer or orthopedics. All these hospitals are regional referral centers and in a few cases national and international referral centers offering the most advanced forms of medical practice available today. In other words, these are places to which physicians in other hospitals often send their sickest patients. And with good reason.

The hospitals profiled in this book are home to many of the most highly regarded medical programs in the nation. Included here are such extraordinary services as the Cleveland Clinic's program in cardiac surgery, the cancer treatment center at the Mayo Clinic, the programs in diabetes at Barnes Hospital in St. Louis, stroke rehabilitation at Columbia-Presbyterian Medical Center in New York, heart transplantation at the University of Alabama, and neonatology at Brigham and Women's in Boston. Other programs, such as the liver transplant program at Presbyterian-University Hos-

1

pital in Pittsburgh, or the bone marrow transplant program at the Fred Hutchinson Cancer Research Center in Seattle, are known throughout the world for their pioneering efforts in these relatively new areas. We've also included many programs that are painstakingly developing new diagnostic procedures and treatments for such little-understood diseases as melanoma (NYU Medical Center), ALS, or Lou Gehrig's disease (University of Chicago), Alzheimer's disease (Johns Hopkins), and many more. In this way, patients suffering from a particular condition can learn of the special programs available to treat that condition, including clinical research projects or experimental treatments not widely known that may offer new hope.

Until recently, this kind of information was the special province of those in the medical profession and the hospital industry. Over the last decade or so, however, the explosion of public interest in all health-care-related issues has created an audience of informed patients who believe in the importance of participating in all decisions relating to one's own medical care. With the information in this book, you will be able, either alone or with a physician, to find outstanding treatment centers for just about any serious illness. The institutions included here are listed by state, so you will be able to select a hospital in your area. However, for certain serious conditions you may be willing to travel to receive the most advanced care. This book can also help you pinpoint the particular hospital or hospitals throughout the country that specialize in the condition you or a family member or friend is suffering from.

Many patients feel that the choice of hospital is far less significant than the choice of doctor. Several recent studies have shown, however, that *where* you are hospitalized can be more important, especially when surgery is involved. Contrary to what most of us have been led to believe, the kind of treatment received from hospital to hospital, even in the same geographic area, is sometimes so dramatically different that choosing a particular hospital can literally determine your medical treatment. Dr. John Wennberg and his colleagues at Dartmouth Medical School have been conducting research in this area for over fifteen years. By examining variations in the frequency rates for common surgical procedures, Dr. Wennberg has demonstrated that most surgeons act in accordance with local medical standards rather than with any understanding of the latest clinical developments. Here are some of his findings for three of the most commonly performed surgical procedures: hysterectomies (over 650,000 are performed annually), tonsillectomies (400,000), and prostatectomies (350,000).

- In one Maine hospital market, women at age seventy had a 50 percent greater likelihood of having had a hysterectomy than women in another part of the *same* state.
- In Vermont the probability of children undergoing a tonsillectomy ranged from a low of 8 percent in one hospital market to a high of nearly 70 percent in another.

- In Iowa the chances that male residents who reach age eighty-five had undergone a prostatectomy range from a low of 15 percent to a high of more than 60 percent in different hospital markets.

Since most of us think of routine operations as, well, routine, figures such as these startle us. We cannot help but be alarmed at this discovery that medicine is not always an exact science. Although Dr. Wennberg notes that once doctors have been shown that their surgical rates are far out of line with regional and national norms they immediately change their approach to these procedures, it is still distressing to observe that the decision to operate is often subjective and sometimes grounded in ignorance.

Dr. Wennberg's research, which also covers variations in the causes of hospital admissions and in diagnostic testing, has recently been used to demonstrate how overutilization of hospitals has been responsible for the soaring costs of hospital care. His contention, in testimony given before Congress in 1984, that hospital costs could be cut by 40 percent if national norms for admissions, surgery, and similar areas could be established has received a great deal of attention and support. But the emphasis on cost cutting should not obscure another savings often more important to hospital patients, the reduction in the mortality rate when unnecessary surgery is eliminated. According to Dr. Wennberg, if, for example, a more conservative approach were taken toward prostatectomy, there would be about 1,900 postoperative deaths as opposed to 6,800 deaths under the more liberal approach.

In other words, many of us fail to realize that all surgical procedures carry some risk, and if we were sufficiently apprised of the magnitude of that risk we might not find it acceptable. Dr. John Bunker, author of *Costs, Risks and Benefits of Surgery*, believes that of the more than 25 million surgical procedures performed each year in our short-stay hospitals perhaps as many as 85 percent are to relieve discomfort or remove a disability or disfigurement, not for conditions that threaten life.

One reason we have so much surgery in this country is that we have so many surgeons, just over 100,000, about twice as many per million of population as in Great Britain, where the per capita rate of surgery is half what it is here. Still, the basic health and life expectancy rates of the British population compare favorably with our own. So even though, as some critics have pointed out, the British system is woefully lacking in its ability to provide open-heart surgery or hemodialysis to patients in need, it's hard to see what Americans have gained by our zealous pursuit of some very expensive medical procedures. In fact, there is strong evidence that we'd be far better off if we eliminated a large portion of the elective surgery that goes on today.

A most telling example of such dangers occurred in Los Angeles in 1976, when many doctors participated in a five-week slowdown, during which only emergency surgery was performed. According to Dr. Bunker, the total population mortality rate for Los Angeles County fell by approximately one-third; it rose again soon after elective surgery was resumed.

In recent years questions about the quality of patient care have gone beyond the area of elective surgery. The professional medical and hospital literature has documented what many doctors and health-care professionals have known for years—that staying in a hospital can sometimes be a dangerous or hazardous experience. In 1983 the Centers for Disease Control estimated that of 38.7 million patients discharged by the nation's hospitals, 1.9 million had acquired new diseases in the hospital, and of those, 96,000 died of causes attributed wholly or in part to these new diseases. In 1984, when there were 1.5 million fewer inpatients, an estimated 75,000 fewer became sick in the hospital, and about 3,700 fewer patients died. Quipped John Rother of the American Association of Retired Persons, "Less hospitalization in most cases is a step forward."

Over the last decade a host of formal studies conducted by doctors, academics, hospital consultants, and insurance companies has only confirmed that statement. Some health-care professionals estimate that *at least* 20 percent of all hospital patients experience some kind of complication or adverse event either not directly related to their disease or not a normal reaction to the prescribed treatment. Furthermore, according to a 1986 report in the *Journal of the American Medical Association*, about 2,000 people die unnecessarily each year as a result of substandard practices in anesthesiology.

Considering, then, both the remarkable achievements and the considerable risks of today's sophisticated medical procedures, technology, etc., the patient is all the more in need of information regarding the quality of care provided by hospitals. Despite the fact that Americans spend over $170 billion a year on hospital care—and that 65 percent of that money comes from public funds—solid, reliable information about hospitals is pitifully scarce. In trying to fill this gap, we did research into the standards set by the industry itself.

Attempts to establish acceptable norms of quality care for hospitals date back to at least 1915, when the American College of Surgeons conducted a survey of the nation's hospitals and discovered such appalling conditions that it refused to release its findings. Gradually over the next thirty years minimum hospital standards evolved. In 1951 all the important national medical groups—the American College of Surgeons, the American College of Physicians, the American Medical Association, and the American Hospital Association—joined to launch an organization that would guarantee the public a high level of quality care in hospitals. Known as the Joint Commission on Accreditation of Hospitals (JCAH), this private, not-for-profit venture was charged with establishing standards for hospital care and conducting on-site surveys to determine whether a hospital is in compliance with those standards. Since then, no other group has been more responsible for constantly improving the quality of care in a rapidly changing field.

Today the JCAH is an enormous organization, occupying two floors of the Hancock Building in Chicago and employing about 400 people. It runs seminars, sponsors a speaker's bureau, and publishes a variety of books and pamphlets for the hospital industry. The heart of the business, however, remains the accreditation process, especially the on-site surveys. Approximately 3,500 hospitals, nursing homes, and other medical facilities are visited each year by a JCAH team consisting of a physician, a registered nurse, and a hospital administrator. The evaluation covers every aspect of operation, from mundane housekeeping matters to rigorous rules about fire safety and disaster planning.

But patient care and treatment are the primary issues in these surveys, and the JCAH has established requirements for the medical staff to ensure its active participation in providing consistent quality care. Since 1979 the JCAH *Accreditation Manual for Hospitals* has included a section called "Quality and Appropriateness Review," which requires the hospital seeking accreditation to have a formal system monitoring every phase of patient care, from admission procedures to infection control. Under these guidelines committees of physicians must meet regularly to review the medical practices of their peers, including the appropriateness of all surgery, blood transfusions, and use of antibiotics.

The process of accreditation is lengthy and costly for any hospital. But few hospitals can afford not to have JCAH approval, since Medicare (which pays a large part of the bill for 40 percent of all hospital patients) as well as many private insurance plans will not cover costs incurred at unaccredited institutions. Moreover, 34 states currently use JCAH accreditation as the norm for their licensing procedures. Today about 5,000 short-stay hospitals rate JCAH accreditation, leaving about 1,500 without it. Some critics believe this high percentage of acceptance proves that the commission's standards are not strict enough.

In the eyes of the layperson, however, JCAH accreditation can be viewed as a *minimum* requirement for any hospital. Actually, whether or not a hospital is accredited is the only thing you can find out from JCAH, since that organization considers its surveys private information. Although all the hospitals in this book are accredited, only a few mentioned to us the results of their JCAH surveys.

For years many hospitals have tried to monitor their quality of care by studying data from other hospitals. The best-known source of such information is the Commission on Professional and Hospital Activities (CPHA), founded in 1955 by the American College of Physicians, the American College of Surgeons, and the American Hospital Association. This commission was designed to provide hospitals with information that would allow them to compare their performances with those of other institutions. The Professional Activity Study of the CPHA now consists of 2 million medical records culled from over 15 million submitted annually by 1,700 member hospitals. The commission has by far the largest data base of patient information in the world, providing physicians and administrators instant access to every conceivable kind of hospital statistic, including such key ones as infection rates (the percentage of patients developing new infections as a result of their stay in the hospital), morbidity rates (the percentage of patients experiencing complications, including new illnesses, as a result of their treatment), and mortality rates (the percentage of patients who die during or after surgery, treatment, or testing).

Through such data administrators can clearly see whether a hospital measures up to regional and national norms in the most vital areas, while physicians can gauge the performance of their peers in relation to a large number of other practitioners. Unfortunately, most physicians and hospital administrators consider such statistics confidential. In their opinion only the medical profession and the hospital industry should determine whether an individual physician or hospital is performing adequately, and only they should establish the criteria to be met.

The collective silence of the hospital industry has produced a tension-filled struggle with consumer groups (often composed of well-informed senior citizens) who are demanding to know more about the actual results of hospital care in specific *institutions*. Some critics cite examples of gross neglect and outright incompetence to prove that neither the medical profession nor the hospital industry monitors the quality of hospital care strictly enough. Others argue that since the taxpayers are funding a large part of the hospital system, statistics vital to patients' welfare cannot rightfully be suppressed. This approach has been gaining momentum over the last few years, and in 1986 the first public disclosure of hospital mortality rates was published in every major newspaper in the country.

Based on a study of 11 million Medicare patients prepared by the Health Care Financing Administration (HCFA)—the unit within the Department of Health and Human Services responsible for administering Medicare and Medicaid—this report gave a detailed picture of mortality rates for many illnesses in thousands of hospitals. It also cited 142 hospitals as having higher-than-expected mortality rates for their Medicare patients. Since some of these were large, well-known hospitals, the potential for embarrassment—or worse—made hospitals determined to keep the report confidential. However, under pressure from the *New York Times*, which threatened to sue under the Freedom of Information Act, the report was released.

As with most news stories, the negative side of the report became the focus of attention: some hospitals that appeared to do poorly were forced to call news conferences and write rejoinders explaining why the HCFA figures were misleading, inaccurate, or both. Lost in all the hubbub were several rather encouraging notes. First, most observers neglected to mention that 127 hospitals were listed in the report as having *lower*-than-expected mortality rates, and in fact 97 percent of the nation's hospitals were, according to HCFA, performing up to par or better.

Unfortunately, after much scrutiny the reliability of the HCFA report was generally conceded to be very poor, even by those who favored its release. We found its information so clumsily assembled and, quite frankly, so misleadingly presented that we decided against using it in this book. Why, for example, would anyone trust a report that cites a hospice for having a high mortality rate, and an orthopedic hospital for having a low one? For the record, however, none of the institutions we describe in this book appeared on the HCFA list of hospitals with higher-than-expected mortality rates, but seven were on the list of those with lower-than-expected rates.

In retrospect, the importance of the HCFA report was that it put hospitals on notice: No longer would public money support them without some kind of public accounting. Just how accurate mortality rates are as a measure of hospital performance may be debatable, but there can be no doubt that they will soon become part of the standard guidelines for all hospitals. At the end of 1986 the Joint Commission on Accreditation of Hospitals stunned the hospital industry with the announcement that by 1990 it would be using surgical mortality rates and complication rates as crucial factors in the accreditation process.

Advocates of strict national standards for hospitals and doctors predict this will have an immediate, positive effect because JCAH accreditation is so essential to hospitals. Over the next decade and certainly by the beginning of the next century, then, we can look forward to a dramatically different system of hospital evaluation by the industry and the medical profession.

## The Criteria for Selection

The criteria we developed for selecting the hospitals and medical centers described in this book were based entirely on the needs and concerns of patients. We sought hospitals that deliver quality care in a wide range of medical categories (or, in some cases, in special areas, such as cancer)* in well-kept facilities employing the most up-to-date medical technology. Most important, we looked for hospitals with high-powered staffs of senior physicians who have national reputations in their fields, with excellent nursing staffs whose quality is maintained through rigorous requirements for acceptance, and with a concern for working conditions.

With these criteria in mind we began to solicit recommendations from physicians in all parts of the country. Not surprisingly—at least not to many people in the hospital and health-care fields—these physicians led us directly to the large teaching hospitals in their areas. A teaching hospital is attached to, or affiliated with, a well-known medical school. They are called teaching hospitals because they provide new doctors with continuing education programs and settings in which to cultivate the practice of medicine. In earlier

---

*We've included only two specialized children's hospitals; our research into the more than 120 children's hospitals convinced us that this topic would require a book of its own. Moreover, most of the major medical centers included in the book have first-rate pediatrics departments; for special needs such as pediatric organ transplantation, most doctors can refer you to the leading hospitals.

days teaching hospitals most often treated indigent patients, whose poverty consigned them to the role of medical guinea pigs. By the 1950s and 1960s, however, many of these hospitals had emerged as prestigious institutions where research and clinical practice were combined, resulting in unprecedented breakthroughs in every area of medical science. Consequently, enormous financial grants from the federal government, corporations, foundations, and wealthy individuals helped place teaching hospitals at the center of American medicine.

All the hospitals and medical centers described in this book have highly respected clinical research programs, the kind that lead to new and better forms of patient care. Many of them have, for example, been specially designated by the National Cancer Institute as regional Comprehensive Cancer Centers or Clinical Cancer Centers and as such receive funding for research, patient care, and in the case of comprehensive centers even community education projects. Most of the 75 hospitals receiving grants through the National Institutes of Health (NIH) General Clinical Research Centers Program are included in this book. Under this program, each selected institution is given sufficient funds to set up a small Clinical Research Center (CRC) within the hospital. Patients with specific, usually difficult-to-handle medical problems receive treatment, and the results of their treatment are made known to the medical community. Funding from the NIH pays for the medical researchers, a specially trained nursing staff, even dietitians and administrative personnel. The combined capacity of these 75 centers is equivalent to that of a 600-bed hospital devoted completely to clinical research and covers the entire spectrum of medical science, from genetic studies in the laboratory to organ transplants in the operating room.

However, we discovered that the impact of a strong research program on the quality of a hospital's care goes far beyond the laboratory. The commitment to support research for finding cures or improving treatment for a broad range of illnesses is a major reason why so many first-rate medical specialists are attracted to the most prestigious teaching hospitals. These men and women frequently pass up the certain financial rewards of a private practice to gain a place in the vanguard of medical exploration. This is not to say that these doctors are not involved in the care and treatment of patients on a daily basis. In fact, of the 1,227 doctors recommended by John Pekkanen in his excellent and well-known 1984 article for *Town and Country*, "The Best Medical Specialists in the United States," over 90 percent are affiliated with hospitals described in this book.

Despite the fine reputation of most teaching hospitals among many doctors and nurses, some people are uncomfortable with the notion that their illness will be scrutinized by neophytes, their bodies made the subject of academic discussion. However, for those who value sophisticated medical care, these are inconveniences worth enduring. It is precisely this commitment to advancing medical knowledge that accounts for the special place teaching hospitals have in our health-care system.

The combination of high-powered research programs and superb medical staffs has made teaching hospitals the repositories of the most advanced styles of medical practice. For this reason, they are frequently asked to treat very sick patients, the ones local community hospitals are simply not equipped to deal with. In other words, these are the hospitals where doctors refer their patients when sophisticated specialized care is required.

Known as tertiary-care hospitals (your physician gives primary care, the local hospital secondary), these hospitals are recognized by the medical community for their expertise in specific areas. (Of course we should note that all the general hospitals described here also offer basic medical services, such as simple obstetrics and general surgery, but that's not the reason they were selected.) These are the hospitals, for example, that perform most organ transplants, utilize the latest experimental cancer drugs, or employ the most up-to-date techniques for treating heart disease. Simply put, they deal with the sickest patients and offer the most complex care.

We have some statistical evidence of this in the so-called case-mix index figures compiled by the Health Care Financing Administration. To allocate payments on an equitable basis to hospitals for Medicare and Medicaid, HCFA devised a system, albeit an imperfect one, that reimburses hospitals handling more complex cases at a higher rate. After examining each hospital's caseload of Medicare patients, HCFA assigns the hospital a numerical rating (with one as the norm). All the hospitals we've chosen have an index number higher than 1.2 (a level reached by only a few hundred facilities in the nation), and most were actually higher than 1.3 in both 1981 and 1984, the only years for which figures are available. These figures confirm that the hospitals recommended to us by physicians are in fact the ones practicing medicine at a degree of difficulty much higher than the overwhelming majority of hospitals.

In investigating each of the hospitals included in this book, we also paid close attention to the quality of the nursing staff. Most patients regard nursing care as only slightly less important than the abilities of their physicians. After all, patients spend more time with their nurses than with their doctors. The hospitals in this book demonstrated that they have created environments that allow nurses a meaningful role in the care and treatment of their patients and that the hospitals encourage them to pursue nursing as a career—these are essential components in nursing excellence, according to the American Nursing Association.

Since most hospitals now do patient surveys to determine the level of patient satisfaction, we were often able to discover whether patients were pleased with the care they received and whether they would return if they required hospitalization in the future. In the few cases where institutions refused to share this information with us, we've noted that fact; prospective patients might want to investigate these institutions more closely on their own.

Finally, we invited each hospital to tell us about their quality-assurance program. While every accredited hospital must have a system of peer review of doctors' performances, we discovered that there is a great deal of variation in the effectiveness of these systems. We've taken note of the hospitals in our survey that seem to pay more attention to this increasingly important dimension of quality control. But we were disappointed to discover that far too many hospitals are unwilling to share such information with the public.

## How to Use This Book

Most of the hospitals we've selected offer a broad array of services, and every entry contains an extensive list of medical specialties available at each hospital. Whenever possible we also provide a list of special clinics and programs. The main body of text for each entry, however, contains a detailed description of each hospital's best-known specialties. These are often in fields where the hospital is a major referral center for the region, or even for the nation, because it has the sophisticated technology and medical expertise to handle the most complex kinds of cases. Very few hospitals offer organ transplants, and fewer still do bone marrow transplants, so we always note when these and other similarly advanced and difficult-to-find services are available.

But we also describe the more common medical services, for cancer, diabetes, heart disease, kidney disease, stroke rehabilitation, and so forth, which have an impact on so many lives. In many of the hospitals included here, the programs for these illnesses are among the most highly regarded in the country. We always note, for example, if a hospital has received special recognition and funding from the National Cancer Institute, or if it has an outstanding program in cardiac surgery, high-risk pregnancy, orthopedic surgery, or Level I trauma services. Level I trauma services, whenever it is used in this book, indicates a sophisticated emergency service administered by a team of specialists—including surgeons—who are on call twenty-four hours a day. A hospital with Level I trauma services offers the highest caliber of services as rated by the American College of Surgeons.

We also mention the availability of advanced medical technology, which of course keeps changing. When we began researching the book, for example, only ten hospitals in the nation had a kidney lithotriptor, a German-built machine that destroys kidney stones with shock waves, thus eliminating the need for surgery. A mere eighteen months later, when this book was ready for the copy editor, almost every acute-care hospital we have written about either had a lithotriptor or had one on order. The same is true of the development of nuclear magnetic resonance imaging, which gives physicians a three-dimensional view of the inside of a patient's body without X rays or other radioactive material. Many of the hospitals described in these pages are contributing to the continuing development of this revolutionary diagnostic tool, which as of this writing was available in only 10 percent of all hospitals in the country.

We also provide a separate section in each entry on special areas of research. Most every hospital in this book has a major research program, and these are always connected to the institution's strengths in clinical medicine. We describe the most important research projects to help our readers find those places that will have the very latest treatments or even experimental programs. (The index at the back of the book can help you pinpoint the hospitals that provide advanced or experimental treatment for a particular condition.)

In addition to this information, we include lists of well-known medical specialists for most hospitals. Our purpose with these lists is to help readers connect their medical needs to a real person, not just a faceless institution. We were surprised to learn that many of these physicians are easily accessible to any sick person seeking their help.

And so, too, are all the hospitals in this book. Early in our research we discovered that many people think that it is necessary to "know someone" to gain entry to these high-powered hospitals. Or that one needs to be under the care of a physician directly affiliated with the hospital. Others think you must have full medical insurance coverage or you won't be admitted. Almost all these assumptions are false, as you will discover in the sections on admission policy for each hospital. Not only can you easily become a patient in these hospitals, but you can do so even if you are one of the 35 million Americans not covered by a health insurance plan. To demonstrate this, whenever possible, we noted hospitals' willingness to help make alternative financial arrangements and the amount of free care each hospital provides annually (this includes charity cases and uncollectible debts). You will be both shocked and impressed by the amount of uncompensated care most of these institutions provide.

Because most of us do pay at least part of our hospital bills, we have also included some figures on the cost of hospitalization in each facility. The differences may astound you. (Compare, for example, the charges at the Mayo Clinic or Barnes Hospital in St. Louis with those at any hospital in Detroit or in the Northeast.) At hospitals where a large number of patients come from out of town, we've also included special hotel rates when they are available.

In short, more information from more hospitals has been gathered here than has ever before been collected for any book or magazine article on this subject. We hope our efforts will stimulate others who seek quality care to take the same steps we did, to ask the hard questions and to urge hospitals and doctors to demonstrate that they can meet the tests of demanding patients. We know that there are hundreds of other first-rate hospitals in the United States, and we hope that this book will be the first of many to provide the public with information about such institutions.

# THE
# HOSPITALS

# The University of Alabama Hospital
# The University of Alabama

**BIRMINGHAM, ALABAMA**

Although this hospital dates back to 1888, when a group of Birmingham citizens opened a one-story facility for charity patients, it is only over the last decade or so that this now vast complex has taken a place alongside the country's best medical institutions. An international leader in both basic and clinical research, The University of Alabama Hospital (UAB) is also a world-renowned organ transplant center and one of America's most highly regarded settings for the diagnosis and treatment of all kinds of illnesses, especially arthritis, cancer, diabetes, heart disease, and kidney disease. In addition, UAB serves the physicians and the people of Alabama and surrounding areas as a regional referral center for neonatal intensive care, spinal cord injuries, and trauma, especially burns. In fact, this hospital ranks second among teaching hospitals and twelfth overall in complexity of care for Medicare patients.

Two services are largely responsible for making UAB attractive to referring physicians outside the Birmingham area and even outside Alabama. One is the Medical Information Service by Telephone (MIST), which has been a model for several similar systems around the country. Specially trained MIST operators can quickly put calling doctors in touch with UAB faculty physicians to answer specific clinical questions at no cost to the caller. (The number is 800-452-9860.)

The second service is the Critical Care Transport Service, which includes a small jet and three ground vehicles, all led by teams of physicians, nurses, and respiratory therapists. These specially outfitted vehicles make nearly obsolete the phrase *too sick to transfer.*

About 3,000 people from outside the state are admitted as patients here each year, and more than half of all patients are from outside Jefferson County, where UAB is located. Many of those who make the trip come for the treatment of kidney failure, which occurs at a noticeably higher rate in Alabama than in most other states. This hospital has one of the four largest dialysis programs in the country, treating almost 300 patients, both at the center and at home, with 26,000 treatments per year. At the Nephrology Research and Training Center patients desiring at-home dialysis can receive full instruction and support from trained personnel. For those needing kidney transplants UAB has one of the most extensive programs in the world (the third largest in the United States); it performed 240 kidney transplants in 1986.

Organ transplantation has played a significant part in solidifying UAB's image as a major referral center in the Southeast. With 129 heart transplants performed since 1981, UAB ranks fifth in the nation in this increasingly important aspect of medicine. Forty-five heart transplants were performed here in 1986 alone. In the same year four liver transplants were performed and over 200 kidney transplants are done here each year. A pancreas transplant program is slated for 1987. These rapidly growing programs are supported by the Alabama Regional Organ Bank, which involves 40 community hospitals and over 100 physicians. The on-site organ retrieval system covers a 75,000-square-mile area, making it one of the largest in the nation.

Hospitals that have extensive heart transplant programs invariably are active in cardiology and cardiac surgery. At UAB an incredible average of 2,800 coronary bypass operations are performed each year. Other surgical programs include treatment for arrhythmias, congenital heart disease, coronary artery disease, and valvular heart disease. Congenital heart disease is of special concern to the highly regarded pediatric cardiologists here; every year over 2,000 children suspected of having this condition are screened at UAB. Children also account for about 400 cardiac diagnostic procedures, 350 cardiac catheterizations, and 500 cardiac surgeries annually.

People from all over the region also travel to UAB for the diagnosis and treatment of cancer. As the site of one of the 20 or so federally designated and funded Comprehensive Cancer Centers, UAB offers the most up-to-date therapies for almost every kind of cancer. Because breast and cervical cancer as well as melanoma are particularly prevalent in Alabama, the center makes special efforts to improve treatment in those areas. Of course, standard chemotherapies and radiation are available, but patients also have access to the newer forms of treatment, including hyperthermia, monoclonal antibodies, and several powerful linear accelerators.

The Multipurpose Arthritis Center at UAB, one of only 12 such federally designated sites, offers the most clinically advanced treatment available in rheumatology, including diagnostic arthroscopy, joint scans, and reconstructive joint surgery (over 350 such operations are done here each year). Physical and occupational therapy are also provided.

Diabetes patients are served by a separate 40-bed hospital and an outpatient clinic. A special Diabetes Research and Training Center provides patient education in the latest forms of insulin injection.

The Comprehensive Community Mental Health Center, a component of the Department of Psychiatry, conducts teaching and research activities and offers diagnostic screening, day treatment, and inpatient services and consultations. The department also includes the Substance Abuse Center and the Substance Abuse Program for Health Professionals.

The UAB Pain Center handles chronic pain problems, including headaches, lower back pain, phantom pain, and pain caused by incurable cancer. Patients are seen on an inpatient or outpatient basis as appropriate. Treatments include acupuncture, behavior modification, biofeedback, electrical stimulation, hypnotherapy, nerve-blocking techniques, and relaxation therapy.

The UAB Center for Aging coordinates educational programs for those who work with older people.

The Sparks Center for Developmental and Learning Disorders trains graduate and postgraduate students in the treatment of children suffering from a variety of handicapping conditions and provides an impressive array of diagnostic and referral services as well as sponsoring research into preventing such diseases.

The Spain Rehabilitation Center treats head injuries, spinal cord injuries, stroke, and other health problems. The center includes a new therapeutic pool, renal scan capabilities, and a biocommunication department with computerized equipment to help deaf people learn to speak, to eliminate hypernasality, and to deal with communication problems following cancer surgery.

Other centers for excellence, as the hospital calls them, include the Cardiovascular Research and Training Center, the Medical Rehabilitation Research and Training Center, the Nutrition Sciences Center, the Urological Rehabilitation and Research Center, and the Vision Science Research Center. Other departments with strong clinical programs include dermatology, infectious diseases, and pediatrics.

The University Hospital is one of seven units composing the University of Alabama Medical Center on the Birmingham campus. Other clinical components of the medical center include the Smolian Psychiatric Clinic, the Engel Psychiatric Day Treatment Center, the Lurleen Wallace Tumor Institute and Radiation Therapy Building, and the Russell Ambulatory Center. The medical center also has strong ties with other governmental and private institutions adjacent to the campus, including the Veterans Administration Medical Center, Children's Hospital, and the Eye Foundation Hospital.

## Specialties

Adolescent Medicine, Allergy, Anesthesiology, Cardiology, Cardiothoracic Surgery, Dermatology, Ear, Nose, and Throat, Endocrinology, Family Medicine, Gastroenterology, General Surgery, Genetics, Geriatric Medicine, Hematology/Oncology, Infectious Diseases, Internal Medicine, Nephrology, Neurology, Neurosurgery, Obstetrics/Gynecology, Oral and Maxillofacial Surgery, Orthopedic Surgery, Pathology, Pediatrics, Perinatology, Plastic Surgery, Preventive Medicine, Psychiatry, Pulmonary Medicine, Radiation Oncology, Radiation (Diagnostic), Rehabilitation Medicine, Rheumatology, and Urology.

Specialized, advanced diagnostic and treatment services are available for allergy, arrhythmia, arthritis, asthma, bone disorders, cystic fibrosis, epilepsy, headache, infertility, in vitro fertilization, juvenile rheumatoid arthritis, medical genetics, metabolic stones, nutritional disorders, replantation, schizophrenia, sex therapy and marital health, sleep-wake disorders, speech and hearing, sports medicine, stroke, substance abuse, thyroid disorders, and other physical impairments and emotional illnesses.

---

**STATISTICAL PROFILE**

Number of Beds: 788
Bed Occupancy Rate: 79%
Average Number of Patients: 629
Average Patient Stay: 7.96 days
Annual Admissions: 28,705
Births: 1,921
Outpatient Clinic Visits: 225,000
Emergency Room/Trauma Center Visits: 30,623

Hospital Personnel:
    Physicians: 550
    Residents: 410
    Registered Nurses: 1,000
    Total Staff: 4,100

---

# Well-known Specialists

Dr. Lionel Bargeron, pediatric cardiology.
Dr. Claude Bennett, clinical immunology and rheumatology.
Dr. Arnold Diethelm, general surgery; specialist in kidney transplants.
Dr. James Kirklin, cardiothoracic surgery; specialist in cardiac transplants, pioneer in open-heart surgery in the late 1950s while at the Mayo Clinic and developer of the surgery program at UAB.
Dr. Albert LoBuglio, hematology/oncology; coordinator of new drug therapies for leukemia, lymphomas, and solid tumors.
Dr. Robert Luke, nephrology.
Dr. Stephen Mahaley, Jr., neurosurgery.
Dr. Albert Pacifico, cardiothoracic surgery; specialist in congenital heart disease.
Dr. Gerald Pohost, cardiovascular disease; specialist in nuclear magnetic resonance imaging of the heart and metabolic studies.
Dr. Hugh Shingleton, obstetrics/gynecology.
Dr. John Whitaker, neurology.

# Research

Research at UAB receives an impressive amount of funding, more than $74 million, among the highest of any institution cited in this book. In fact, of all the federal money coming into Alabama, about 67 percent goes to UAB for research. The university is in the top four southeastern universities receiving support from the NIH (behind Johns Hopkins, Duke, and North Carolina at Chapel Hill), and it is twenty-third among all universities in the nation in terms of federally supported research in the life sciences. The medical center is the site of a federally funded Clinical Research Center.

The Comprehensive Cancer Center is UAB's largest research unit; it receives over $20 million a year. One important program is testing the use of specially developed cellular material to deliver anticancer drugs to cancer sites without harming surrounding healthy cells. Interleukin-2 studies are being conducted here, along with research into immunologic disorders.

Major research projects are also in place to combat conditions such as arthritis, cystic fibrosis, diabetes, gastrointestinal system disorders, heart disease, herpes, hypertension, immunodeficiency in children and transplant patients, and the effects of damage such as spinal cord injury and burns.

---

**ROOM CHARGES (per diem)**
Private: $355–$372
Semiprivate: $345–$353
Ward: $339–$353
ICU: $625–$1,120
Room charges at the University Inn: $27 per day for patients and
  visitors of inpatients (Call 205-933-9000)

**AVERAGE COST PER PATIENT STAY:** $7,946

**AVERAGE COST OF ORGAN TRANSPLANTATION**
Heart Transplant: $65,000
Kidney Transplant: $27,000
Liver Transplant: $125,000

**MAILING ADDRESS**          **TELEPHONE**
619 South 19th Street        205-934-4011
Birmingham, AL 35233

---

# Admission Policy

Patients can be admitted to the hospital without a doctor's referral through the emergency room or one of the clinics. Anyone can make an appointment by calling 205-934-4000. There is a special number for doctors to call for either referral or consultation: 800-452-9860.

Patients are required to show proof of insurance coverage or some other indication of their ability to cover their financial obligation to the hospital. But special arrangements can be made on a case-by-case basis. In fact, UAB gives $25 million worth of uncompensated care per year, almost entirely to Alabama residents.

# University Medical Center
# Arizona Health Sciences Center
# University of Arizona
**TUCSON, ARIZONA**

Enormous public attention was focused on University Medical Center (UMC) at the University of Arizona Health Sciences Center in August 1985, when Dr. Jack Copeland used the Jarvik-7 artificial heart to allow a twenty-five-year-old man to live long enough to receive a donor heart. It was the first federally authorized use of the artificial heart as a bridge to transplant. The operation came thirteen days after Dr. Copeland received permission from the Food and Drug Administration (FDA) to use the Jarvik-7 as a temporary measure. Dr. Copeland had performed a similar procedure in March 1985 using an artificial heart that had not received government approval and set off a vigorous ethical debate in the medical establishment. (The procedure later was given the sanction of the FDA as having been justified by the emergency situation.)

This program is only one part of UMC's full cardiac program, which also includes procedures such as coronary artery bypass, balloon angioplasty, Doppler echocardiography, an active rehabilitation program, transplants, and specialized neonatal and pediatric treatment and surgery. Dr. Hugh Allen is one of only a handful of doctors in the nation who can use the Fontán procedure to correct a congenital malfunction of the heart in newborns.

Other programs in neonatology and pediatrics also go well beyond the ordinary, including UMC's maternal and neonatal transport, which brings critically ill infants and expectant mothers to the center's intensive care units from all over the southern part of Arizona. This service has resulted in a dramatic reduction of the state's neonatal mortality rate.

The center's intensive care unit for high-risk mothers is the only such center in southern Arizona. Currently, an average of 160 mothers deliver their babies at UMC each month. The expertise of UMC obstetricians is reflected in the center's low percentage of cesarean sections despite the number of high-risk mothers. It is also reflected in the number of mothers who have had cesarean sections and then have a vaginal delivery at UMC.

The center's pediatric lung disease program is nationally recognized for its care of children with asthma, bronchopulmonary dysplasia, and cystic fibrosis and of infants at risk of sudden infant death syndrome. Outstanding programs exist in pollen allergies, childhood cancer, child abuse, eating disorders of adolescents, hemophilia and other bleeding disorders, infectious diseases, nutritional problems of newborns and young infants, and the relationship of familial stress to illness in children. These programs, combined with specialists in a variety of pediatric areas, offer a full range of care, rounded out by support from a play therapist and social workers, who help children and their families.

Major breakthroughs in cancer treatment and research have taken place at the Arizona Health Sciences Center in the last several years, including development of the procedure for growing a patient's cancer cells in the laboratory so that various drugs and drug combinations can be tested to determine the most effective treatment for a given tumor.

The Arizona Cancer Center is an integral part of UMC's oncology program. Because this major research facility is housed in the same complex as UMC, the hospital benefits in many areas, including the availability of drugs not generally in use. Treatment is provided for and research conducted in, among others, breast cancer, adult leukemia, melanoma, multiple myeloma, and ovarian cancer. Ninety-five percent of those treated at the cancer center are outpatients. A multimillion-dollar care and research center was opened in October 1986.

University Medical Center provides a full range of orthopedic services, including diagnosis, hand surgeries, total joint replacements, pediatric orthopedics, customary and difficult reconstruction orthopedics, replantation of severed parts, and a sports medicine clinic. Dr. Robert Volz has been instrumental in developing an artificial hip, knee, and wrist. In fact, his artificial wrist was the first of its kind in the nation. Dr. Volz's efforts, combined with those of rheumatologist Dr. Eric Gall, geriatrician Dr. Jack Boyer, and physiatrist Dr. Pedro Escobar have resulted in a full program of treatment and rehabilitation for arthritic and handicapped individuals. Special emphasis is placed on geriatric rehabilitation, particularly in the areas of amputations, fractures, osteoporosis, rheumatism, and stroke.

Medical care at UMC is monitored through a quality-assurance program that is one of the best of its kind. The center is one of only six hospitals in the nation that is piloting a new, highly regarded—and very complex—quality-assurance computer software program. With this system UMC is able to review all its patients' records using generic screening criteria with ongoing peer reviews by department. Referrals, denials, and cost summaries are also systematically monitored.

Constructed between 1968 and 1971, University Medical Center became Arizona's first major resource for clinical teaching in medicine, nursing, pharmacy, and health-related fields. It is also the primary teaching hospital for the University of Arizona College of Medicine.

## Specialties

Cardiology, Emergency and Trauma Service, Intensive Care, Neonatology, Obstetrics, Oncology, Organ Transplantation, Orthopedics and Rehabilitation Medicine, Pediatrics, Radiology, and Urology.

**STATISTICAL PROFILE**

Number of Beds: 300
Bed Occupancy Rate: 72%
Average Number of Patients: 185
Average Patient Stay: 5.5 days
Annual Admissions: 12,192
Births: 1,852
Outpatient Clinic Visits: 112,967
Emergency Room/Trauma Center Visits: 21,482

Hospital Personnel:
    Physicians: 260 active; 215 associate
    Residents: 330
    Registered Nurses: 593
    Total Staff: 1,600

Other special services and programs include a regional allergy center, cystic fibrosis treatment and research, a regional hemophilia center, joint replacement surgery, muscular dystrophy treatment and research, a pediatric pulmonary disease center, sleep disorders treatment, sudden infant death syndrome research and care, and a valley fever center.

## Well-known Specialists

Dr. Hugh Allen, pediatric cardiology; specialist in neonatal cardiac surgery.
Dr. Jack Boyer, geriatrics.
Dr. Paul Capp, radiology.
Dr. C. Donald Christian, obstetrics/gynecology.
Dr. Jack Copeland, cardiothoracic surgery; specialist in heart transplants.
Dr. George Drach, urology.
Dr. Pedro Escobar, physiatry.
Dr. Gordon Ewy, cardiology.
Dr. Vincent A. Fulginiti, pediatrics.
Dr. Eric Gall, rheumatology.
Dr. Evan Hersh, hematology/oncology.
Dr. Frank Marcus, cardiology.
Dr. Sidney Salmon, cancer treatment and research.
Dr. Robert Volz, orthopedics; specialist in joint replacement.
Dr. Tony Vuturo, family and community medicine.

# Research

Research funding at the Arizona Health Sciences Center totals close to $40 million and is divided between the College of Medicine ($34 million), the College of Nursing ($576,000), and the College of Pharmacy ($4.5 million). Major areas of research and treatment include cardiology, oncology, and pediatrics.

The Arizona Cancer Center offers clinical trials of advanced treatment methods, including biological response modifiers, improved delivery systems, new anticancer drugs, drug combinations, hyperthermia, and computer-enhanced radiation therapy.

Internationally recognized research programs relating to children have been developed in many areas, including cancer, cardiac abnormalities, child abuse, hemophilia, infectious diseases, lung disorders such as asthma and cystic fibrosis, nutritional disorders of the newborn, school health, and sudden infant death syndrome. The center is currently developing further research programs in gastroenterology, genetics, immunology, metabolic disorders, and nutrition disciplines.

Cardiac research includes studies in areas such as the effects of various cardiac medicines on clotting mechanisms and clinical trials for patients under treatment for heart failure and for patients with heart arrhythmias who may have had unsatisfactory responses to presently available drugs.

Gerontology, restorative medicine, and geriatrics are also areas of investigation. Clinical research is being conducted in management of depression, disease prevention, pain, sleep disorders, and many other areas relating to the elderly.

# Admission Policy

Any person who comes through UMC's emergency department will be admitted if the attending physician deems it appropriate, regardless of ability to pay.

There is a policy regarding ability to pay, but the hospital says that no one in need of medical care for an illness or injury that would threaten life or limb is denied admission. Noninsured patients seeking elective procedures are required to make a deposit before admission. However, if such patients cannot meet the financial requirements, their cases are referred to the medical director, who will work with the physicians in charge of the cases to determine whether admission can be delayed until financial questions are resolved. If the medical director feels that medical reasons preclude delay, the patients are admitted.

**ROOM CHARGES** (per diem)
Private: $215
Semiprivate: $200
Ward: $195
ICU: $405–$775

| MAILING ADDRESS | TELEPHONE |
| --- | --- |
| 1501 North Campbell Avenue | 602-626-0111 |
| Tucson, AZ 85724 | |

# Cedars-Sinai Medical Center

**LOS ANGELES, CALIFORNIA**

In southern California the level of concern about health care, wellness—call it what you will—is probably higher than in any other part of the country. The large number of first-rate hospitals in the Los Angeles area is striking evidence of this. Within a fifty-mile radius one can find hospitals with leading national reputations in a variety of specialties, including orthopedics (The Orthopedic Hospital), pediatrics (The Los Angeles Children's Hospital), cardiology (St. Vincent's Medical Center), and oncology (University of Southern California Medical Center). An impressive array of well-known teaching hospitals offering a wide range of medical services can also be found: Good Samaritan Hospital in Los Angeles, Harbor-UCLA Medical Center in Torrance, Huntington Memorial Hospital in Pasadena, and the Medical Center in Loma Linda.

The two best-known medical facilities are the University of California, Los Angeles, Medical Center (see page 46) and Cedars-Sinai Medical Center. UCLA, of course, has gained an international reputation in many specialties and its research programs often produce headline-making results. At Cedars-Sinai, however, fame arrived for different reasons.

Much to the consternation of the people who work here, Cedars-Sinai Medical Center has the reputation of being the "hospital to the stars." Indeed, it seems as though whenever a movie star or television personality enters the hospital in Hollywood he or she is admitted to Cedars-Sinai.

Part of this reputation is based on the more glamorous aspects of health care provided here. For example, there are no semiprivate rooms or wards; all patients have private rooms. Consequently, the per diem cost of care here is higher than at many other hospitals. However, the rich and famous are not attracted to Cedars-Sinai solely because of the accommodations. People come because this is one of the world's most diversified and sophisticated medical centers, delivering high-quality medical and surgical care.

At Cedars-Sinai the relation between the commitment of the nursing staff and the quality of patient care is especially significant. Cedars-Sinai's annual turnover rate for nurses is only 1 percent, the lowest in California. The dedication of the nursing staff is reflected in patient satisfaction. In a recent hospital questionnaire, nurses received a 95 percent positive evaluation from former patients. Another questionnaire, distributed in March 1986, showed that 95 percent of Cedars-Sinai's former patients would recommend the hospital for patient care.

An acute-care tertiary center for southern California and the West, Cedars-Sinai is capable of handling virtually any kind of medical problem. Over the past ten years the center has treated over 1 million patients in all specialties of medicine and surgery.

An impressive portion of the patient population at Cedars-Sinai is composed of expectant mothers and newborns. A birthing center offers tours of the maternity facilities, childbirth education classes, and classes in the care of newborns. The Department of Obstetrics/Gynecology is geared to identify and treat high-risk mothers through prepregnancy counseling that uses the latest maternal-fetal surveillance procedures (including chorionic villi sampling). Cedars-Sinai has the lowest infant mortality rate in California. This may be partly because of its neonatology intensive care unit, a referral center for southern California.

The medical center is also designated a pediatric intensive-care center. The Department of Pediatrics treats newborns to adolescents in all areas of medicine and surgery, including surgical subspecialties, cardiology, endocrinology, hematology/oncology, and nephrology. The nurses in this department are especially sensitive to children's needs. Visiting hours are more flexible, and special measures are taken to help alleviate children's apprehensions. Parents or family members are encouraged to stay with their children whenever possible. As part of this department, the Amie Karen Cancer Center treats cancer and blood disease and is associated with Camp Rainbow, a summer facility for children with cancer.

The Department of Medicine is the parent department for many specialties. Among them, Cedars-Sinai offers inpatient care for adults with cancer and is developing variations in the treatment of gynecologic malignancies. An outpatient comprehensive cancer center provides advanced diagnostic and therapeutic care, enabling patients to avoid prolonged hospitalizations.

The Division of Cardiology is internationally recognized for care and rehabilitation of heart patients. It includes electrocardiographic and nuclear cardiology divisions, a coronary care unit, a cardiac catheterization laboratory, an echocardiographic service, and cardiac stress testing.

Located in a community densely populated with senior citizens, Cedars-Sinai recently inaugurated a multidisciplinary treatment and research program dealing with all aspects of geriatrics and gerontology. One of its initial projects has been the Senior Resource Center, which provides members of the community with free information on and referral to services available to seniors and their families.

The medical center has specialized capabilities in pulmonary therapy, including laser bronchoscopy; inpatient treatment of diabetes; and treatment of biliary disease and kidney disease, including dialysis. Cedars-Sinai boasts one of the most advanced facilities nationwide for gallstone surgery and has developed as a major center for kidney transplantation. The center is also preeminent in the West for cardiovascular and thoracic surgery—from simple operations to the most complex coronary artery bypass grafting, valve replacement, and valve repair.

The Arthur and Eleanor Ellis Eye Center treats people of all ages for a variety of ophthalmic conditions. Treatments and diagnostic procedures include cryosurgery, electrophysiological procedures, eye photography, fluorescein angiography, lens calculations, visual field studies, and treatments utilizing argon and neodymium-YAG lasers. Research in eye surgery and disease is conducted at a newly designated facility in the Cedars-Sinai Research Institute.

The Chronic Pain Management Program, under the auspices of the Department of Physical Medicine and drawing on ten disciplines, uses an integrated team approach. The program leads patients through a specific series of behaviors, increasing the amount of activity they can perform and developing their pain-coping skills so that they can eliminate (or at least decrease) their reliance on pain medication. An adjunct to this program is biofeedback therapy, offered on both inpatient and outpatient bases.

The hospital also provides a full range of services in the Ambulatory Care Department, a comprehensive twenty-four-hour emergency unit, and a complete psychiatric program in the Thalians Mental Health Center. The Trauma Center, located in the emergency area, along with the heliport, which was formally dedicated in June 1984, have given Cedars-Sinai Class A status in treating emergencies. The Level I Trauma Center can handle up to 750 cases per year.

In 1984 numerous services were added, including a detoxification program for adult and adolescent victims of alcohol and drug abuse, and the Swallowing Clinic, which, as part of the Department of Surgery, treats all disorders relating to the swallowing mechanism.

Cedars-Sinai offers extensive programs of community education, medical education, and research. It is a major teaching hospital affiliated with the University of California at Los Angeles School of Medicine. Nurses' training is also conducted here on many levels with an increasing number of school and cooperative programs. And a broad program of inservice training is offered to professional and nonprofessional employees.

## Specialties

Cardiology (adult and pediatric), Diagnostic Radiology and Nuclear Medicine, Emergency Medicine, Endocrinology (adult and pediatric), Gastroenterology, Gynecologic Oncology, Hematology/Oncology (adult and pediatric), Infectious Diseases, Maternal-Fetal Medicine, Medicine, Neonatology, Nephrology, Obstetrics/Gynecology, Ophthalmology, Pathology and Laboratory Medicine, Pediatric Intensive Care, Pediatrics, Physical Medicine and Rehabilitation, Psychiatry, Pulmonary Medicine, Radiation Therapy, Reproductive Endocrinology and Infertility, Rheumatology, Surgery, and Thoracic and Cardiovascular Surgery.

Specialized services and facilities include the Autologous Blood Program, the Diabetes Outpatient Training and Education Center, the Genetics Center, the Home Care Program, the Hospice Unit, the Medical Genetics Birth Defects Center, the Regional Arrhythmia Center, the Reproductive Endocrinology Center, and the Weight Control Program.

---

**STATISTICAL PROFILE**

Number of Beds: 1,201
Bed Occupancy Rate: 73%
Average Number of Patients: 878
Average Patient Stay: 6.7 days
Annual Admissions: 38,346
Births: 6,442
Outpatient Clinic Visits: 27,608
Emergency Room/Trauma Center Visits: 38,859 (106 per day)

Hospital Personnel:
   Physicians: 2,020
   Residents: 239
   Registered Nurses: 1,057
   Total Staff: 5,723

---

# Well-known Specialists

All doctors listed are directors of their respective departments.

Dr. Michael Bush, director of the Diabetes Outpatient Training and Education Center, codirector of the Weight Control Program.
Dr. Meyer Davidson, diabetes.
Dr. Burton Fink, pediatric cardiology.
Dr. Calvin Hobel, maternal-fetal medicine and obstetrics/gynecology.
Dr. Carol Hurvitz, pediatric hematology/oncology.
Dr. Alan Jasper, director of the Respiratory Intensive Care Unit.
Dr. Leo Lagrasse, gynecologic oncology; associate director of obstetrics/gynecology.
Dr. Jack Matloff, thoracic and cardiovascular surgery.
Dr. Richard Meyer, infectious diseases.
Dr. Glenn Murata, general internal medicine.
Dr. Gary Oakes, perinatal outreach and obstetrics and antenatal care.
Dr. Jeffrey Pomerance, neonatology and pediatrics.
Dr. Eugene Richards, physical medicine and rehabilitation.
Dr. David Rimoin, pediatrics; director of the Medical Genetics Birth Defects Center.

Dr. Sima Sconyers, director of the Pediatrics Intensive Care Unit.
Dr. Myron Stein, pulmonary medicine.
Dr. H. J. Swan, cardiology.
Dr. Robert Taub, director of the Hospice Unit.
Dr. Ronald Thompson, radiation therapy.
Dr. Maclyn Wade, obstetrics/gynecology.
Dr. Frank Williams, family and child psychiatry.

## Research

Basic biomedical and clinical research programs are an integral part of Cedars-Sinai. The medical center presently has more than 100 active projects, which involve over 70 principal investigators. The center receives approximately $6 million annually in support of its research activities from federal, state, corporate, and foundation sources. The NIH accounts for two-thirds of this support.

Among studies under way are investigations of diagnosis and treatment of heart disease by innovative tests, including tests with the Excimer laser; pediatric diseases such as cancer, juvenile diabetes, and growth disorders; diabetes detection and treatment; blood apheresis treatment for arthritis; treatment of gallbladder disorders by noninvasive procedures; treatment of corneal infections and ocular herpes; variations in the treatment of gynecologic malignancies; advanced surgical techniques, including, for example, spleen surgery; and refined endoscopic procedures.

## Admission Policy

Patients may be admitted to Cedars-Sinai through the Emergency Department, where they are assigned a physician, or through the Ambulatory Care Clinic, where they make an appointment, are screened, and then are assigned a physician from that clinic.

There is a financial requirement for admission. Patients are expected to provide proof of insurance or to pay a deposit. In 1985 Cedars-Sinai absorbed $4.6 million in free care.

---

**ROOM CHARGES (per diem)**
Private: $375–$590 (All rooms are private.)
ICU: $1,035

**MAILING ADDRESS**      **TELEPHONE**
8700 Beverly Boulevard    213-855-5000
Box 48750
Los Angeles, CA 90048

# The Medical Center at the University of California, San Francisco (UCSF)

## SAN FRANCISCO, CALIFORNIA

The hospital industry in California includes over 450 short-term facilities, 80,000 beds, and 330,000 employees, which makes it not only big business but an important part of the state's economy. Californians in fact spend a vast amount of money on hospital care—around $20 billion annually. California hospitals lead the nation with the highest average daily room rates and the highest average cost-per-patient stay. But if California has the most expensive hospital system in America, it also has one of the best.

About 65,000 doctors live and work in California, far more than in any other state, and their incomes are among the highest in the nation. Nurses' salaries, too, are at the very top of the pay scale, especially in the Bay Area, and hospital workers in general receive better wages than almost anywhere else. Moreover, the very intense competition among hospitals has not led to a lowering of rates but to a race to acquire all the latest medical technology so patients will remain loyal. In other words, costs escalate quickly in hospitals here, but so too does the level of care.

As a result, in the high-income areas of Silicon Valley and San Francisco one can even find community hospitals and private hospitals recommended without hesitation or reservation by many doctors (El Camino in Mountain View and Alta Bates in Berkeley are two that were brought to our attention). This area is also home to several nationally prominent children's hospitals, including Children's Hospital of San Francisco, Stanford Children's Hospital, and the Children's Hospital of Northern California in Oakland. Several fine teaching hospitals—including Presbyterian Hospital of the Pacific Medical Center, St. Mary's, the Kaiser Foundation Hospital, and Mount Zion—are located in San Francisco. In addition, two of the world's leading academic medical centers are located here: Stanford University Medical Center (see page 41) and the less publicized Medical Center at the University of California, San Francisco, which includes Moffitt and Long hospitals, the UCSF Children's Medical Center, Langley Porter Psychiatric Hospital, Herbst Emergency Service, and the UCSF Ambulatory Care Service. The School of Medicine at UCSF is responsible for patient care, teaching, and research at the affiliated, city-owned San Francisco General Hospital, which handles 300,000 outpatients annually, provides one of the finest trauma services in the country, and is the foremost AIDS treatment center in the West.

Some 75 medical specialties and subspecialties are practiced at UCSF, and the hospital is the major referral center for northern California and parts

31

of Idaho and Nevada. About one-third of all its patients come from outside the five-county Bay Area, many from across the country and some from overseas. Here are some of the reasons.

Over 2,700 kidney transplants have been done at UCSF, more than at any other hospital in the world; currently, over 250 are done each year, many on children. UCSF is also an international leader in the field of pediatric cardiology; more than one-half of all newborns in this area requiring heart surgery are brought to UCSF. In fact, according to the hospital, of the 5,000 patients a year admitted to the 72-bed pediatric unit, less than 10 percent have what could be considered a common condition or ailment. Cancer, so-called craniofacial anomalies, cystic fibrosis, growth disorders, hemophilia, neurological tumors, and puberty disorders all have special treatment centers at UCSF.

In addition, for 700 or more newborns each year who may be at risk or whose mothers may be, the medical center is a leading referral institution in neonatology and high-risk pregnancy, and it offers both in-utero treatment and fetal surgery. UCSF is also the home of the Northern California Comprehensive Center for Sickle Cell Disease, which includes screening, treatment, and research facilities.

For cancer treatment, UCSF sees 2,000 new patients each year, more than any other hospital in the Bay Area except for Stanford. It is a regional referral center for gynecologic cancers, leukemia, brain tumors, and for the latest therapies, such as bone marrow transplant, including procedures in which the donor and the recipient are not related.

In cardiology, UCSF's physicians and surgeons have access to the most up-to-date clinical research through the Cardiovascular Research Institute. Every form of treatment, including surgery and balloon angioplasty, and the latest drug therapies are available.

UCSF pioneered use of the latest diagnostic equipment—including magnetic resonance imaging, lasers for surgery, and lithotriptors for dissolving kidney stones. Its researchers recently developed the most advanced cochlear implant for aiding the deaf and a bladder pacemaker.

But more than the technology, it is the quality of the staff, both physicians and nurses, that is a major reason UCSF is considered one of the best medical facilities in the country. Every national survey published in the past decade has listed many UCSF physicians as among "the best." In a recent survey that asked department heads and chiefs of clinical services throughout the country to identify the 120 physicians "outstanding in the U.S.," ten of the 120 names were at UCSF.

There are 700 physicians on the active medical staff, all of whom are on the faculty of the School of Medicine, most of them full time; many are authors of authoritative textbooks in their various fields and editors of the most prestigious journals. In fact, faculty physicians are so highly regarded nationally that according to the standard survey of medical schools, UCSF has ranked among the top five medical schools in the country for the past ten years.

In addition, the hospital employs 820 full-time nurses—about 70 percent have bachelor's and master's degrees and 20 are clinical nurse specialists. In a recent nationwide survey undertaken by the American Academy of Nursing, UCSF was cited (with only 40 others) as a "magnet" hospital, one that attracts and retains professional nurses in a manner far above the average. These hospitals were found to be superior places for nurses to work because they involved nurses in patient care in a meaningful way.

The physical facilities at UCSF are relatively new or have been modernized, like the Herbert C. Moffitt Hospital, built in 1955. The Joseph M. Long Hospital was completed in 1983, and even more recently a surgical pavilion, a radiation oncology pavilion, and an emergency service pavilion were opened.

## Specialties

Ambulatory Care, Anesthesiology, Cardiology, Chronic Illness, Dentistry, Dermatology, Emergency Medicine, Endocrinology, Gastroenterology, Genetics, Hematology, Infectious Diseases, Internal Medicine, Kidney Transplantation, Neonatal and Perinatal Medicine, Nephrology, Neurology and Neurological Surgery, Nuclear Medicine, Obstetrics/Gynecology, Oncology, Ophthalmology, Orthopedics, Orthopedic Surgery, Otolaryngology, Pathology, Pediatrics, Plastic Surgery, Psychiatry, Pulmonary Medicine, Radiation Oncology, Radiology, Replantation Surgery, Rheumatology, Surgery, Tropical Medicine, Urology, Vascular Surgery.

A selected listing of clinics and centers includes: Adolescent Medicine,

---

**STATISTICAL PROFILE**

Number of Beds: 560
Bed Occupancy Rate: 67%
Average Number of Patients: 377
Average Patient Stay: 7.3 days
Annual Admissions: 18,970
Births: 1,561
Outpatient Clinic Visits: 201,597
Emergency Room/Trauma Center Visits: 21,406

Hospital Personnel:
  Physicians: 700
  Residents: 240
  Registered Nurses: 820
  Total Staff: 2,800

Adult Bone Marrow Transplant Service, Adult Immunodeficiencies, Allergy, Alzheimer's Center, Arthritis Clinic, Behavioral and Developmental Pediatrics, Breast Screening Clinic, Cardiology, Chest Disease (Pulmonary Medicine), Children's Renal Center, Cystic Fibrosis Treatment Center, Diabetes Center, Ear, Nose, and Throat Clinic, Eye Clinic, Gastrointestinal Clinic, Genetic Counseling, High-Risk Obstetrics, Infectious Disease and Tropical Medicine Clinic, In Vitro Fertilization, General Internal Medicine, Hematology-Oncology Clinic, Gynecology Clinic, Lipid Clinic, Male Infertility Clinic, Obstetrics Clinic, Occupational Medicine, General Pediatrics, Pediatric Specialties Clinic, Plastic and Reconstructive Surgery Clinic, Psoriasis Day Care, Psychiatric Clinic (Adults), Renal Clinic, Screening and Acute Care Clinic, Thyroid Clinic.

## Well-known Specialists

Dr. R. Palmer Beasley, epidemiologist and infectious-disease specialist.
Dr. Marek Bozdech, director of Adult Bone Marrow Transplant Service.
Dr. Edwin Cadman, director of the UCSF Cancer Research Institute.
Dr. Kanu Chatterjee, well-known cardiologist.
Dr. Morton Cowan, director of the Pediatric Bone Marrow Transplant Unit.
Dr. Haile Debas, head of the Department of Surgery.
Dr. Mitchell Golbus, director of the prenatal diagnosis program.
Dr. Melvin Grumbach, pediatric endocrinology.
Dr. Creig Hoyt, pediatric ophthalmology.
Dr. Robert Jaffe, chief of obstetrics/gynecology and reproductive sciences, reproductive endocrinology.
Dr. Steven Kramer, chairman of ophthalmology, director of the Beckman Vision Center, specialist in corneal diseases.
Dr. Alexander Margulis, chairman of radiology.
Dr. William Murray, chairman of orthosurgery.
Dr. Roderic Phibbs, chief of neonatology.
Dr. Theodore Phillips, chairman of radiation therapy.
Dr. Richard Root, chairman of the Department of Medicine, specialist in infectious diseases.
Dr. Abraham Rudolph, pediatric cardiology.
Dr. Oscar Salvatierra, chief of kidney transplant service.
Dr. Marvin Sleisenger, gastroenterology, vice-chairman of medicine.
Dr. Emil Tanagho, chairman of urology.
Dr. Charles Wilson, chairman of neurosurgery.

## Research

In 1985, UCSF research projects received $94 million from NIH, second only to those of Johns Hopkins. The UCSF School of Medicine alone has an annual research budget in excess of $33 million, and in the past fifteen years, the school has been awarded more funds from NIH than any other medical school in the country.

UCSF is one of the world's major centers for biomedical research. Several discoveries have had widespread effects. The discovery of "cancer genes"— oncogenes—for example, was made by microbiologists at UCSF several years ago; they have received many awards as a result, including the Lasker Basic Medical Research Award. Molecular geneticists at UCSF have developed safe and accurate methods for the prenatal identification of sickle cell anemia. Other basic research programs exist in behavioral sciences, developmental and cell biology, human development and aging, immunology, neurobiology, parasitic disease, psychiatry, reproductive sciences, and toxicology.

The multichannel cochlear implant that allows profoundly deaf people to hear was developed by UCSF physicians and scientists. Procedures to inhibit the immune reaction that causes transplanted kidneys to be rejected by the body were developed here. The millisecond Cine CT scanner, which for the first time made it possible to scan the beating heart, and one of the most advanced versions of magnetic resonance imaging were also developed here.

An experimental bladder pacemaker, which gives "normal" function to paraplegics and quadriplegics, was recently invented at UCSF. So too was a new method of treating ocular cancer without removing the eye, new surgical techniques for formerly inoperative retinal detachments, and a dozen different ways of using lasers, microsurgery, and ultrasound.

UCSF clinicians and investigators have made an enormous, multidisciplinary contribution to the fight against AIDS, both locally and nationally. The work of 150 investigators, conducting research through the UCSF AIDS Clinical Research Center, ranges from epidemiological studies into the ways AIDS is spread to developing a model for care that is both humane and cost-effective, from preventive public health education to basic studies of the immune system.

Major clinical research grants from NIH have been given to physician-researchers working in plastic surgery, pulmonary medicine, the treatment of malignant brain tumors, cardiovascular responses to stress, arteriosclerosis, and sickle cell disease. The hospital is also the site of two NIH-funded Clinical Research Centers, one for adults and one for children.

Among the many special research facilities at UCSF are the Rosalind Russell Research Center for Arthritis, the Cardiovascular Research Institute, the Cystic Fibrosis Research Center, the Koret Vision Center, the Brain Tumor Research Center, the Senator Jacob Javits Center for Excellence in Neurosciences, and the UCSF Cancer Research Institute.

## Admission Policy

Most patients are referred by their physicians, usually for advanced diagnostic or surgical procedures. Patients who wish to refer themselves to outpatient faculty practice clinics may call 415-476-2285 for more information. UCSF also has a Screening and Acute Care Clinic, open six days a week, and an emergency room for those needing immediate care.

---

**ROOM CHARGES (per diem)**
Private: $465
Semiprivate: $456
Ward (four beds): $442
ICU: $991–$1,508

**AVERAGE COST PER PATIENT STAY:**   $6,723

**MAILING ADDRESS**          **TELEPHONE**
505 Parnassus Avenue      415-476-1000
San Francisco, CA 94143

# Scripps Clinic and Research Foundation

## LA JOLLA, CALIFORNIA

Scripps Clinic and Research Foundation is one of the oldest private medical centers in the United States. It is a nonprofit institution dedicated to quality patient care, biomedical research, and specialized medical education. Founded almost sixty years ago by Ellen Browning Scripps, the Scripps Metabolic Clinic functioned as part of the Scripps Memorial Hospital, specializing in the beginning in diagnostic services and research, primarily for diabetes. The clinic separated from the hospital in 1951, and its present name was adopted in 1956.

Under the leadership of Dr. Charles C. Edward, who assumed the presidency of Scripps in 1977, a major shift in the clinic's philosophy of health care began. To contain costs while providing high-quality medical services, Scripps began to emphasize preventive medicine and outpatient care over the traditional hospital-oriented practice of medicine. The Anderson Outpatient Pavilion was opened in 1983. Another step in this direction was the creation of a network of smaller clinics throughout San Diego County. In addition to the Anderson Pavilion and the Cecil and Ida Green Hospital, there are 11 regional Scripps Clinic medical centers, in Borrego Springs, Chula Vista, Escondido, Jamul, Lake San Marcos, Rancho Bernardo, Rancho San Diego, San Diego, San Jacinto, Solana Beach, and Welk Village. Affordable general family-care medical services are available at each facility, with comprehensive specialty care provided at Chula Vista, Rancho Bernardo, Rancho San Diego, and San Diego. General family care is also offered at the main Torrey Pines facility, where the largest number of specialists practice.

The Scripps Clinic Medical Group has nearly 300 members offering services in over 50 fields of medicine and surgery, together with specialized centers.

The Alcohol/Chemical Dependency Center offers screening evaluation, assessment, and treatment on an outpatient basis. In addition, education and treatment are provided for family members and friends.

The Diabetes Center offers complete medical services as well as extensive ongoing educational, counseling, and behavior modification programs designed to help patients live with their disease as easily and comfortably as possible. Each patient's program is personalized.

The Eating Disorders Clinic treats compulsive eating or food addiction patterns. Patients are admitted through self- or physician referral and, although participants are asked to commit themselves for one year, treatment time varies according to individual needs. Bariatrics programs use physiological techniques to help people lose weight and maintain their new weight.

Emergency Services treats emergency medical problems other than major trauma on an unscheduled walk-in basis.

The Fertility Center includes evaluation, treatment, ongoing data collection, and research using a team of physicians from many specialties.

The Low Vision Service, the only medically supervised facility of its kind in the county, offers an inventory of optical and nonoptical aids and appliances, including spectacle-mounted telescopes and microscopes, lamp magnifiers, and sophisticated electronic devices such as a closed-circuit television system. The service also offers writing aids, stands, special tables, and counseling on activities available to the visually disabled.

The Medical Genetics Program includes genetic counseling, prenatal diagnosis, and research.

In the Pain Treatment Center laboratories concentrate on technologies for the evaluation, treatment, and management of chronic pain. Staff members also conduct research on intractable pain.

Preventive Medicine provides a series of programs designed to identify and modify life-threatening risk factors and to improve the quality of life through more healthful habits. The center offers individual counseling in life-style intervention and exercise, nutrition, stress management, and other areas. Programs for business and industry are available to help improve employee productivity through enhancing physical health.

The Sleep Disorders Clinic diagnoses sleep-related disorders, evaluates patients with specific sleep pathologies, assesses medical conditions in which sleep plays a crucial role, and devises treatment plans.

The Sports Medicine Center offers assistance to sports enthusiasts in achieving proper condition, maintaining fitness, and preventing injuries through consultation, medical evaluation, sports physical therapy, and education. Treatment and aggressive rehabilitation of injuries are also part of the program.

The Urgent Care Centers, located in the Anderson Outpatient Pavilion, Chula Vista, Rancho Bernardo, and San Diego, provides treatment for urgent medical problems such as minor childhood diseases, colds, flu, fever, lacerations, sprains, and other non-life-threatening situations.

Other specialty centers include the Allergy and Allergic Disease Center and the Kidney Stone Treatment Center.

Scripps offers advanced educational opportunities to future biomedical researchers and clinical specialists through its postdoctoral fellowship program and provides continuing medical education for physicians across the country.

# Specialties

Allergy and Immunology, Cardiac Surgery, Cardiovascular Diseases, Chest Medicine, Community Medicine, Dermatology, Diabetes, Endocrinology and Nephrology, Family and General Practice, Gastroenterology, General Internal Medicine, General Surgery, Head and Neck Surgery and Otology, Hematology and Oncology, Infectious Diseases, Neurology, Neurosurgery, Obstetrics and Gynecology, Oral Medicine and Stomatology, Ophthalmology, Optometry, Orthopedic Surgery, Pathology, Pediatrics and Adolescent Medicine, Plastic and Reconstructive Medicine, Psychiatry and Behavioral Medicine, Radiation Oncology, Radiology, Rheumatology, Thoracic and Vascular Surgery, and Urology.

---

**STATISTICAL PROFILE (Green Hospital)**

Number of Beds: 158
Bed Occupancy Rate: 60%
Average Number of Patients: 95
Average Patient Stay: 5 days
Annual Admissions: 6,500
Outpatient Clinic Visits: 471,000 (all 12 clinics)

Hospital Personnel (all 12 clinics):
   Physicians: 320
   Residents: 9
   Registered Nurses: 233
   Total Staff: 714

---

# Well-known Specialists

Dr. Eugene Bernstein, thoracic and vascular surgery.
Dr. Ernest Beutler, chairman of Basic and Clinical Research, head of the Hematology and Oncology Division.
Dr. Clifford Colwell, head of the Orthopedic Surgery Division.
Dr. Donald J. Dalessio, specialist in neurology, chairman of the Department of Medicine.
Dr. Ralph Dilley, head of the Thoracic and Vascular Surgery Division.
Dr. Ruben F. Gittes, specialist in urology, chairman of surgery.
Dr. Ruth Grobstein, head of the Radiation Oncology Division.
Dr. Allen Johnson, head of the Cardiovascular Diseases Division.
Dr. Gustavo Kuster, general surgery.
Dr. Joseph Michelson, ophthalmology; director of the Retina-Uveitis Division.

Dr. Robert M. Nakamura, chairman of the Department of Pathology.

Dr. James Oury, cardiac surgery.

Dr. Donald Stevenson, head of the Allergy and Immunology Division.

Dr. Eng Tan, head of the Research Rheumatology Division and the Autoimmune Disease Center.

Dr. Richard Timms, director of Sleep Disorders, head of the Chest Medicine Division.

Dr. Thomas Waltz, neurosurgery.

## Research

With $56 million in federal, corporate, and private funding, the Research Institute at Scripps Clinic has become the largest private medical research facility in the world not affiliated with a university; its professional and technical staff of over 1,000 conducts investigations into the biological underpinnings of disease. The institute has made noteworthy contributions to the understanding and treatment of alcoholism and chemical dependency, anemia, cancer, circulatory conditions leading to stroke and heart attacks, infectious diseases, kidney disease, various neurological conditions, and viral disorders.

Since 1974 Scripps has operated a Clinical Research Center within Green Hospital. It is one of 75 such facilities designated by the NIH and the only one not affiliated with a medical school. A small number of beds are set aside in this facility for the development and evaluation of new and experimental therapeutic procedures, especially for autoimmune diseases, such as rheumatoid arthritis and systemic lupus erythematosus.

## Admission Policy

Appointments with Scripps Clinic physicians can be made by contacting the clinic directly or by recommendation of one's personal physician. Prospective patients or referring physicians should call the Appointment Scheduling Office at 619-455-8770. The office will either book the appointment or refer the caller to the appropriate division.

---

**ROOM CHARGES (per diem)**
Private: $315
Semiprivate: $295

**MAILING ADDRESS**         **TELEPHONE**
10666 North Torrey Pines Road   619-455-9100
La Jolla, CA 92037

# Stanford University Medical Center
# Stanford University Hospital
# Stanford University Clinic

**STANFORD, CALIFORNIA**

We doubt that any best hospital list compiled over the last twenty years would have excluded this extraordinary institution. In fact, almost every department at Stanford is consistently rated among the best in the country, probably because of the high caliber of people who come to work, study, do research, and practice medicine here. Several Stanford researchers have won prestigious international awards, including the Nobel Prize and the Lasker Award, for their work in cancer. Physicians such as Dr. Norman Shumway, the world-famous heart transplant surgeon; Dr. Saul Rosenberg, an expert in the treatment of Hodgkin's disease and other lymphomas; Dr. Philip Sunshine, a neonatologist; and Dr. Hugh McDevilt, an immunologist, have won professional and public acclaim. In recent years 14 members of the Stanford faculty have been elected to the National Academy of Sciences and fourteen to the Institute of Medicine.

The spirit of excellence also affects the way people are admitted to or hired by Stanford on every other level. The struggle to secure a place in Stanford's residency programs is legendary, and the medical school annually receives 6,000 applications for fewer than 100 openings. From the patient's perspective, however, a perhaps more important measure of Stanford's commitment to employing the best people can be found by reviewing some facts about the nursing staff, certainly among the most impressive we discovered while researching this book.

Stanford has created an environment in which nurses want to work. In a profession whose major problem over the last decade has been keeping skilled personnel, Stanford has virtually no turnover. Only a handful of hospitals in the country come close to its retention rate of 98 percent. Moreover, there is a waiting list of several hundred nurses who wish to work here.

Qualifications for nurses are high. Just over half of Stanford's registered nurses hold bachelor's degrees, far above the national average, and there are 12 Ph.D's as well. Stanford is nationally famous for conducting seminars on many aspects of nursing research and management (several staff members have written a book on this topic) as well as in specialized medical areas where the hospital in collaboration with the school of medicine faculty has led the way in developing patient-care techniques, especially cardiovascular and perinatal nursing.

The caliber of its medical staff enables Stanford to deliver high-tech medicine at its best. In 1985, for example, the staff performed 48 heart transplants, more than any other hospital.

The medical center has three components: the Stanford University School of Medicine; the Stanford University Hospital, a teaching and research facility with patients from Palo Alto, nearby communities, and around the world; and the Stanford University Clinic, a collection of more than 80 outpatient clinics staffed by medical school faculty members.

The medical school, founded in 1858, is the oldest in the West. It was started in San Francisco as the medical department of the University of the Pacific and moved to the Stanford University campus in 1959.

The hospital is a university-owned sister corporation. Like the medical school, it is a nonprofit organization operated without public funding or subsidy from the university.

The clinic serves as "doctor's office" for faculty members; its group practice for Stanford's full-time faculty physicians is called the Faculty Practice Program, and it is governed by a faculty committee. It offers medical students, residents, and postdoctoral fellows an opportunity to become familiar with outpatient problems under faculty supervision. Clinic revenue is a source for faculty salaries and general operating costs of the medical school.

---

**STATISTICAL PROFILE**

Number of Beds: 583
Bed Occupancy Rate: 72%
Average Number of Patients: 419
Average Patient Stay: 6.6 days
Annual Admissions: 23,233
Outpatient Clinic Visits: 144,000
Emergency Room/Trauma Center Visits: 26,966

Hospital Personnel:
  Physicians: 1,150
  Residents: 416
  Registered Nurses: 1,217
  Total Staff: 4,230 (including part-time employees)

---

## Specialties

**Clinic**: Anesthesia (Pain Service), Cardiovascular Surgery, Dermatology, Medicine, Obstetrics/Gynecology, Neurology, Pediatrics, Psychiatry, Radiology, and Surgery.

**Hospital**: Acute Respiratory Care, Anesthesia, Basic Emergency Medical Care, Cardiovascular Surgery, Coronary Care, Intensive Care, Intensive Care/Newborn, Medicine, Nuclear Medicine, Oncology, Pediatrics, Perinatal Care, Physical Therapy, Psychiatry, Radiation Therapy, Radiology, Rheumatology, Speech Pathology, and Surgery.

Regional medical services include the Coronary Intervention Program, the Home Care Program, Life Flight (Critical Care Transport Program), the Perinatal Outreach Program, the Trauma Center, and the Washington-Stanford Radiation Oncology Center in Fremont, California.

## Well-known Specialists

Dr. William Stewart Agras, behavioral medicine; specialist in eating disorders and phobias.

Dr. Michael Amylon, pediatric oncology; specialist in bone marrow transplantation.

Dr. Malcolm Bagshaw, radiation therapy.

Dr. John Baldwin, cardiovascular surgery; specialist in heart-lung transplantation.

Dr. David Baum, pediatric cardiology.

Dr. Eugene Black, orthopedic surgery.

Dr. Robert Chase, hand surgery and microsurgery.

Dr. John Collins, surgery; specialist in traumatic shock.

Dr. William C. Dement, sleep disorders.

Dr. Willard Fee, otolaryngology; specialist in head and neck cancer.

Dr. Stuart Flechner, renal transplantation.

Dr. Bertil Glader, pediatric oncology.

Dr. Don R. Goffinet, radiotherapy; specialist in head and neck cancer.

Dr. Gary Gray, gastroenterology.

Dr. John W. Hanberry, neurosurgery.

Dr. William Hancock, cardiology.

Dr. Halsted Holman, arthritis and lupus erythematosus.

Dr. Michael Jacobs, primary care/internal medicine.

Dr. Paul Jacobs, dermatology.

Dr. Emmet Lamb, infertility.

Dr. Iris Litt, adolescent medicine.

Dr. Hugh McDevitt, immunology.

Dr. James B. D. Mark, thoracic surgery.

Dr. Michael Marmor, ophthalmology.

Dr. Thomas C. Merigan, infectious diseases.

Dr. Gerald Reaven, diabetes and metabolism.

Dr. Saul Rosenberg, oncology; specialist in Hodgkin's disease and lymphomas.

Dr. John S. Schroeder, cardiology.

Dr. Norman Shumway, cardiovascular surgery; specialist in cardiac transplantation.

Dr. Blair Simmons, otorhinolaryngology; specialist in cochlear implants.

Dr. Thomas A. Stamey, urology.

Dr. Lawrence Steinman, pediatric neurology.

Dr. Samuel Strober, allergy/immunology.

Dr. Philip Sunshine, neonatology.

Dr. Kent Ueland, obstetrics/gynecology; specialist in perinatology and high-risk pregnancy.

## Research

Stanford's reputation as one of the premier research institutions in the world has been justly earned. Beginning with one of the first kidney transplants in 1960, the first human heart transplant in the United States in 1968, and the first successful human heart-lung transplant in the world in 1981, the medical center has received international acclaim.

In 1984 faculty members at the School of Medicine received grants and contracts totaling more than $80 million in support of research, teaching, and patient care. The federal government is a major contributor, and the hospital has been designated a General Clinical Research Center by the NIH. Under this grant some Stanford doctors and researchers are conducting investigations into a variety of problems, including hypertension and antiarrhythmic drugs, in vitro fertilization, liver disease therapy, premature infants, psoriasis, and sleep disorders. The following is a partial list of ongoing projects in major areas.

Arthritis—providing research and education in areas including new irradiation treatments, innovative self-care methods, and ARAMIS, a national data bank on medical and social aspects of the disease.

Cancer treatment—studying hyperthermia, radiosensitizers, new approaches to solid tumors of the head and neck and to tumors of the genitourinary system, radiation therapy and chemotherapy to treat Hodgkin's disease, monoclonal antibodies, DNA replication, and other recombinant DNA research to understand how cancer cells grow.

Cardiology—investigating new drugs and devices for treating heart disease, including laser vaporization of clogged arteries, agents for preventing heart attacks and abnormal heart rhythms, and implantable devices that shock an ailing heart into a normal pumping pattern.

Expert systems—developing computer programs to help in the diagnosis and treatment of disease.

Interferon—testing the antiviral agent's power to fight a variety of diseases, including some types of cancer, the common cold, and hepatitis.

Biological basis of mental illness—studying neurotransmitters, the chemicals responsible for communication between cells in the brain.

Neonatal intensive care—researching nutritional deficiencies, respiratory distress syndrome, and sudden infant death syndrome.

# Admission Policy

Strictly speaking, patients are admitted to Stanford only by the hospital's medical staff, which is composed of medical school faculty and physicians in private practice. But since anyone can make an appointment for consultation or treatment through the Stanford University Clinic, admission to the hospital is not difficult for patients who are really sick. In fact, patients admitted through the clinic make up more than half of the 153,000 patients' days of care at Stanford University Hospital. For information call Clinic-Patient Relations at 415-723-6903.

While there is no official financial requirement for admission, advance deposits are requested for some of the more difficult procedures.

---

**ROOM CHARGES (per diem)**
Private: $451
Semiprivate: $388
Ward: $365
ICU: $979–$2,345
Patients who receive around-the-clock medical supervision by
    residents incur additional charges of $30 to $50 a day.
In 1987 Stanford University Hospital, in conjunction with the Santa
    Clara Chapter of the National Assistance League, opened a 42-
    unit "hometel" providing short-term, low-cost housing for out-of-
    town patients and their families. The cost of stay in the hometel is
    $10 a day.

**AVERAGE COST PER PATIENT STAY**
    $9,576 (excludes normal newborns)

**MAILING ADDRESS**          **TELEPHONE**
300 Pasteur Drive            Hospital: 415-723-4000
Stanford, CA 94305           Clinic: 415-723-5631 or
                                     800-982-5784

# University of California, Los Angeles, (UCLA) Medical Center

**LOS ANGELES, CALIFORNIA**

The excellent nursing service at the UCLA Medical Center is one of the reasons that 96 percent of the patients responding to a recent patient-discharge survey conducted by the hospital said they would recommend it. Ongoing education for nurses is strongly emphasized. They are encouraged to receive certification, to take advantage of the medical center's affiliation with two baccalaureate nursing programs, and to participate in projects in their research department. Continuing education programs have also been established to help acute-care and intensive-care nurses further their skills.

This attention to the nursing staff has paid off handsomely. Nurses at UCLA have been responsible for at least 20 publications in the past year, including a chemotherapy manual that has been nationally recognized. Nurses have also made presentations on a variety of topics, including cardiac nursing, critical-care techniques, oncology, and transplants.

Humanistic patient care is emphasized throughout the medical center. Monthly awards are given to employees who demonstrate extra concern for patients. A grant from the Borun Foundation supports the development of a variety of programs encouraging employees to be sensitive and empathetic to patients.

The UCLA Medical Center is the primary teaching hospital for the School of Medicine at UCLA. The center provides inpatient and outpatient services in nearly all medical specialties; it offers both primary and tertiary care for adults and children.

The center's heart and liver transplant programs have helped scores of patients. Bone marrow, kidney, and pancreas transplants are also performed here. The Regional Organ Procurement Agency, housed at UCLA, centralizes the collection and allocation of donated organs used in transplant programs throughout southern California.

The Jonsson Comprehensive Cancer Center, adjacent to the medical center, is one of 20 such centers in the country designated by the NIH. It includes the largest clinic in the world for the treatment of melanoma. Oncologists at UCLA are leaders in treating cancer with hyperthermia and immunotherapy. An innovative surgical technique in which cancerous bone and muscle are replaced with metallic implants eliminates the need to amputate limbs that contain cancerous tumors and greatly increases patients' chances for survival. Bone marrow transplantation techniques continue to be improved at UCLA.

Treatment for infertility through in vitro fertilization is another specialization of UCLA. Physicians sometimes use a noninvasive ultrasound technique to guide the removal of eggs from the patient's ovaries. The success rate here for achieving pregnancy through in vitro fertilization is among the highest in the nation.

Infants, children, and adults with congenital and acquired heart problems are treated by a team of cardiac-care experts. The UCLA Adult Congenital Heart Program is one of the few in the country designed for patients who were born with heart defects and have survived to adulthood.

A comprehensive geriatric medicine program offers services ranging from a special inpatient care unit to community outreach. Staff members include geriatricians, social workers, geropsychiatrists, and nurse practitioners. The Sylvia Olshan Health Center, a community service facility affiliated with the geriatrics program, has become a model for community-based health-care centers.

In the UCLA School of Dentistry's Oral and Maxillofacial Clinic, prosthodontists sculpt and fit patients with nearly exact replicas of facial features lost primarily through the removal of tumors. The nearby Rehabilitation Center houses special facilities for outpatient physical and occupational therapy and clinics for the treatment of arthritis, collagen disease, Paget's disease, and scleroderma. Pediatric amputee programs and a lab for making and fitting artificial limbs are also located here.

The Pain Management Center treats patients with chronic pain, including headaches and asthma. Treatments range from traditional medications to ancient methods such as acupuncture.

The medical center is equipped with the most advanced technology available, including a lithotriptor, magnetic resonance imaging units, a PET scanner, CAT scanners, and the MEG (magnetoencephalography), a device used to pinpoint areas of abnormal brain function in patients with epilepsy. A clinical neutron therapy facility, one of only four in the country, bombards tumors with neutrons, offering new treatment opportunities for certain kinds of slow-growing or inoperable tumors. The UCLA MedStar is the only helicopter service in the area staffed by a physician and an intensive-care flight nurse. Digiplan, a unique computerized system that provides directions to more than 200 locations within the medical center, was installed in 1985. To find a particular clinic, visitors push a button on the screen and receive a printout with detailed map and directions.

Two floors of the medical center cater to patients who request special amenities. Established in 1969, the 60-bed Wilson Pavilion has larger rooms with special furnishings and serves gourmet meals on fine china. In addition, it has its own admitting service and laboratory, and electrocardiograms are performed in patients' rooms.

The UCLA Medical Center operates on a nonprofit, self-supporting basis. It was constructed in 1955 on the southern portion of the University of California, Los Angeles, campus. Other components of the UCLA Center for Health Sciences include the schools of Medicine, Nursing, Dentistry, and Public Health; the Neuropsychiatric Institute and Hospital; the Clarence Reed Neurological Research Center; the Brain Research Institute; the Biomedical Cyclotron; and the Jerry Lewis Neuromuscular Research Center.

## Specialties

Anesthesiology, Cardiology, Dentistry, Emergency Medicine, Geriatrics, Immunology, Infectious Diseases, Intensive Care, In Vitro Fertilization, Neonatal Intensive Care, Neurology, Obstetrics/Gynecology, Oncology, Ophthalmology, Organ Transplantation, Orthopedics, Pathology, Pediatrics, Psychiatry, Radiation Oncology, Radiology, Rehabilitation, Sports Medicine, Surgery, and Urology.

In addition to inpatient services, the medical center houses the outpatient ambulatory care clinics, where patients are seen by specialists in more than 80 areas, including arthritis, cancer, adult congenital heart defects, infertility, kidney stones, and lupus.

---

**STATISTICAL PROFILE**

Number of Beds: 711
Bed Occupancy Rate: 66%
Average Number of Patients: 466
Average Patient Stay: 7 days
Annual Admissions: 23,399
Births: 2,155
Outpatient Clinic Visits: 250,000
Emergency Room/Trauma Center Visits: 40,229

Hospital Personnel:
   Physicians: 657 full-time
   Residents: 472
   Registered Nurses: 891
   Total Staff: 3,388

---

## Well-known Specialists

Dr. Donald Becker, chief of neurosurgery.
Dr. Ronald Busuttil, surgery; specialist in liver transplantation.
Dr. Stephen Feig, pediatric hematology/oncology.
Dr. David Golde, hematology/oncology; specialist in leukemia, lymphoma, and hematology.

Dr. Hillel Laks, specialist in heart surgery and transplantation, chief of cardiothoracic surgery.

Dr. Donald Morton, specialist in melanoma and other skin cancers. chief of surgery/oncology.

Dr. Joseph Perloff, cardiology; specialist in adult congenital heart disease.

Dr. Michael Phelps, specialist in the PET scanner, professor of biophysics and radiological sciences.

Dr. Kenneth Shine, cardiology; specialist in ischemic heart disease, former president of American Heart Association.

Dr. Bradley Straatsma, ophthalmology; specialist in cataracts and intraocular lens transplants.

# Research

It would be impossible to list all the subjects under investigation at UCLA, but even a quick overview of selected topics will demonstrate the range.

In infectious diseases UCLA is a leader in herpes research and the first to have studied the effect of the oral drug acyclovir on an initial episode of genital herpes. Immunologists at UCLA were the first to recognize AIDS in 1981, and they continue to investigate the virus. Immunotherapy and antiviral therapies for AIDS are being developed, and research on the AIDS virus blood test is being conducted.

Cancer researchers are investigating the link between distinct families of cancer-causing viruses that may shed light on the changes in cells that lead to cancer.

In researching cardiovascular problems, scientists are studying how the body manufactures cholesterol, how its amount is regulated in the body, and what causes an overabundance of the substance. Techniques to improve damaged heart muscle and expand the use of coronary revascularization (which bypasses diseased arteries by grafting) are also being investigated.

Indocin, a medication that had been used to treat arthritis, is now being used to treat patent ductus arteriosus, a heart defect common among premature infants that previously was treated with heart surgery.

Researchers are studying the use of bone marrow transplantation to treat certain inherited central nervous system disorders.

Researchers and surgeons are focusing on improving the outcome of patients who have suffered serious brain injuries, such as stroke or head trauma. One neurological project is studying how partially damaged brain cells can recover.

# Admission Policy

Patients can be admitted to UCLA without a doctor's referral through the clinic or emergency room.

Patients are responsible for the expenses associated with their care. Payment most commonly comes from the patient's insurance or other provider arrangements or coverage. A limited number of patients qualify to have their bills paid because they participate in a research program or newly developed treatment program funded by another source. Specially trained financial counselors are available.

**ROOM CHARGES** (per diem)
Private: $458
Semiprivate: $342
Ward: $324
ICU: $811

**AVERAGE COST PER PATIENT STAY:**    $9,226

**MAILING ADDRESS**          **TELEPHONE**
10833 Le Conte Avenue    213-825-9111
Los Angeles, CA 90024

# University of California, San Diego, (UCSD) Medical Center

**SAN DIEGO, CALIFORNIA**

The UCSD Medical Center is one of five health sciences centers of the University of California. It serves as the primary teaching and research facility for the UCSD School of Medicine. Since its inception in 1966, the medical center has become world renowned for its work in diabetes control, endocrine disorders, high-risk pregnancy, kidney transplantation, laser surgery, newborn care, nuclear medicine, stroke prevention, and treatment of trauma. The first successful treatment of the childhood killer Reye's syndrome and the use of human surfactant to prevent respiratory distress syndrome in premature infants were developed here. Over 150 general and specialty clinics are held at several outpatient locations, including the Theodore Gildred Cancer Center. The UCSD Medical Center was selected by *Business Week* as one of the 24 best hospitals in the United States.

The UCSD Cancer Center is one of around 20 so-called Comprehensive Care Centers designated by the NIH. Patients who cannot be helped by conventional treatments receive here experimental drugs and therapies not generally available. A promising treatment for ovarian cancer infuses chemotherapy agents directly into the abdominal cavity for greater impact and considerably lessened side effects. Intensive laboratory and clinical research with monoclonal antibodies is also under way.

The UCSD Level I Trauma Center, the only one in San Diego, and its blue-and-white Life Flight helicopters are the keystone of the San Diego Regional Trauma System, which has cut preventable death from trauma in the two-county area by 85 percent. The medical center's critical-care service also includes the Regional Burn Center and the Comprehensive Emergency Medical Hyperbaric Medicine Center, the only ones in the San Diego area. The Neurosurgical Intensive Care Unit is a leader in head trauma treatment, and the innovations of the Neonatal Intensive Care Unit are internationally known. Ambulance planes transport critically ill babies from distant points.

The Diabetes Center teaches diabetics how to reduce or eliminate the need for insulin through control of blood sugar levels. A Diabetes Pregnancy Program in conjunction with the Reproductive Medicine Department is aiding diabetic women to carry healthy babies to term.

The Medical Center Comprehensive Geriatrics Program started in 1982 with SOCARE, Seniors Only Comprehensive Assessment and Retirement Evaluation. Complete physical and psychobehavioral examination by a multidisciplinary team includes a home visit to check on safety and personal factors. If needed, the SOCARE staff will set up a linkage with requisite community services. The program strives to maintain independent living for the patient as long as possible.

Patients who display symptoms of memory disorders are referred to the Alzheimer's Disease Diagnostic and Treatment Center. The UCSD Alzheimer's Disease Research Center is one of only a handful in the United States funded by the NIH. The world's first brain bank is also located at the medical center.

The UCSD Laser Center encompasses the services of dermatologists; gynecologists; neurosurgeons; ophthalmologists; pulmonary, nose, and throat specialists; and urologists who are employing laser surgery on otherwise untreatable conditions of the skin, reproductive organs, brain, spinal cord, eye, pulmonary organs, throat, and kidneys.

Infant corneal transplants, hormone pumps to induce pregnancy without the risk of multiple births posed by fertility drugs, dissolution of gallstones under local anesthetic, and restoration of partial hearing through an "electronic ear" are among the other advanced treatment services for which the medical center is known.

The center emphasizes the personal side of medical care along with advanced technology. Interpreters are available for non-English-speaking patients. Primary nursing, instituted in 1984, provides the security of a continuing relationship between patient and nurse. Visiting hours are generous.

A dozen miles north of the medical center, on the UCSD campus in La Jolla, are the internationally recognized UCSD Eye Center, the Lipid Research Facility, and the Internal Medicine Group. Other clinics are located in various parts of the city. A second hospital, on the La Jolla campus, which will treat primary and secondary illnesses, is in the planning stage. The medical center pediatrics faculty also is affiliated with nearby Children's Hospital under an agreement amalgamating neonatal and other pediatric services of the two institutions.

## Specialties

Departments in Anesthesiology, Community and Family Medicine, Medicine, Neurosciences, Ophthalmology, Pathology, Pediatrics, Psychiatry, Radiology, Reproductive Medicine, and Surgery.

Specialties in Adolescent Medicine, AIDS, Allergy/Immunology, Alzheimer's Disease, a Birth Defects Program, a Burn Center, Cardiac Services, Clinical Research, Cochlear Implants, Complex Neurosurgery (adult and pediatric), Cornea Implants, Dermatology, Diabetes, Endocrinology, Epilepsy, Gastrointestinal Surgery, Genetics, Geriatrics, Glaucoma Surgery, Gynecology, Hand Surgery and Rehabilitation, High-Risk Obstetrics, Industrial Health, Kidney Transplant, Laser Surgery, Lithotripsy, Lung Cancer, Magnetic Resonance Imaging, Neonatal Intensive Care, Nuclear Medicine, Oncology, Orthopedics, Plastic and Reconstructive Surgery, Pulmonary Rehabilitation, Reproductive Endocrinology, Spine Surgery and Rehabilitation, a Stroke Program, and a Trauma Center.

---

**STATISTICAL PROFILE**

Number of Beds: 437
Bed Occupancy Rate: 82%
Average Number of Patients: 336
Average Patient Stay: 5.8 days
Annual Admissions: 20,664
Births: 3,356
Outpatient Clinic Visits: 192,546
Emergency Room/Trauma Center Visits: 42,568

Hospital Personnel:
  Physicians: 310 faculty (salaried); 700 attending
  Residents: 420
  Registered Nurses: 1,008
  Total Staff: 3,520

---

## Well-known Specialists

Dr. Wayne H. Akeson, orthopedic surgery.
Dr. Stuart Brown, ophthalmology; specialist in infant corneas.
Dr. Irma Gigli, dermatology.
Dr. Mark Green, oncology.
Dr. Jon Isenberg, gastroenterology.
Dr. Michael Kaback, pediatrics; specialist in Tay-Sachs disease.
Dr. Robert Katzman, neurology; specialist in Alzheimer's disease.
Dr. George Leopold, radiology.
Dr. Larry Marshall, head trauma surgery.
Dr. A. R. Moossa, gastrointestinal surgery.
Dr. Kenneth Moser, specialist in the lung, particularly in embolisms.
Dr. William Nyhan, pediatrics; specialist in Lesch-Nyhan syndrome.
Dr. Jerrold Olefsky, diabetes research.
Dr. Robert Resnik, reproductive medicine; specialist in high-risk pregnancy.
Dr. Samuel S. C. Yen, reproductive endocrinology.
Dr. Nathan Zvaifler, rheumatology.

# Research

In the Association of American Medical Colleges' most recent survey, the UCSD School of Medicine ranked first of 122 medical colleges in percentage of faculty directing federally supported research projects, with 42 percent of the faculty listed as principal investigators. At the end of 1986, 519 active research grants were in progress, totaling nearly $80 million.

Research centers of excellence established at UCSD by the NIH include the AIDS Treatment Evaluation Unit, the Alzheimer's Disease Research Center, the UCSD Cancer Center, and the Diabetes Control and Complications Trial. The NIH has also committed millions of dollars in funding to designated Specialized Centers of Research in atherosclerosis, heart disease, hypertension, and pulmonary physiology.

The Institute for Research on Aging, headquartered on the School of Medicine campus, coordinates research on age-related conditions in conjunction with the active clinical program in geriatric medicine.

A long-term population study of Rancho Bernardo, a suburb of San Diego, is investigating environmental and life-style factors contributing to health and longevity. Observations on topics ranging from the connection between "secondhand" smoke and heart disease to the risks and benefits of estrogen replacement therapy for women are now cited as landmark studies.

Basic research being conducted in molecular biology and genetics, supported by federal funding and by the Howard Hughes Medical Institute, will lead to advances in the treatment of depression, immunology, language and learning disorders, metabolic and congenital defects in children, and reproductive disorders such as infertility and premenstrual syndrome.

Many of these programs have a clinical component and serve patients through the NIH-supported Clinical Research Center.

# Admission Policy

Patients are admitted by UCSD Medical Center physicians through clinics and the energency room as well as by private community physicians.

Patients are required to pay 50 percent of their estimated bill upon admission, but this payment is not a condition of admission for emergency cases.

---

**ROOM CHARGES (per diem)**
Private: $310
Semiprivate: $290
Ward: $285
ICU: $950

---

**AVERAGE COST PER PATIENT STAY:**   $1,200–$1,300 per day

**MAILING ADDRESS**               **TELEPHONE**
225 Dickinson Street              619-543-6222
San Diego, CA 92103-9981

# National Jewish Center for Immunology and Respiratory Medicine

DENVER, COLORADO

In 1984 the National Jewish Center for Immunology and Respiratory Medicine (the new name for the institution previously known as the National Jewish Hospital/National Asthma Center) instituted LUNG LINE®, a nationwide toll-free telephone number (800-222-LUNG, 303-398-1477 for Colorado residents) providing answers to callers concerned about lung disease, allergies, and immune system disorders. In its first year of operation, LUNG LINE received nearly 11,000 calls from every state. Today LUNG LINE averages 127 calls a day, and more than 75,000 people have dialed the service, talked with a nurse, and received more than 120,000 brochures, pamphlets, and informational mailings from the center.

LUNG LINE is only one of many services provided by National Jewish, one of the world's outstanding institutes for the study and treatment of lung disease, allergies, and immunology, which account for a large percentage of cases of chronic illness. National Jewish is the largest treatment and research center for both adult and childhood asthma in the world.

Patients come for treatment of diseases such as allergies, asthma, chronic bronchitis, emphysema, autoimmune and immune-deficiency disease, occupational and environmental lung disorders, tuberculosis, and others. Experts from many fields are involved in patient care—physicians; nurses; psychiatrists; psychologists; social workers; physical, recreational, and occupational therapists; and teachers in the accredited school on the medical center campus. An intensive "whole person" approach is taken to each case, with attention given to all aspects of the patient's well-being. National Jewish has, for example, the only inpatient facility in the United States geared exclusively to providing medical/psychosocial support for children and adolescents with chronic respiratory and immunologic diseases.

An unusual aspect of the clinical program here is the emphasis on teaching patients to manage their chronic diseases so as to prevent or reduce costly emergency room visits and hospital stays after discharge. Data reported nationally early in 1986 established that the center's programs are highly cost effective, saving many of its patients thousands of dollars in annual health expenditures after they return home.

As part of its educational function, National Jewish has been selected by the U.S. Department of Health and Human Services to conduct training programs for health professionals on juvenile rheumatoid arthritis.

National Jewish is also a prestigious teaching hospital. More than 25 percent of the pediatric allergists now practicing in the United States received their training at the institute, which is affiliated with the University of Colorado Health Sciences Center. University fellows in allergy, clinical immunology, and pulmonary medicine spend four months of their first year on clinical service at National Jewish. All residents in the internal medicine program also rotate through National Jewish for experience with its special patient populations. And all members of the National Jewish professional staff hold teaching appointments at the university.

Founded in 1899 as the National Jewish Hospital for Consumptives, the hospital was a nonsectarian treatment center helping the thousands of tuberculosis victims who poured into Denver because of the dry air and sunny climate. In 1925 the hospital was designated a training center in tuberculosis and chest medicine for the University of Colorado School of Medicine. In the 1950s, with tuberculosis in retreat, the hospital began to look in new directions, especially asthma and allergic illnesses. However, National Jewish now has one of the few major programs in the world treating patients suffering from drug-resistant tuberculosis and related diseases.

Among the most important achievements of National Jewish immunologists have been the isolation and study of major parts of the immune system; investigation of the basic mechanisms of allergic, autoimmune, and immune-deficiency diseases; and development of new methods to diagnose and treat these conditions.

---

**STATISTICAL PROFILE**

Number of Beds: 94
Bed Occupancy Rate: 86%
Average Number of Patients: 81
Average Patient Stay: 26 days
Annual Admissions: 1,100
Outpatient Clinic Visits: 12,000

Hospital Personnel:
   Physicians: 95 (38 senior physicians, 57 fellows)
   Registered Nurses: 107
   Total Staff: 1,034 (including research personnel)

---

## Specialties

Allergic Conditions, Allergies, Asthma, Bronchitis, Cystic Fibrosis, Emphysema/Chronic Obstructive Pulmonary Disease, Immune System Diseases, Juvenile Rheumatoid Arthritis, Occupational and Environmental Lung

Diseases, Pneumonia, Sarcoidosis, Sinusitis, Tuberculosis, Drug-resistant Tuberculosis and Atypical Mycobacterial Infections, Vocal Cord Dysfunction, and other respiratory ailments and disorders of the immune system.

## Well-known Specialists

Dr. Erwin W. Gelfund, specialist in immunology and rheumatology, chairman of the Department of Pediatrics.

Dr. Michael Grunstien, specialist in pulmonary diseases of newborns and older children.

Dr. J. Roger Hollister, pediatric rheumatology; specialist in juvenile rheumatoid arthritis.

Dr. Michael D. Iseman, internal and pulmonary medicine; specialist in drug-resistant tuberculosis and related illnesses, head of the Clinical Mycobacterial Service.

Dr. James F. Jones, immunology/allergies; author of many textbooks on infection and resistance.

Dr. Talmadge E. King, pulmonology; specialist in interstitial lung disease, medical director of the outpatient clinic.

Dr. Charles Kirkpatrick, clinical immunology; pioneer in research on immune deficiency disorders.

Dr. Kathleen Kreiss, internal and preventive medicine; head of the Occupational Health Program.

Dr. Gary L. Larsen, pediatric pulmonology; director of a study of the relation between inflammation and asthma.

Dr. Richard J. Martin, pulmonology; director of the Sleep Disorders Program.

Dr. Robert Mason, pulmonology; chairman of the Department of Medicine.

Dr. Bruce D. Miller, pediatric psychiatry.

Dr. David A. Mrazek, psychiatry; researcher in the risk factors of children developing asthma.

Dr. Stanley J. Szefler, clinical pharmacology; specialist in drug treatments for asthmatics under six years old.

## Research

National Jewish is funded by more than $22 million in research money. While more than $9 million of this amount comes from federal funding, the remainder is raised through donations. In one of the most advanced and highly regarded programs of its kind in the world, researchers here are defining and analyzing the components of the immune system.

John Kappler, Ph.D., and Philippa Marrack, Ph.D., have pioneered research on the key immune system protein, the T-cell receptor. The Howard Hughes Medical Institute will provide major funding for their research for the next seven years.

In the department of pediatrics, Dr. James Jones, one of the discoverers of chronic Epstein-Barr virus syndrome, is researching a serious illness involving virus infection of lymphocytes.

National Jewish is a Specialized Center of Research designated by the NIH to investigate immunologic and interstitial lung diseases. The center studies inflammation and its effects on respiratory function and has received a $4.9-million NIH grant to study the relation of inflammation and asthma. Additional research focuses on subjects as diverse as the mechanisms of asthma and emphysema, drug-resistant tuberculosis, occupational lung disease, food allergy, respiratory-related sleep disorders, and clinical pulmonary testing.

## Admission Policy

The most efficient way to become an inpatient at National Jewish is through physician referral. During treatment and after discharge, close contact is maintained with the patient's home physician to assure consistency of care. Outpatients may refer themselves to the Cohen Clinic by calling the patient referral representative at 303-398-1565.

National Jewish accepts coverage by Medicare, Medicaid, and most private insurance programs. Financial assistance from the center is also available in some cases on an ability-to-pay basis. The hospital provides about $2 million of indigent care annually.

---

**ROOM CHARGES (per diem)**
Private: $285
Semiprivate: $275

**AVERAGE COST PER PATIENT STAY**
$20,150, although the amount varies widely according to length of stay and severity of disease.

| MAILING ADDRESS | TELEPHONE |
|---|---|
| 1400 Jackson Street | 303-388-4461 |
| Denver, CO 80206 | |

---

# University Hospital
# University of Colorado

**DENVER, COLORADO**

Although Denver ranks only twenty-fifth in the nation in terms of population, its half-million inhabitants have ready access to some of the best medical services available anywhere. "Ninety-nine percent of problems people have can be treated in Denver," claims Dr. Alden Harken, chairman of the Department of Surgery at University Hospital. "I've worked in Washington, Philadelphia, and Boston, and I don't think any of those centers offers the breadth of specialized medical treatment available here. There tend to be areas in the country where everyone seems to be asking new questions and doing new things at once. I think Denver is one of those places right now."

There are 17 acute-care hospitals in the Denver area, most of them highly regarded. Several have nationally known programs in specialized fields; for example, Craig Hospital for spinal cord injuries and the National Jewish Center for Immunology and Respiratory Medicine (see page 56). Denver's major tertiary-care hospital, however, is University Hospital, located at the University of Colorado. As one doctor from Denver told us, "When you talk about a major referral center for the region, every hospital is a junior partner compared to University Hospital."

About 80 percent of all patients here come from metropolitan Denver, which includes seven counties and encompasses a large geographic area and much of the state's population. The remaining 20 percent come to University Hospital from quite a distance. The Adult Burn Center serves a five-state region and attracts patients with its specially designed Intensive Care Unit; the hospital is a designated Level I Trauma Center. It is also a regional referral center for neonatal prolems; more than half of the 2,600 births here each year involve high-risk pregnancies. In addition, over 300 low-birth-weight or extremely ill babies are cared for annually in the neonatal intensive care unit.

Heart transplants were begun at University Hospital only a few years ago, but kidneys have been transplanted here for over a decade. Over 60 patients a year now receive kidneys at University Hospital. Kidney disease in both adults and children is one of the hospital's more active areas. Over 1,000 kidney disease patients have been treated here, and in 1985 the NIH gave $10 million to continue research and development of the program.

The University Hospital Cancer Care Center treats brain, gastrointestinal tract, gynecologic, head and neck, heart, liver, lung, and prostate cancers. A referral center for individuals with melanoma uses new technology and experimental drugs. The South East Oncology Group is a referral center for patients with breast cancer, leukemia, lymphomas, and other tumors. Interferon and monoclonal antibodies are studied at a separate center in the Department of Medical Oncology.

In cardiology University Hospital is one of only a handful of medical centers in the country equipped to perform the operation required to correct arrhythmia. The University Cardiovascular Care Center also includes an electrophysiology laboratory and facilities for pediatric cardiology and cardiac surgery, peripheral vascular disease, and cardiac rehabilitation.

The Center for Neurological Diseases/Rocky Mountain Multiple Sclerosis Center includes basic laboratory research, clinical patient-oriented research, patient care, and education. The patient-care division offers acute and ongoing care, rehabilitation and specialized therapy, stress management, biofeedback, and counseling services. Since its creation in 1978, the center has become the largest, most comprehensive multiple sclerosis facility in the country. Patients can be referred here by their private physician or can contact the center directly for diagnostic testing, therapy, consultation for special problems, or close monitoring during acute attacks. (The phone number is 303-394-8866.)

The C. Henry Kempe National Center for the Prevention and Treatment of Child Abuse provides a wide array of educational, research, and clinical programs. Services range from a therapeutic preschool for sexually abused children (ages three to six) to the Hope for the Children family, an evaluation and treatment program for families in which physical abuse, sexual abuse, and other problems have been documented or evaluated for courts. The center's Child Protection Team was started in 1958; now there are more than 900 such teams in the country. The team includes a pediatrician, a child health associate, a social worker, and a coordinator. It evaluates and provides intervention for 400 suspected victims of child abuse per year.

The Colorado Psychiatric Hospital/Davis Pavilion treats patients who are mentally ill or have sleep disorders or neurophysiological dysfunctions. Programs include addiction research and treatment, an anxiety and phobic disorders clinic, and psychiatric emergency services. A mother and child clinic for schizophrenic mothers and their preschool children is the only such facility in the region. The Denver Institute for Psychoanalysis maintains an analytic clinic providing low-cost psychoanalysis for Colorado residents.

Other special clinics treat almost every kind of ailment, including allergies, arthritis, cleft palate, cystic fibrosis, diabetes, epilepsy, infertility, liver disease, chronic lung disease, lung tumors, osteoporosis, pain, sickle-cell anemia, spina bifida, and venereal disease. All the specialty departments have clinics as well. In addition, University Hospital has developed a number of specialized programs and is affiliated with the Webb-Waring Lung Institute, the Barbara Davis Institute for the Treatment and Research of Childhood Diabetes, the Eleanor Roosevelt Institute for Cancer Research, and the John F. Kennedy Child Development Center, which offers help for dyslexic, emotionally disturbed, and physically handicapped children.

An essential question for any major teaching hospital is how well such high-powered services are being delivered. A recent extensive survey sponsored by the hospital indicates that satisfaction among former patients is high. About 80 percent said they would definitely recommend University Hospital, and almost 75 percent of those who had been hospitalized elsewhere indicated that the treatment they received here was better (over 40 percent called it "much better"). One reason for the positive response must surely be the nursing staff, which is composed entirely of registered nurses, almost 70 percent of whom have a bachelor's degree or above.

## Specialties

Anesthesia, Cardiology, Clinical Immunology, Clinical Pharmacology, Dermatology, Emergency Medicine, Endocrinology, Family Medicine, Gastroenterology, Hematology, Infectious Diseases, Internal Medicine, Medicine, Medical Oncology, Neurology, Neurosurgery, Obstetrics/Gynecology, Ophthalmology, Orthopedics, Otolaryngology, Organ Transplantation, Pathology, Pediatrics, Plastic Surgery, Psychiatry, Pulmonary Sciences, Radiology, Rehabilitation Medicine, Renal Medicine, Rheumatology, Surgery, and Vascular Surgery.

---

**STATISTICAL PROFILE**

Number of Beds: 352
Bed Occupancy Rate: 72%
Average Number of Patients: 244
Average Patient Stay: 5.8 days
Annual Admissions: 15,649
Births: 2,642
Outpatient Clinic Visits: 208,624
Emergency Room/Trauma Center Visits: 60,437

Hospital Personnel:
  Physicians: 373
  Residents: 550
  Registered Nurses: 638
  Total Staff: 2,309

---

## Well-known Specialists

Dr. Frederick Battaglia, pediatrics; specialist in neonatology.
Dr. Paul Bunn, oncology; specialist in lung cancer.
Dr. David Campbell, pediatric cardiothoracic surgery and cardiac transplantation.

Dr. Peter Chase, pediatric diabetes.

Dr. David Clarke, pediatric cardiothoracic surgery.

Dr. William Clewell, fetal medicine.

Dr. Ernest Cotton, pediatric pulmonary medicine.

Dr. David Crawford, chief of urology, governor of the Southwestern Oncology Group.

Dr. Tommy Evans, obstetrics/gynecology; specialist in reconstructive vaginal surgery.

Dr. Alden Harken, cardiac surgery; specialist in arrhythmia surgery, chairman of the Department of Surgery.

Dr. Lawrence Horwitz, cardiology.

Dr. Bruce Jafek, otolaryngology; specialist in head and neck surgery.

Dr. Michael Johnson, surgery; specialist in lung cancer.

Dr. Fred Kern, gastroenterology.

Dr. Laurence Ketch, craniofacial and plastic surgery.

Dr. Richard Krugman, pediatrics; specialist in work with battered children.

Dr. John Lilly, pediatric surgery.

Dr. Edgar Makowski, obstetrics/gynecology; specialist in intrauterine growth retardation.

Dr. Ernest Moore, trauma surgery and prehospital care.

Dr. Thomas Petty, pulmonary medicine; one of the team of physicians sent to Bhopal, India, to treat victims of the Union Carbide disaster.

Dr. William Robinson, oncology; specialist in melanoma.

Dr. Robert Rutherford, author of the standard textbook in vascular surgery.

Dr. Robert Schrier, specialist in kidney disease, chairman of the Department of Medicine.

## Research

Each year the faculty and staff of the University of Colorado School of Medicine and University Hospital receive approximately $40 million in research grants. The NIH funds two Clinical Research Centers at the hospital, one for adults and one for children. Among the major areas of investigation are studies of children with cystic fibrosis, juvenile diabetes, and various neonatal problems and of adults with diabetes, herpes simplex, hypertension, lupus, multiple sclerosis, chronic obstructive pulmonary disease, and scleroderma.

Other areas of investigation are funded by the American Cancer Society, the Leukemia Society, several major pharmaceutical companies, the NIH, and other well-known foundations. Aging, immunology, kidney disease, lupus, metabolism, multiple sclerosis, oncology, and pediatrics are just a few of the subjects under study here. A Hepatobiliary Research Center, funded by the NIH, studies and treats diseases of the liver and biliary tract.

# Admission Policy

A patient can be admitted to University Hospital without a physician's referral. Admission through a clinic or the emergency room is also possible. Clinic admissions can be made by calling 303-329-3066. A referral coordinator will direct the caller to the appropriate clinic and possibly set up an appointment.

All patients are expected to provide evidence of insurance or sufficient personal financial resources upon admittance. However, the hospital claims that all emergency patients are accepted. Colorado citizens can be admitted if medically indigent, but elective procedures are permitted for them only when medically indigent funds are adequate. Over $20 million worth of indigent care is provided annually.

---

**ROOM CHARGES (per diem)**
Private: $276
Semiprivate: $250
ICU: $444–$643

**AVERAGE COST PER PATIENT STAY:**  $4,835

**MAILING ADDRESS**             **TELEPHONE**
4200 East Ninth Avenue     303-394-8446
Denver, CO 80262

---

# Alfred I. duPont Institute
## WILMINGTON, DELAWARE

Although the Alfred I. duPont Institute maintains only 97 inpatient beds, there's no question that this children's hospital ranks among the best in the country, particularly in pediatric orthopedics. DuPont has an international reputation for patient care, research, and education.

Delaware's only hospital for children, the institute was established in 1940 under the will of Alfred I. duPont, a Delaware philanthropist. Funded by the Nemours Foundation, the institute has served more than 80,000 children from not only Delaware but many parts of the world. Other specialties include developmental medicine, genetics, neurology, pediatric surgery, rehabilitation, rheumatology, and sports medicine.

The institute offers the latest technological advances in pediatric care. For example, it was the first children's hospital in its region to introduce a myoelectric prosthetics program. For children born without fully developed arms, this prosthesis is cosmetically attractive and electronically powered. Working with a team consisting of a prosthetist, an orthopedist, and an occupational therapist, the child learns to send brain messages to arm muscles which, by means of a microchip, tell the battery-operated arm to open and close the hand.

The Rehabilitation Program is one of a limited number of programs in the country that focus on pediatrics. Individuals through age twenty-one receive comprehensive inpatient and outpatient services. For over a decade, duPont has specialized in treating traumatic brain injury; spinal cord injury; congenital and acquired neuromuscular disorders; musculoskeletal dysfunction following trauma, illness, or congenital anomalies; and dependence on mechanical ventilation.

In 1984 the institute became the nation's first children's hospital to acquire digital (low-dose) computerized radiography, which reduces a child's exposure to radiation. This is particularly helpful to children with scoliosis, who require frequent radiological checks. Children scanned by this machine receive approximately 1 percent of the radiation required for the same study done by a conventional X-ray machine.

The institute's Neurophysiology Laboratory enables pediatric neurologists to perform on-site services for children who once had to travel to other hospitals for such tests. Children can undergo an electroencephalogram, an examination that monitors brain waves for a child with epilepsy; somatosensory auditory and visual evoked potential testing, which helps diagnose conditions such as acoustic neuromas, multiple sclerosis, and spinal cord tumors; and an electromyogram, used to measure electrical activity and to determine the cause of a child's weakness.

A wide variety of specialty clinics are available at the institute. At the Seating and Mobility Clinic, orthopedics and rehabilitation engineering combine to enable physically disabled individuals to become more functionally independent. The clinic serves disabled patients who need specialized seats and mobility devices, basic needs for the child with moderate or even severe physical disability. The latest techniques and equipment are also available for children with cerebral palsy, muscular dystrophy, spina bifida, spinal and head injuries, and other disabilities.

Other pediatric disorders of the central and peripheral nervous system are evaluated and treated at the Child Neurology Clinic. Epilepsy, headaches and other pain syndromes, learning disorders and other developmental disabilities, muscular dystrophy, disorders of the spinal cord, and general neurological disorders including cerebral palsy and spinal lesions are all treated here on an inpatient basis or in the Ambulatory Care Center.

The Recreation and Sports Medicine Clinic provides services for young athletes. In addition to comprehensive evaluation and diagnosis, treatment programs return athletes safely to a preinjury level of sports functioning and educate them in techniques of conditioning that guard against future injury. Clinical research is currently involved in a screening program to identify local "at-risk" athletes. Progressive treatment programs are under investigation to improve clinical methods.

In 1984 the institute opened a $150-million state-of-the-art hospital facility adjoining the original hospital building. And each July the institute sponsors Camp Manito for 100 handicapped children of New Castle County. "The hospital's location on the beautiful 300-acre Nemours estate is a delight in the summer," says Marian George, a child life therapist. "It enables us to have many more activities with the children than we could if we were in a more urban setting."

---

**STATISTICAL PROFILE**

Number of Beds: 97
Average Number of Patients: 60
Average Patient Stay: 13 days
Annual Admissions: 1,384
Outpatient Clinic Visits: 23,939

Hospital Personnel:
  Physicians: 24 full-time; 71 affiliated part-time
  Residents: 14
  Registered Nurses: 144
  Total Staff: 531

## Specialties

Anesthesiology, Child Psychiatry, Dentistry, Developmental Medicine, Medical Genetics, Neurology, Ophthalmology, Orthopedics, Pathology, Pediatrics, Plastic Surgery, Radiology, Rehabilitation, Rheumatology, Sports Medicine, Surgery, Thoracic Surgery, and Urology.

## Well-known Specialists

Dr. J. Richard Bowen, orthopedics.
Dr. William P. Bunnell, orthopedics.
Dr. Robert A. Doughty, rheumatology/immunology.
Dr. H. Theodore Harcke, medical imaging.
Dr. Harold G. Marks, neurology.
Dr. Peter D. Schindler, psychiatry.
Dr. Charles I. Scott, genetics.
Dr. Angela Smith, sports medicine/orthopedics.
Dr. Douglas M. Spencer, pediatrics.

## Research

Research at the duPont Institute is conducted from the cellular to the clinical patient study level. Continuing research studies concentrate on seven basic pediatric areas: the central nervous system, genetics, histology/histochemistry, immunology, medical research computations, metabolic bone disease, and muscles.

Control mechanisms of the central nervous system and neural control of peripheral functions are the primary concerns of the Central Nervous System Research Program. Major emphasis is also placed on spinal trauma and the potential prevention of extensive spinal cord damage during immediate post-accident periods.

Diseases resulting from gene abnormalities account for a large percentage of the institute's patients. Thus, the Genetics Research Program uses material from this population base to characterize chromosomal linkage, breaks, and other abnormalities and to develop diagnostic tools.

A diagnostic and basic research immunology program was developed when the institute expanded pediatric services in arthritis, with special emphasis on rheumatoid arthritis. Clinical trials will be developed to aid in the diagnosis of rheumatoid diseases in children.

The efforts of the Medical Research Computations Program are directed at aiding the physician in retrospective and prospective studies concerning patients' diagnosed conditions. Specially designed data base methods and statistical analysis are applied to patient information. Animal studies of bone growth, healing processes, and surgical procedures also fall within this area.

The Metabolic Bone Disease Research Program provides a clinical service and research effort in calcium metabolism in relation to vitamin D. Much effort is directed toward the study of bone formation and remodeling.

The Muscle Research Program seeks to determine pathological changes in muscles at the histochemical and biochemical levels. Primary emphasis is on studying the regeneration of skeletal muscle. The role of electrical stimulation to prevent muscle atrophy from immobilization is being studied.

## Admission Policy

Children can be referred to the duPont Institute by their physicians or other health-care professionals, or parents can call direct and request an appointment. All services are performed on an appointment basis. For an appointment or information in any of the following areas call:

Clinic: 302-651-4200
Developmental Medicine: 302-651-4504
Muscle Histochemistry: 302-651-5930
Neurophysiology Laboratory: 302-651-5930
Pediatric Imaging: 302-651-4620
Seating and Mobility Clinic: 302-651-4243
Sports Medicine: 302-651-5905

After making an appointment, parents are mailed an application for examination. A portion is to be completed by the child's physician, and the form returned to the institute before the child's first visit.

Financial assistance is provided. In fact, the foundation's policy is that no child who needs medical care at the institute will be refused treatment for lack of ability to pay. A financial assistance program funded by the Nemours Foundation is available to help families pay for hospital and physician services. To receive more information contact the Financial Assistance Office at 302-651-4243.

---

**ROOM CHARGES (per diem)**
Private or Semiprivate: $395
Rehabilitation: $445 (private or semiprivate)

**MAILING ADDRESS**     **TELEPHONE**
1600 Rockland Road       302-651-4000
Box 269
Wilmington, DE 19899

---

# Shands Hospital
# University of Florida
## GAINESVILLE, FLORIDA

In the Southeast Shands Hospital at the University of Florida is the referral center for transplants of all kinds—bone, bone marrow and tissue, corneas, hearts, kidneys, and livers. Since Shands's first kidney transplant in 1966, people throughout the Southeast and from as far away as South America have been coming here for this procedure. "Shands is at the forefront of transplantation," says Dr. Richard Howard, a renal surgeon who has performed more than 400 kidney transplants. "Under one roof, we have a team of technical experts and the ongoing research necessary to support transplant efforts."

Shands Hospital is the patient-care and clinical education unit of the Health Science Center at the University of Florida. It is also one of 75 NIH-funded Clinical Research Centers nationwide and the only one in Florida. In addition to conducting research, Shands is a referral hospital for health professionals in Florida and the Southeast. Patients who are referred to Shands benefit from many special diagnostic and clinical services that are not always available in their communities.

Shands's bone transplant program is one of only ten or so in the country specializing in fresh-frozen bone transplants. The University of Florida Department of Orthopedics is recognized around the world for its contribution in osteoarticular (large joint) and intercalary (large bone segments) allograft transplantation. "Bone transplants offer a permanent and biologic replacement for diseased bone," explains Dr. Dempsey Springfield, associate professor of orthopedics. "This is especially important for the young patient, who has decades of life ahead." Approximately 20 percent of bone transplants are accepted without problems; 60 percent will eventually be successful, but will have delayed incorporation; and 20 percent are totally rejected. In an effort to understand better the rejection phenomenon and predict the outcome of transplants, physicians in the Department of Orthopedics are participating in a $2.5-million NIH study with Harvard University, Yale University, and the Mayo Clinic.

Shands is one of only several university medical centers in the country using immunomagnetic purging, or the cancer magnet, for patients who are difficult to match for bone marrow transplants. So far the technique has been used solely for children who suffer from neuroblastoma, but doctors hope it eventually will be able to help victims of various types of leukemia. The Bone Marrow Transplant Unit at Shands is the only one of its kind in Florida.

Another important service is the in vitro fertilization program, which began at Shands in January 1986 and is the first of its kind in northcentral Florida. In October 1986 the program celebrated its first live birth.

The Neonatal Intensive Care Unit is one of the largest of ten centers in Florida, treating 750 infants annually. Less critically ill infants are treated in the Neonatal Intermediate Care Unit. Technology for treating newborns has so advanced that infants weighing less than three pounds now have an 80 to 85 percent chance of survival. The Neonatal Center accepts infants from anywhere in the state when a closer unit is full; the unit receives admissions from 50 of Florida's 67 counties.

Other intensive care units at Shands include Bone Marrow Transplant, Burn, Cardiac, Medical/Coronary, Pediatric, and Surgical.

Children's health care in much of Florida and the surrounding areas has always been linked to Shands, where almost 100 physicians, dentists, and health professionals for children work as a team. In conjunction with the University of Florida Science Center staff, Shands offers a full range of children's subspecialty services, including the only program of its kind in the Southeast for children suffering from respiratory ailments.

Other special pediatric services include a cardiology/cardiovascular program, genetics and diabetes units, and a renal transplantation center. Shands is one of the major centers in the Southeast for the treatment of children with spina bifida. Pediatricians here established the first camp for children with cancer, a camp for children with diabetes, the first associate arts degree cardiovascular/pulmonary technical program in conjunction with a local community college, and the first neonatal program in pharmacokinetics.

An even more unique specialty at Shands is hyperbaric medicine, which is performed in a recompression chamber; its best-known use is for scuba divers suffering from "the bends." However, hyperbaric medicine can also be used to treat ailments such as carbon monoxide and cyanide poisoning, gas gangrene, chronic nonhealing wounds, and chronic osteomyelitis and to help the body accept skin grafts. While most recompression chambers can accept only one person, the chamber at Shands, built to NASA specifications, can accommodate up to three patients, an attendant, and a physician, and it can be set up as a self-contained intensive care unit. NASA uses the chamber as a backup for the space shuttle program.

Shands medical staff members are also faculty in the University of Florida College of Medicine and are active in teaching, patient care, and research. Shands also provides outreach clinics in primary through tertiary care for adults and children in many areas of northcentral Florida.

Shands Hospital opened in 1958 as a state agency and was named for the late state Senator William A. Shands of Gainesville, who was instrumental in the development of the hospital and the medical complex. Shands became a private, not-for-profit corporation in 1980.

# Specialties

Anesthesiology, Communicative Disorders, Community Health and Family Medicine, Immunology, In Vitro Fertilization, Internal Medicine, Neurological Surgery, Neurology, Neuroscience, Obstetrics and Gynecology, Oncology, Ophthalmology, Oral and Maxillofacial Surgery, Orthopedics, Otolaryngology, Pathology, Pediatrics, Physiology, Psychiatry, Pulmonary Medicine, Radiation Therapy, Radiology, and Surgery.

---

**STATISTICAL PROFILE (1984–85)**

Number of Beds: 476
Bed Occupancy Rate: 85.8%
Average Number of Patients: 396
Average Patient Stay: 7.8 days
Annual Admissions: 18,429
Births: 2,955
Outpatient Clinic Visits: 161,203
Emergency Room/Trauma Center Visits: 27,402

Hospital Personnel:
  Physicians: 289
  Residents: 363
  Registered Nurses: 708 full-time; 82 part-time
  Total Staff: 2,536 full-time; 393 part-time

---

# Well-known Specialists

Dr. Michael Carmichael, adult cardiothoracic surgery.
Dr. Edward Copeland, surgery; specialist in breast and colon cancer, contributing author of *Surgical Oncology.*
Dr. William F. Enneking, orthopedic surgery; specialist in bone tumors and bone transplantation.
Dr. Birdwell Finlayson, urologic surgery; specialist in kidney stones.
Dr. Eduard Georg Friedrich, Jr., obstetrics and gynecology; specialist in vulvovaginal diseases, author of the most comprehensive textbook in this field.
Dr. Ira Gessner, pediatric cardiology.
Dr. James McGuigan, specialist in peptic ulcers.
Dr. Thomas J. Merimee, endocrinology; specialist in diabetes mellitus and endocrine problems.
Dr. Carl Pepine, cardiology; specialist in balloon angioplasty.

Dr. William Pfaff, renal transplant surgery; has performed more than 815 kidney transplants.

Dr. Albert Rhoton, neurosurgery; specialist in tumors in the brain and spinal cord.

Dr. Arlan Rosenbloom, pediatric endocrinology; specialist in childhood diabetes.

Dr. Melvin Rubin, ophthalmology; specialist in diseases of the retina.

Dr. George Sypert, neurosurgery; specialist in spinal cord injuries and certain types of epilepsy.

Dr. James L. Talbert, pediatrics and surgery; specialist in problems that affect the windpipe.

## Research

Shands medical staff conduct research at the NIH-funded Clinical Research Center. "We have patients who have come all the way from Montana, even South America, because they have heard of specific research studies that are going on here," says Heather Barbour, CRC nursing administrator. Like other such centers across the country, the unit at Shands operates as a minihospital within a hospital, enabling researchers to carry out protocols in a controlled environment that they couldn't pursue any other way. Every patient involved in a clinical study receives a detailed description of the research protocol and the potential risks. The informed consent explains why the experiment is important and what benefits to the patient, or to society in general, the researcher hopes to realize. So that patients know what to expect, they also receive a copy of their day-to-day protocol. Furthermore, a patient is free to withdraw from a study at any time.

Currently over 100 different clinical studies are being conducted at Shands. Over the last five years this research has been supported with nearly $4 million from the NIH. Some major fields of study include cardiac surgery, cholesterol, diabetes, a new drug for herpes, cures for impotence in male diabetics, large-bone transplants, and a new test for pancreatic disease.

## Admission Policy

Patients can be admitted to Shands without a doctor's referral through the Emergency Center or one of the outpatient clinics.

Financial arrangements must be made for all admissions, but admissions for urgent or emergent conditions will not be delayed. Programs administered by the state of Florida's Health and Rehabilitation Services provide assistance to patients with limited financial resources. State programs pay for hospitalization and clinical visits for select patients and help patients obtain prescriptions and medical supplies.

**ROOM CHARGES** (per diem)
Private: $246
Semiprivate: $235
Ward (pediatric): $234
ICU: $450–$575

**AVERAGE COST PER PATIENT STAY**
$5,626 (*Note*: This is the cost to Shands per admission.)

**MAILING ADDRESS**       **TELEPHONE**
Gainesville, FL 32610    904-395-0111

# University of Miami
# Jackson Memorial Medical Center

**MIAMI, FLORIDA**

In Florida most of the newspaper stories about the University of Miami/ Jackson Memorial (UM/JM) Medical Center concern its financial problems and its need for increased state funding. A public hospital, the UM/JM Medical Center handles 12 percent of Florida's Medicaid patients. Unfortunately, its role in treating the needy often overshadows its national reputation as a center for research and treatment, such as in the Bascom Palmer Eye Institute and as a leading center for research in blood diseases.

Even more unusual for a public hospital, these services are protected by one of the strictest quality-assurance programs of all the hospitals we reviewed for this book. The program here is recognized by the Joint Commission on Accreditation of Hospitals as innovative, comprehensive, and result oriented. And, in the hospital's most recent evaluation by former patients, 91.6 percent of the respondents said they would choose Jackson Memorial Hospital again.

One of the largest public teaching hospitals in the nation, the UM/JM Medical Center now serves up to 59,000 inpatients a year.

The following is a brief review of some of the facilities at the UM/JM Medical Center.

The Center for Neurological Diseases earned the medical center international acclaim for its work in Alzheimer's disease, multiple sclerosis, Parkinson's disease, diseases of peripheral nerves and muscles, and stroke. This center handles a broad spectrum of neurological diseases, from sleep disorders and headaches to Lou Gehrig's disease, and each year treats 13,000 patients.

The Rehabilitation Center is a designated regional spinal cord research center, providing acute and rehabilitative care. It has been accredited in hospital-based rehabilitation, vocational education, job placement, and the spinal cord injury program.

The UM/JM Medical Center also has a designated Comprehensive Cancer Center providing a multidisciplinary team approach. Recently merged with the Papanicolaou Cancer Research Institute, the center is one of the 20 or so federally designated centers nationwide. Services are offered in breast cancer, dermatologic oncology, gastrointestinal oncology, gynecologic oncology, head and neck cancers, hematologic oncology, lung cancer, medical oncology, neurosurgical oncology (brain and spinal cord tumors), oncological intractable pain, ophthalmic oncology, orthopedic oncology, pathology, pediatric cancer, radiation therapy, surgical oncology, and urologic malignancies.

Ophthalmology services are handled at the Bascom Palmer Eye Institute/ Anne Bates Leach Eye Hospital, a part of the University of Miami School of Medicine, which provides education, patient care, and research particularly in vitreoretinal diseases. The recently created Laser Research Center, one of only a few such experimental laboratories in the United States, investigates laser use for a variety of ophthalmologic uses. A major referral center for the southeastern United States and Central and South America, this institute treats over 6,000 inpatients annually. Outpatient clinics provide specialists in external diseases, glaucoma, macula, neuroophthalmology, pediatric ophthalmology, retina, and vitreous, attending to more than 60,000 patient visits each year. All the latest diagnostic and therapeutic equipment is available to treat any kind of eye problem. The Children's Eye Clinic, the Low Vision Clinic, the Contact Lens Clinic, and the Florida Lions Eye Bank are all part of the institute.

In the past several years the medical center has developed an outstanding array of services for children and adolescents, which are now unified in the Children's Hospital Center. Services include the largest adolescent unit in south Florida, extensive facilities for treatment of heart disease and pediatric open-heart surgery, child and adolescent psychiatry, the Comprehensive Children's Kidney Center, The Deed Club's Children's Cancer Clinic, newborn intensive care, a pediatric rehabilitation center, treatment for behavioral and learning disorders, and developmental evaluation.

The Women's Hospital Center's services are equally comprehensive. Women with pelvic cancers and benign gynecologic disorders are attended by a wide array of medical and surgical specialists. In fact, this is the largest gynecologic oncology facility in the southeastern United States. Almost 11,000 babies are delivered every year at the hospital; more than 50 percent are high-risk cases. And Florida's first in vitro fertilization program is located here.

Emergency and trauma care are provided at Jackson's Level I Trauma Center, the largest in the Southeast and the fifth busiest in the nation. More than 100,000 cases are handled here annually, in addition to pediatric walk-in and psychiatric emergencies.

Over 96 specialized outpatient clinics deliver health care in a wide range of services from allergy treatment to wound checking. Two of the most unique are the Patient/Family Education Clinic and the Mood Disorders Clinic. In twice-weekly meetings at the Patient/Family Education Clinic, discharged patients with problems such as limb amputations, diabetic foot ulcers, spina bifida, and spinal cord injuries are taught to care for themselves. Family members are also instructed in how to help the patients. The Mood Disorders Clinic treats patients suffering from inexplicable exhaustion, aches and pains, sleeplessness, sadness, and a loss of interest and pleasure. Manic-depressive disorders are also treated.

Other outpatient clinics offered by the Mental Health Department include Anorexia/Bulimia, Evaluations, Follow-up, Intakes (Aftercare), Lithium,

Medication Adjustment, Monthly Groups, Psychotherapy, Therapy (Individual), and Weekly Groups.

Jackson Memorial Hospital is the teaching hospital for the University of Miami School of Medicine, a private institution and Florida's largest medical school. The clinical chiefs are chairmen of the departments at the School of Medicine, and clinical staff are on the medical school faculty.

## Specialties

Almost every medical specialty is offered at UM/JM Medical Center, with special emphasis on Adolescent Medicine, Cardiology, Cardiothoracic Surgery, Dermatology, Endocrinology, Emergency and Trauma Care, Gastroenterology, Genetics, Gynecology, Hematology, Intensive Care, Juvenile Diabetes, Neonatal Intensive Care, Nephrology, Neurology, Neurosurgery, Obstetrics, Oncology, Ophthalmology, Orthopedics/Rehabilitation (especially back disorders and hand injuries), Pediatric Cardiology, Pediatrics, Psychiatry, Radiology, Transplantation, and Urology.

Outpatients are treated in areas such as allergy, arthritis, burns, family medicine, infertility, oral surgery, plastic surgery, sickle-cell transfusion, spinal cord injuries, strokes, tumor surgery, and urology.

---

**STATISTICAL PROFILE (1985–86)**

Number of Beds: 1,250
Bed Occupancy Rate: 89%
Average Number of Patients: 1,160
Average Patient Stay: 7.1 days
Annual Admissions: 59,421
Births: 10,545
Outpatient Clinic Visits: 253,655
Emergency Room/Trauma Center Visits: 129,093

Hospital Personnel:
  Physicians: 1,300 admitting; 700 full-time attending
  Residents: 395
  Registered Nurses: 1,393
  Total Staff: 5,880

---

## Well-known Specialists

Dr. Hervy E. Averette, gynecologic oncology.
Dr. Mark D. Brown, orthopedics.
Dr. Carl Eisdorfer, aging and Alzheimer's disease.

Dr. Henry Gelband, pediatric cardiology.
Dr. Barth A. Green, spinal cord injury.
Dr. William H. Harrington, internal medicine; specialist in hematology.
Dr. Gerard Kaiser, thoracic surgery.
Dr. Alfred S. Ketchum, oncology.
Dr. J. Maxwell McKenzie, thyroid disease.
Dr. Ralph Millard, plastic surgery.
Dr. D. Daniel H. Mintz, juvenile diabetes.
Dr. Edward W. D. Norton, ophthalmology.
Dr. Victor A. Politano, urology.
Dr. Peritz Scheinberg, neurology.
Dr. Eugene R. Schiff, liver disease.
Dr. Robert Zeppa, surgery.
Dr. C. Gordon Zubrod, oncology.

# Research

The UM School of Medicine received a total of $48 million in research grants in 1986, representing more than a 20 percent increase over the previous year.

The school receives about $6 million for pharmaceutical studies, most of which are conducted at Jackson. An example of this research is anticancer drug analysis in which a drug is added to the standard chemotherapy. Because of its location in an area where AIDS is a problem, the medical center has been granted $5 million each year over the next five years to study drugs and the treatment of AIDS.

With over 10,000 babies delivered at Jackson this year, pediatric research, especially neonatal projects, receives considerable support. The National Institute of Child Health and Human Development has provided a five-year base grant of $1.3 million to make the medical center one of seven participants in a clinical research network of neonatal medicine. One of eight participating centers in the Infant Health and Development Program, the medical center was awarded a $2.6-million grant to continue its study of the effectiveness of services designed to reduce the health and developmental problems often experienced by low-birth-weight babies.

The internationally renowned UM Center for Blood Diseases is headed by Dr. William Harrington, one of the heroes of the book *Human Guinea Pigs*, who inoculated himself with a mystery blood disease called ITP (idiopathic thrombocytopenic purpura) to prove his theory that it was caused by the body rejecting its own platelets.

The medical center is also known for the pioneering work of Dr. Daniel Mintz in transplanting the cells of the pancreas that produce insulin and the success of Dr. Hubert Rosomoff in the UM Comprehensive Pain Center with reducing back pain.

Experimental laser research is conducted in neurosurgery, obstetrics/

gynecology, ophthalmology, and otolaryngology. Other areas of research include dermatologic studies, hematologic diseases, radiological studies, stress testing, triaging of trauma patients, and wound healing.

## Admission Policy

Patients can be admitted to the UM/JM Medical Center without a referral through a clinic or the emergency room, at which time an attending physician is assigned. A private patient referral number (305-547-5757) is available to assist patients in finding the appropriate physician to treat a particular problem or to make an appointment.

Once emergency care is given, patients are responsible for their bills. A deposit toward full charges less any payments expected to be made by insurance or a third-party payer is required. Self-paying patients must pay an estimate of full charges. Any waiver of deposit must be approved by the director or vice-president of finance. The center provides an extraordinary $50 million in indigent care annually.

---

**ROOM CHARGES (per diem)**
Private: $295–$315
Semiprivate: $265–$295
ICU: $800

| **MAILING ADDRESS** | **TELEPHONE** |
|---|---|
| 1611 Northwest Twelfth Avenue | 305-325-7429 |
| Miami, FL 33136 | |

---

# Emory University Hospital
# The Emory Clinic

**ATLANTA, GEORGIA**

A private multispecialty referral clinic, The Emory Clinic was formed as a partnership of physicians, all of whom are members of the faculty of the Emory University School of Medicine. After examination at the clinic, patients who need hospitalization may be referred to the Emory University Hospital or one of several affiliated hospitals.

Emory University Hospital is a major center for advanced tertiary care and research. The NIH funds a 12-bed clinical research unit within the hospital. A Center of Rehabilitation Medicine and a separate psychiatric center are also part of the hospital.

The treatment of heart disease through coronary bypass surgery, heart valve replacement, and coronary angioplasty makes Emory one of the five busiest cardiac centers in the nation. Emory is well known for coronary bypass surgery, with more than 1,000 operations performed every year and one of the lowest mortality rates in the nation (according to the Health Care Financing Administration, the federal agency that operates the Medicare program). Emory was also one of the first institutions in America to offer heart valve replacement.

Another special heart program first offered at Emory is coronary angioplasty. Since 1980 more than 5,000 physicians have studied this procedure at Emory's Gruentzig Cardiovascular Center, founded by the late Dr. Andreas Gruentzig, who first performed this procedure in Zurich in 1977. In addition, Emory has been selected by the NIH to be the single site of a five-year, $8 million comparative study of the effectiveness of angioplasty and bypass surgery in patients with multivessel heart disease.

Well-known specialists in hematology and medical/surgical oncology provide a strong base at Emory for the treatment of cancer and its complications. In addition to bone marrow transplants, Emory physicians are making great strides in the treatment of bladder cancer, colorectal cancer, melanoma, and other cancers.

The Emory Eye Center is one of the nation's largest corneal transplant centers and one of the few where transplants can be scheduled months in advance. Outside NIH, Emory has one of the few labs in America with the capability to perform high-level tissue-matching studies. Its sophisticated lasers provide treatment for uveitis and diseases of the retina associated with diabetes. And immune system research is being done here on ocular herpes.

Emory's 56-bed Center for Rehabilitation Medicine is a freestanding facility built exclusively for treatment of people with disabilities resulting from illness or injury; it includes an eight-bed module specifically designed for patients with head injuries. Other patients in the center include those with problems related to amputation, arthritis, spinal cord injury, stroke, and other neuromuscular or musculoskeletal conditions. A comprehensive program in cardiac rehabilitation is also available.

In 1986 Emory University Hospital expanded its services in psychiatry with a new 47-bed facility. In addition to general psychiatry, a large medical psychiatric unit has been created. The unit is particularly well suited to the elderly (who constitute the majority of patients) because most patients with both medical and psychiatric problems are over sixty-five. Severe depression, superimposed on dementia, like Alzheimer's disease, is a typical problem treated here.

The Emory Transplant Center performs bone marrow transplants, corneal transplants, and kidney transplants. Its heart transplant program, begun in 1985, is one of the nation's most successful; after one and a half years, only two out of 36 patients have died. A liver transplant program is planned, as is transplantation of the pancreas.

Other areas of expertise at Emory include cleft palate repair, embolization, an extracorporeal lithotriptor for kidney stones, laser surgery, flap reconstruction of damaged limbs, liver surgery, and other microsurgery.

Both The Emory Clinic and Emory University Hospital are part of The Robert W. Woodruff Health Sciences Center of Emory University. Other divisions of the Health Sciences Center include the Crawford Long Hospital; the Schools of Medicine, Nursing, and Dentistry; and the Yerkes Regional Primate Research Center. In addition, seven independent agencies are affiliated with the Health Sciences Center: Henrietta Egleston Hospital for Children, Jesse Parker Williams Hospital, Grady Memorial Hospital, Wesley Homes Health Services, Atlanta Veterans Administration Hospital, the U.S. Public Health Service Centers for Disease Control, and the Georgia Mental Health Institute.

## Specialties

Anesthesiology, Cardiology, Dentistry, Dermatology, Endocrinology, Gastroenterology, General Surgery, Hematology, Infectious Diseases, Internal Medicine, Nephrology, Neurology, Neurosurgery, Oncology, Ophthalmology, Orthopaedic Surgery, Orthoptics, Otolaryngology, Obstetrics/Gynecology, Pathology, Pediatrics, Plastic Surgery, Psychiatry, Pulmonary Disease, Radiation Therapy, Rehabilitation Medicine, Rheumatology, Thoracic Surgery, and Urology.

Ancillary services at The Emory Clinic include audiovisual testing, breast imaging, cardiac catheterization, diabetes counseling, genetics counseling, lithotripsy, nuclear medicine, nutritional counseling, pulmonary function testing, speech pathology, and ultrasound.

**STATISTICAL PROFILE**

Number of Beds: 604
Bed Occupancy Rate: 76%
Average Number of Patients: 461
Average Patient Stay: 7 days
Annual Admissions: 21,640
Outpatient Clinic Visits: 400,000

Hospital Personnel:
   Physicians: 353
   Residents: 150
   Registered Nurses: 700
   Total Staff: 2,950

# Well-known Specialists

Dr. John T. Galambos, gastroenterology.
Dr. Robert A. Guyton, surgery; specialist in cardiac surgery.
Dr. Charles R. Hatcher, surgery and cardiology.
Dr. J. Willis Hurst, cardiology; author of *The Heart*.
Dr. Ellis L. Jones, surgery; specialist in cardiac surgery.
Dr. M. J. Jurkiewicz, surgery; specialist in plastic surgery.
Dr. Spencer B. King, radiology; specialist in angioplasty, professor of medicine.
Dr. Juha Kokko, nephrology; chairman of the Department of Medicine.
Dr. Luella Klein, chairman of the Department of Obstetrics/Gynecology.
Dr. Garland D. Perdue, vascular surgery.
Dr. Robert Smith, surgery; specialist in vascular surgery.
Dr. Paul Sugarbaker, surgery; specialist in colorectal cancer.
Dr. W. Dean Warren, chairman of the Department of Surgery.
Dr. John D. Whelchel, surgery; specialist in renal transplantation.
Dr. Thomas E. Whitesides, orthopedics.

# Admission Policy

Outside physicians may refer patients to The Emory Clinic by phone or by mail for diagnosis or treatment of an already diagnosed problem. Admission to Emory University Hospital is through a physician in The Emory Clinic.

Patients will not be denied care for medical emergencies regardless of their ability to pay.

**ROOM CHARGES** (per diem)
Private: $235
Semiprivate: $230
ICU: $660–$756

**AVERAGE COST PER PATIENT STAY:**   $6,000

**MAILING ADDRESS**          **TELEPHONE**
1364 Clifton Road, N.E.      404-727-3456
Atlanta, GA 30322            Clinic: 404-321-0111

# Northwestern Memorial Hospital

**CHICAGO, ILLINOIS**

There are 15 major teaching hospitals in the immediate Chicago area. Several are specialty hospitals with impressive national reputations (Schwab Rehabilitation Center and The Children's Memorial Hospital, for example). Others such as Michael Reese Hospital, the University of Illinois Hospital, and the Loyola Medical Center provide vital tertiary-care services in several fields. Loyola's program in cardiac surgery, for example, is considered one of the most successful in the nation, its surgeons regularly performing heart transplants in addition to hundreds of bypass operations with a mortality rate of less than 2 percent. Add to these the extraordinary work done at Cook County Hospital (with its 400,000 outpatient visits a year) and the services offered at the three Chicago facilities we've included in this book and you can understand why the city's hospital system is so highly regarded.

Northwestern Memorial Hospital (NMH) is a comprehensive tertiary-care facility receiving referrals from throughout the Midwest and the United States and offering a full range of adult, geriatric, maternal, fetal, and perinatal medicine. Pediatric care is provided by the related Children's Memorial Hospital. Northwestern Memorial is a private, nonprofit institution that serves as the principal teaching hospital of Northwestern University Medical School.

Despite its name NMH is not connected to Northwestern University in the same way that UCLA and Columbia are to their universities. The hospital and the school are both members of the McGaw Medical Center of the university, a charitable, research, and educational consortium that also includes Northwestern University Dental School and three other private teaching hospitals: Evanston Hospital Corporation, Children's Memorial Hospital, and Rehabilitation Institute of Chicago.

Northwestern Memorial and the medical school are on adjacent campuses along Chicago's downtown lakefront and share a number of facilities and resources. All NMH's attending physicians hold appointments in the medical school. Approximately one-third of the hospital's physicians are full-time faculty in the medical school; the remaining two-thirds have part-time teaching responsibilities and practice privately in the community.

With nearly every modern medical and surgical specialty represented, NMH is one of the major academic medical centers in the Midwest. A few of its more prominent departments are detailed in the following paragraphs.

Northwestern Memorial is one of the major centers for high-risk pregnancies in the Midwest and is a designated Perinatal Center in Illinois. A team headed by Dr. Richard Depp has performed intrauterine surgery and is familiar with gestational diabetes and hydrocephalus. The Prentice

Women's Hospital, a part of NMH, has an active reproductive endocrinology and infertility program, which includes in vitro fertilization, genetic screening, and counseling programs and is also the site for gynecologic cancer treatment at NMH. A new Menopause Center focuses on clinical and counseling assistance to older women and provides estrogen replacement, treats osteoporosis, and addresses the psychological aspects of midlife maturation.

The Cancer Center, a joint project of NMH and Northwestern University, has subspecialists in gynecologic oncology, hematology/oncology, laser procedures, oncology nursing, and radiation therapy. Tbe hospital also sponsors support groups for cancer patients and their families.

As part of its cardiac/cardiovascular program, NMH is one of a small number of hospitals in the United States using an advanced blood conservation technique during heart surgery, which reduces the need for transfusions. The Blood Flow Laboratory permits diagnosis of arterial occlusive disease and venous problems. The hospital pioneered same-day admission for cardiac surgery, made possible by extensive outpatient preadmission testing.

The Spinal Cord Injury Care Center, an official trauma center for the entire Midwest, treats patients from Illinois, Indiana, Iowa, Michigan, and Wisconsin; in 1986 there were 260 patients at the center. The program includes basic and clinical research into the treatment and vocational rehabilitation of patients with spinal cord injuries.

The Institute of Psychiatry, located in the Stone Pavilion, offers a broad range of emotional health services, treating mental illness on both an inpatient and an outpatient basis. "We're looking for ways to help people identify stress in their lives before it requires drastic action," reports Dr. Harold Visotsky, director of the institute. Programs are available in all major nonpediatric psychiatric disciplines, such as adolescent psychiatry, short-stay adult psychiatry, chemical dependence, eating disorders, emergency intervention, older adult and geriatric psychiatry, and outpatient psychotherapy. The institute serves 1,800 patients on an inpatient basis annually, and outpatient visits number 100,000 per year.

Orthopedic physicians at NMH perform a large number of joint replacement procedures annually and are currently investigating alternative approaches (such as cement and mechanical techniques) to securing the prostheses. The Reconstructive Orthopedic Center offers reconstructive surgery after injury or crippling arthritic disease. Procedures include hip replacements and finger and knee joint repairs. The Medical Program for Performing Artists treats musicians, singers, dancers, and other performers. There is also a program focusing on sports medicine.

A Geriatric Evaluation Service provides a comprehensive evaluation of medical condition, psychological state, social functioning, and daily living activities by a multidisciplinary staff including an internist, a nurse practitioner, and a social worker; it also draws on backup services from many other departments. The Alzheimer's Disease Assessment Program makes diagnoses and develops treatment plans.

The Diabetes Center sponsors workshops, individualized counseling, and other programs. Patients must be referred by their personal doctor, but those without a physician can contact the center for referral. For information call 312-908-7822.

The Human Services Department helps patients deal with the emotional difficulties, such as depression and feelings of hopelessness, that can prolong hospitalization, and is aimed at treating the total person. Under the direction of a psychiatrist, the program combines services of the Departments of Consultation/Liaison Psychiatry, Discharge Planning, Pastoral Care, Social Work, and Supportive Care (for the terminally ill). In operation since 1983, the program has been so successful at providing cost-efficient physical/psychosocial care that it may well become a model for hospitals across the country.

The NMH Quality-Assurance Program, focusing on the evaluation and improvement of clinical care, is overseen by members of the medical staff. Sections of the program have been singled out for praise by the Joint Commission on Accreditation for Hospitals as models for other institutions.

Northwestern Memorial Hospital was created in 1972, when two of Chicago's oldest and most respected health-care institutions—Chicago Wesley (founded 1848) and Passavant Memorial (founded 1865)—merged. Prentice Women's Hospital and Maternity Center became part of NMH in 1975, as did the Institute of Psychiatry. In 1979 the Olson Pavilion was completed, housing the NMH-NU Cancer Center, coronary care, the emergency de-

---

**STATISTICAL PROFILE**

Number of Beds: 714
Bed Occupancy Rate: 78%
Average Number of Patients: 554
Average Patient Stay: 7.8 days
Annual Admissions: 25,988
Births: 4,252
Outpatient Clinic Visits: approximately 210,000
Emergency Room/Trauma Center Visits: 33,448

Hospital Personnel:
  Physicians: 800
  Residents: 280
  Total Staff: 3,800

partment, intensive care, operating rooms, and radiology facilities. In 1984 a building was constructed to contain the hospital's new magnetic resonance imaging scanner.

## Specialties

Allergies, Ambulatory Care, Anesthesia, Arthritis, Cardiology, Cardiothoracic Surgery, Clinical Pharmacology, Community Health, Critical Care Medicine, Dentistry, Dermatology, Emergency Medicine, Endocrinology, GI, General Medicine, Head and Neck Tumors, Hematology, Human Genetics, Infectious Diseases, Nephrology, Neurology, Neurosurgery, Obstetrics/Gynecology, Oncology, Ophthalmology, Orthopedic Surgery, Otolaryngology, Pathology, Pediatrics, Plastic Surgery, Psychiatry, Pulmonary Medicine, Radiology, Rehabilitation Medicine, Surgery, Urology, and Vascular Surgery.

## Well-known Specialists

Dr. Henry Betts, rehabilitation medicine.
Dr. Edward Brunner, anesthesia.
Dr. Alan Dyer, community health.
Dr. John Grayhack, urology
Dr. Donald Harter, neurology.
Dr. Peter Hurst, dentistry.
Dr. Lee Jampol, ophthalmology.
Dr. David Nahrwold, surgery.
Dr. Roy Patterson, medicine.
Dr. Henry Roenigk, dermatology.
Dr. Lee Rogers, radiology.
Dr. Dante G. Scarpelli, pathology.
Dr. Michael Schafer, orthopedic surgery.
Dr. John Sciarra, obstetrics/gynecology.
Dr. George Sisson, otolaryngology.
Dr. James Stockman, pediatrics.
Dr. Harold Visotsky, psychiatry.

## Research

A Clinical Research Center, funded by an NIH grant, enables NMH to maintain a small patient-care unit for treatment using research protocols.

Several clinical specialties have received special emphasis and research support. The Cancer Center, for example, does basic and clinical research into cancer causes and treatment. A team of NMH researchers is one of five in the United States studying the use of a vaccine made from a patient's own tumor (monoclonal antibodies) to prevent the recurrence of colon cancer. Other projects focus on an implantable infusion pump for continuous administration of a new combination chemotherapy and new forms of treatment for head and neck tumors.

Research projects in the Prentice Women's Hospital and Maternity Center focus on high-risk pregnancies, fetal medicine, drug use in pregnancy, perinatal risk and treatment, vitamin supplementation in neural tube defects, and preterm delivery. In psychiatry a major study is currently being funded by the National Institute of Alcohol Abuse and Alcoholism.

Cardiac/cardiovascular research programs include a three-hospital joint venture in heart-lung transplantation and a myocardial infarction study.

## Admission Policy

Patients may be admitted to NMH through several routes. A patient may already have an established relationship with an internist or specialist on NMH's staff or be referred to an NMH physician, often a specialist, by another physician in the community. Patients may also refer themselves to NMH physicians. The hospital maintains the Telephone Referral Service (312-908-6464) to assist patients in identifying an appropriate physician. Finally, patients may enter the hospital through the Emergency Room, a designated Level I Trauma Center.

The hospital provides approximately $5 million annually in free care to patients who cannot pay for treatment. This is funded in part by philanthropy and in part by revenues from paying patients.

---

**ROOM CHARGES (per diem)**
Private: $395
Semiprivate: $375

**MAILING ADDRESS**                       **TELEPHONE**
Superior Street and Fairbanks Court    312-908-2000
Chicago, IL 60611

---

# Rush–Presbyterian–St. Luke's Medical Center

**CHICAGO, ILLINOIS**

People in Chicago refer to Rush–Presbyterian–St. Luke's Medical Center simply as Rush. One of the city's busiest hospitals, it is also a nationally known tertiary-care teaching institution with a highly respected research program. Among doctors and health-care personnel in the Chicago area, Rush has a distinguished reputation, and it would qualify for inclusion in this book by almost any standard. When we spoke to nonmedical people, however, the image of Rush that emerged was quite different. Unlike Chicago's other fine teaching institutions and major research centers, Rush is seen first and foremost as a patients' hospital, one that provides excellent patient care along with advanced medicine. Some facts and figures we uncovered strongly support this view.

Patient satisfaction with Rush is extraordinarily high. A recent survey by the hospital reported that 97 percent of former patients rated the overall quality of nursing care good/very good; 98 percent gave the same rating to the quality of care from their physicians, and, most impressive, 100 percent of the patients surveyed said they would recommend the center to their family and friends.

Much of the credit for these responses must go to the highly skilled nursing staff at Rush, almost 80 percent of whom hold at least a bachelor's degree. Today all new nurses must have at least a bachelor's, and those in leadership positions must have a master's degree. Because nursing at Rush functions in a self-governing way, with its own quality-assurance program and with nurses being assigned responsibility for individual patients (the so-called Primary Model), there seems to be a sense of pride and accomplishment among the staff here. The turnover rate has been less than 20 percent in recent years. Rush is often chosen as a reference point for other facilities seeking to upgrade their nursing services—some even come from overseas to study its nursing program.

Founded over 150 years ago, Rush is one of Chicago's oldest health-care institutions. Located on the Near West Side of the city, it offers programs in health care, education, and research. Its principal components are Presbyterian–St. Luke's Hospital, The Johnston R. Bowman Health Center for the Elderly, The Sheridan Road Hospital, and Rush University.

The medical center is the heart of a health-care network of 18 hospitals and health-care agencies in Illinois and Indiana, and of an educational network of 16 colleges and universities in six states. Through its own programs and in conjunction with affiliated institutions, Rush is the main component of a cooperative health organization designed to provide care for some 1.5 million people in northern Illinois.

Presbyterian–St. Luke's Hospital provides primary and tertiary care to its immediate community and secondary and tertiary care to patients from across the country. Along with The Sheridan Road Hospital and The Johnston R. Bowman Health Center for the Elderly, its medical staff sees an estimated 350,000 patients annually.

The following paragraphs offer brief highlights of some of Rush's programs and medical specialties.

The Bone Marrow Transplant Center has a capacity of six beds and a staff of physicians, scientists, and specially trained nurses as well as nutritionists and social workers. In the past year there were 24 harvestings of bone marrow and 17 transplants. The center staff also concentrates on research to improve the success rates of transplants for people with leukemia and certain cancers. Several other transplant programs, including cornea, kidney, and liver, have been established. The medical center did the first heart transplant in Chicago in 1968.

Oncology is one of the major departments at Rush. Almost 20 percent of all Rush admissions are cancer patients, and 30,000 outpatients are treated for some form of the disease. Twenty-two of the 36 departments at Rush are involved in cancer treatments; they include specialized areas such as the Pigmented Lesion Center, the first of its kind in the Midwest, which opened in 1985. The center offers a multidisciplinary approach to the diagnosis and treatment of skin cancer. A comprehensive center for diagnosis and treatment of breast cancer combines the expertise of surgeons, radiation therapists, and oncologists, who evaluate each case and present a joint recommendation on the most appropriate treatment.

The Pediatric Critical Care Unit provides for patients' physiological needs through careful monitoring of vital functions and for developmental needs by encouraging families to visit. Critical care for over 1,000 premature babies is given in the Special Care Nursery; over 300 high-risk pregnancies are referred here annually.

The Rush pharmacy department operates the Poison Control Center for the nine northeastern counties of Illinois; it is one of three such centers designated by the state. This twenty-four-hour emergency service may be contacted at 312-942-7063.

Areas of surgical expertise include cardiovascular surgery, open-heart surgery, spine surgery for scoliosis, and, for chemonucleolysis, a specialized disc surgery. In neurosurgery Rush physicians perform intracranial pump implantations and epilepsy surgery.

Other areas of expertise include orthopedics, in which physicians have established a reputation for successful complex joint replacement, and the psychiatry department, which is known for its work in forensic psychiatry, dissociative disorders, and child psychiatry.

Rush is particularly proud of its in vitro fertilization specialists, who have brought about several births, as well as of the Field Foundation Emergency Treatment Center, which consists of 15 adult and five pediatric acute-care cubicles and two cardiac and major trauma areas.

The Johnston R. Bowman Health Center for the Elderly is a unit hospital of Rush designed to serve as a national model for hospital-based geriatric care. It offers a comprehensive range of inpatient and outpatient services and includes acute care, rehabilitation, psychiatric treatment, and physical, occupational, speech, and hearing therapies. In addition to patient-care rooms, the center offers modern apartments for residents capable of independent living.

Rush is a pioneer in community medicine: it has a continuing relationship with Mile Square Health Center; it created its own health maintenance organization, ANCHOR; and it offers expanding services in Chicago and beyond. At present there are medical center offices and facilities at 31 locations throughout the Chicago metropolitan area.

In addition to providing such a wide range of medical services, Rush is responsible for educating and training an enormous number of students from the health professions. Rush University has approximately 1,160 students enrolled in Rush Medical College, the College of Nursing, the College of Health Sciences, and the Graduate College. Twenty of the 1985 Rush Medical College graduates did their residency at the medical center in 1986.

---

**STATISTICAL PROFILE (Presbyterian–St. Luke's Hospital)**

Number of Beds: 903
Bed Occupancy Rate: 75.5%
Average Number of Patients: 884
Average Patient Stay: 8.6 days
Annual Admissions: 30,271
Births: 3,558
Outpatient Clinic Visits: 150,028
Emergency Room/Trauma Center Visits: 31,814

Hospital Personnel:
  Physicians: 730
  Residents: 440
  Registered Nurses: 1,361
  Total Staff: 7,197

# Specialties

Thirty-six departments cover every medical specialty. Centers for specific diseases and special requirements include the Adolescent Family Center, Alcohol and Drug Abuse, Arthritis, Birth Defects, Bone Marrow Transplantation, Breast Cancer, Cancer Treatment, Cardiac and Pulmonary Rehabilitation, Child Abuse, Epilepsy, Kidney Stones, Multiple Sclerosis, Ophthalmology, Organ Transplantation and Procurement, Osteoporosis Prevention and Treatment, Pain Management, Parkinson's Disease, Perinatal Care, Pigmented Lesions, the Rape Victim Advocate Program, and the Sleep Disorders Research Center.

# Well-known Specialists

Dr. Roger C. Bone, pulmonary medicine; specialist in adult respiratory distress syndrome.
Dr. Richard E. Buenger, diagnostic radiology.
Dr. Steven G. Economou, general surgery and surgical oncology.
Dr. L. Penfield Faber, thoracic surgery; specialist in lung cancer.
Dr. Jan Fawcett, psychiatry; specialist in depression.
Dr. Jorge O. Galante, orthopedic surgery; specialist in joint replacement surgery.
Dr. Jules E. Harris, internal medicine; specialist in medical oncology/immunology.
Dr. Harold Klawans, neurology; specialist in parkinsonism.
Dr. Hassan Najafi, cardiovascular surgery.
Dr. Elva Poznanski, child psychiatry; specialist in affective disorders.

# Research

In 1985 Rush received over $12.5 million in research funding from outside sources. While this might seem a small sum when compared with the amounts given to major medical school programs, Rush's research is almost all clinical, whereas much of the funding for research in larger institutions is given to basic life science research projects.

Research is an increasingly important aspect of the medical center's mission; over 1,000 projects are currently in progress. The four top areas of research are cancer, with more than 200 projects; cardiovascular disease, with 150; and neurological sciences and immunology, with about 100 each.

Cancer researchers are involved in continued evaluation of cancer drug effects on patients' suppressor cells, immunologic effects on tumor growth and rejection, and blood-group-related antigens in human bladder cancer.

Among the new cancer treatments being tested clinically are intraoperative radiation therapy, total-body electron beam irradiation, treatment of brain tumors by interstitial irradiation, and hyperthermia.

Cardiovascular research involves studies of noninvasive techniques for diagnosing coronary disease as well as investigations into the effects of various medical and surgical techniques. Among these studies was a new, noninvasive recording technique for identifying patients at high risk for sudden cardiac death and an investigation of the role of anticoagulants in coronary bypass surgery. The department of preventive medicine was one of several centers to participate in a study that not only evaluated the safety and effectiveness of antihypertensive medications but also, for the first time, analyzed their impact on users' quality of life.

Among the major areas of investigation in neurological research are aging, epilepsy, memory, movement disorders, multiple sclerosis, and stroke. Studies are also under way to evaluate the use of programmable drug pump implants in treating patients with cancer pain and Alzheimer's disease and of electrical stimulation to help those with motor control problems.

Research in the department of psychiatry continues on depression, suicide prevention, and the mentally ill offender; new interests are childhood depression and dissociative disorders.

Research in the orthopedic surgery department focuses on basic growing and healing processes. Projects include development of the titanium fibermetal surface of artificial joints, a bone staple gun for treatment of grafts and fractures, use of computers to develop techniques to custom-make artificial parts, and use of bone grafts in the treatment of bone cancer of the arms and legs.

Among many other recent research projects are investigations related to the development of an experimental vaccine against herpes, the development of male contraceptives, biomechanical aspects of total knee replacement and gait analysis, the effects of alcohol on male sexual development, and electrical stimulation of nerve regeneration.

## Admission Policy

Patients can be admitted to Rush without a physician's referral through the emergency room or through an inner-city community health center with which Rush has a relationship. Patients are assigned a Rush physician upon admission.

According to medical center policy, patients should show adequate insurance coverage upon admittance. A deposit is required for those who are uninsured or underinsured. However, patients who lack the ability to pay will not be turned away if they need urgent care. In fiscal year 1985 Rush provided over $9 million worth of free care.

**ROOM CHARGES (per diem)**
Private: $374
Semiprivate: $370
Ward: $370 (three-bed room)
ICU: $653

**AVERAGE COST PER PATIENT STAY:**    $9,124.86

**MAILING ADDRESS**             **TELEPHONE**
1753 West Congress Parkway    312-942-5488
Chicago, IL 60612

# University of Chicago Medical Center

**CHICAGO, ILLINOIS**

The University of Chicago is preeminent in just about every field of academic endeavor. Fifty-three Nobel Prizes have been won by faculty members here, including 11 in the biological sciences and two in medicine. Over the last sixty years the school of medicine, the biological research laboratories, and the hospitals have all played important parts in establishing the university as a leading medical research institution. This is the way most people in Chicago and even most doctors seem to perceive what is now called the University of Chicago Medical Center, but after some investigation we discovered that research is not the medical center's only strength.

Since more than 200,000 patients from the Chicago area alone are treated here each year, the University of Chicago Hospitals must also be regarded as important providers of health-care services. They are the home of several regional emergency care centers (including a first-rate burn center and a perinatal unit treating over 1,500 high-risk pregnancies every year); they are also the site of an emergency helicopter service. The hospitals offer nationally known federally funded programs for the treatment of a host of illnesses including cancer, diabetes, digestive diseases, heart disease, mental retardation, and multiple sclerosis. Programs are available to prospective patients through more than 80 specialty clinics dealing with everything from asthma and cystic fibrosis in children through back pain and obesity in mature adults to the ailments of old age in the newly founded Geriatrics Clinic. The medical center recently opened the Windermere Health Center, a facility in the Hyde Park community specializing in the treatment of older people.

So the University of Chicago is a premier research institution, but the scope, quality, and accessibility of its patient services also make it a vital medical resource for the people of the Chicago area. Since 1983 most of these services have been offered in brand-new facilities, including the 480-bed Bernard Mitchell Hospital; Chicago Lying-In Hospital, offering women's health care; an adjacent ultramodern 48-bed intensive care tower; and a surgical wing that includes 15 operating rooms. These buildings are part of a ten-year comprehensive modernization plan. One result of the plan has been a change in the way people perceive the quality of the services here.

We're told that about ten years ago native Chicagoans generally felt that while one could obtain fine, sophisticated medical treatment at the University of Chicago, the level of patient amenities there was somewhat below those available at several other area hospitals. In recent years this feeling appears to have changed, and in the center's latest surveys of discharged patients 96 percent indicated that they would choose the University of Chicago again if they needed hospitalization.

The medical center offers services in just about every specialty as well as a wide range of subspecialties. We can only highlight a few departments here.

The University of Chicago is a nationally famous organ transplantation center, the most important in its region. Over 100 kidney transplants and 10 to 12 heart transplants are done each year in the center, which is headed by Dr. Frank Stuart, a kidney surgeon. Recently, the medical center emerged as one of the leading hospitals for liver transplantation, and between 30 and 40 liver transplants a year are performed here under the direction of Dr. Christoph Broelsch, a well-known transplant surgeon from West Germany. Approximately 50 bone marrow transplants are done here annually, mostly for victims of leukemia and a few other types of cancer.

The diagnosis and treatment of cancer is a major concern here, and the hospital is a regional referral center that sees over 1,200 new cancer patients a year. Almost every department has specialists in cancer treatment. In fact, there seems to be no form of cancer that cannot be treated here with the most up-to-date equipment. There is the 24-bed Hematology/Oncology Unit for patients undergoing radiation or chemotherapy as well as a number of specialty clinics, including those for gynecologic cancer and head and neck cancer. There is also a special screening center for the detection of prostate cancer.

In neurology Chicago has had a strong reputation for many years. Today programs cover the full range of neurological problems, including autoimmune disease, brain tumors, dementia, epilepsy, and myasthenia gravis. The department also runs a Sleep Disorders Center, an Alzheimer's Disease Referral Center, a Multiple Sclerosis Clinic sponsored by the Illinois Chapter of the National MS Society, and an ALS clinic and research program (for Lou Gehrig's disease) that is one of only four in the country sponsored by the National ALS Foundation.

Other major specialties include cardiology, which has many programs and clinics, for both the prevention of heart failure and the treatment of heart disease; endocrinology, through one of the country's best-known diabetes research and treatment programs; gastroenterology, in which Chicago is well known for its work with inflammatory bowel disease, liver disease, complex nutrition problems, and obesity; and surgery, which offers every kind of service.

As is often the case at major medical centers, the strengths of Chicago's other departments are reflected in pediatrics. Housed in the 134-bed Wyler Children's Hospital (next to the main facility), the pediatric group has specialists in congenital heart disease, juvenile diabetes, oncology, psychiatry, rheumatology, and urology, among others. Of course, allergies, asthma, and other common childhood problems are dealt with here, as are cystic fibrosis and sickle-cell disease. The center's expertise in organ transplantation, open-heart surgery, and almost all other kinds of surgery is also available to children. (Those who need rehabilitation and management of long-term illness are treated at nearby La Rabida Children's Hospital.)

Chicago Lying-In Hospital opened a century ago as a storefront with the goal of offering free obstetric care. Today it provides family-centered maternity care with expertise in gynecologic disease and special programs in cancer detection and treatment, genetic counseling, high-risk pregnancies, infertility and endocrinology, and gynecologic surgery. The new inpatient facility includes a newborn unit; an intensive-/intermediate-care nursery; and labor, delivery, operating, and recovery suites. The hospital operates the Regional Perinatal Network with Michael Reese Hospital and Medical Center; it offers special care to high-risk mothers and infants.

## Specialties

Allergy, Anesthesiology, Cardiac Surgery, Cardiology, Dentistry, Dermatology, Emergency Medicine, Endocrinology, Gastroenterology, Genetics and Genetic Counseling, Hematology/Oncology, Infectious Diseases, Internal Medicine, Neonatology, Nephrology, Neurology, Neurosurgery, Obstetrics/Gynecology, Ophthalmology, Organ Transplantation, Orthopedics, Otolaryngology, Pathology, Pediatrics, Plastic and Reconstructive Surgery, Psychiatry, Pulmonary Medicine, Radiology, Rheumatology, Surgery, Thoracic Surgery, Urology, and Vascular Surgery.

---

**STATISTICAL PROFILE**

Number of Beds: 600
Bed Occupancy Rate: 81%
Average Number of Patients: 450
Average Patient Stay: 8.4 days
Annual Admissions: 21,500
Births: 2,500
Outpatient Clinic Visits: 230,000
Emergency Room/Trauma Center Visits: 55,000

Hospital Personnel:
  Physicians: 400
  Residents: 400
  Registered Nurses: 720
  Total Staff: 3,400

---

# Well-known Specialists

Dr. Barry G. W. Arnason, neurology; specialist in multiple sclerosis, chairman of the Department of Neurology and director of the Brain Research Institute.

Dr. George Block, surgery; specialist in gastrointestinal disease, chief surgeon.

Dr. Christoph Broelsch, surgery; specialist in liver transplantation.

Dr. Frederic Coe, kidney disease; specialist in the cause of kidney stones.

Dr. Leslie DeGroot, endocrinology; specialist in thyroid disease.

Dr. Donald Ferguson, surgery; specialist in breast cancer.

Dr. Harvey Golomb, hematology/oncology; specialist in leukemia and lung cancer, chief of the Section of Hematology/Oncology.

Dr. Arthur Herbst, obstetrics/gynecology; specialist in gynecologic cancer, chairman of obstetrics/gynecology.

Dr. Leonard Johnson, pediatrics; specialist in bone marrow transplants for children.

Dr. Robert Karp, surgery; specialist in cardiac transplantation, chief of the Section of Cardiac Surgery.

Dr. Barbara Kirschner, pediatrics; specialist in gastrointestinal disorders of childhood, codirector of the Section of Gastroenterology/Hepatology.

Dr. Joseph Kirsner, gastroenterology; specialist in inflammatory bowel disease.

Dr. Thomas Krizek, specialist in reconstruction after thermal burns and injuries to the hands and extremities, chief of the Section of Plastic and Reconstructive Surgery.

Dr. Atef Moawad, obstetrics; specialist in high-risk pregnancy, chief of the Section of Fetal-Maternal Medicine.

Dr. John Mullan, chief of neurosurgery.

Dr. William Panje, surgery; specialist in reconstructive surgery of neck and head and voice rehabilitation for cancer patients.

Dr. Leon Resnekov, cardiology.

Dr. Robert Rosenfield, pediatric endocrinology; director of the Children's Clinical Research Center.

Dr. Arthur Rubenstein, endocrinology; specialist in diabetes.

Dr. Harry W. Schoenberg, urology; specialist in adult and childhood bladder cancer, chief of the Section of Urology.

Dr. David Skinner, thoracic surgery; specialist in surgical oncology.

Dr. Frank Stuart, surgery; specialist in kidney transplantation, chief of the Transplantation Service.

Dr. John Ultmann, oncology; specialist in Hodgkin's disease and lymphoma, director of the Cancer Research Center.

# Research

Each year more than $45 million in research grants from public, corporate, and nonprofit foundation sources enables the faculty and staff at Chicago to conduct over 700 research projects. Cardiology (there is a special Center for Research in Ischemic Heart Disease), endocrinology (especially diabetes), gastroenterology, and neurology all have nationally recognized programs. But cancer research, which receives over 30 percent of all funds, is far and away the largest single field of study. A recent 300-page annual report on cancer research at the university described 124 separate studies including 45 clinical investigations centering on cancers such as those found in the brain, esophagus, head and neck, liver, lung, ovaries, and prostate. The focal point of these investigations is the National Cancer Research Center, which utilizes the expertise of more than 400 physicians and scientists to increase basic knowledge about cancer and to find better methods of early diagnosis and treatment.

This dedication to cancer research dates back many years and has resulted in important developments in treating cancers of the bowel and the liver as well as gynecologic cancer, Hodgkin's disease, and leukemia. In 1966 a University of Chicago physician won the Nobel Prize in medicine for his work in prostate cancer.

In 1985 a $9-million grant from a charitable foundation to the neurosciences enhanced the already famous research studies into ALS, multiple sclerosis, and myasthenia gravis, which have also been going on here for some time. Alzheimer's disease, Parkinson's disease, and the entire spectrum of diseases linked to the immune system are part of the multidisciplinary research programs at the Brain Research Institute.

Research at Chicago in organ transplantation dates back to 1904, when a large number of transplants were performed on animals. Today researchers here are trying to find an antirejection drug to replace cyclosporine, which still has many drawbacks. Another project entails the development of "banks" for storing bones, corneas, and tissues for use when needed.

The NIH funds two Clinical Research Centers here, one at Wyler Children's Hospital, another for adults. Congenital heart disease, hypertension, juvenile diabetes, and Reye's syndrome are a few areas of investigation in the children's center. For adults, work includes clinical studies of the role of diet and food allergies in emotional disorders, new therapies for hypertension, the chemotherapy of leukemia, and Lou Gehrig's disease.

The NIH also funds the Joseph P. Kennedy, Jr., Mental Retardation Research Center, where physicians and scientists are studying the causes of retardation as well as finding ways to improve the care of retarded children.

In 1986 the university received $7.2 million to build a Howard Hughes Medical Institute research unit, one of only 22 to be contracted throughout the country, which will specialize in biomedical research.

# Admission Policy

Given the nature of the services offered at Chicago, most patients are referred by their physicians. Doctors who are not familiar with the medical center can call the UC MedPhone toll-free for either consultations or referrals at 800-572-3692 (Illinois) or 800-482-6917 (out of state). Prospective patients can also be admitted through the emergency room or through one of the many specialty clinics. Appointments at the clinics can be made by calling the Physicians Appointment Service: 312-702-9200.

There are minimum financial or insurance requirements for admission, but decisions regarding admission rest solely with the medical staff. If a patient does not meet financial admissibility requirements, the physician determines whether to admit, transfer, or postpone admission after evaluating the patient's medical condition. In recent years the center has also provided about $14 million worth of indigent care annually.

---

**ROOM CHARGES (per diem)**
Private: $460
Semiprivate: $445
ICU: $960

**AVERAGE COST OF ORGAN TRANSPLANTATION**
Heart: $112,000
Kidney: $44,000
Liver: $110,000

| MAILING ADDRESS | TELEPHONE |
|---|---|
| 5841 Maryland Avenue | 312-702-1000 |
| Chicago, IL 60637 | (main phone number) |

# Indiana University Medical Center

**INDIANAPOLIS, INDIANA**

While most hospitals profess concern about patient satisfaction, Indiana University Medical Center actively seeks to learn whether patients are pleased with the quality of care received here. The medical center initiates quarterly opinion polls, which involve aggressive telephone interviews asking former patients if they would recommend the facilities to a friend. Most recently, from 94.0 to 96.4 percent responded yes to recommending University Hospital, with 96.3 to 97.0 percent saying they would recommend Riley, the center's children's hospital.

In other areas former patients rated the medical center equally high. On a scale where 4 points equals "absolute excellence," ratings for physician skills ranged from 3.71 to 3.75 for University Hospital; from 3.76 to 3.83 for Riley Hospital. Ratings for nurse skills for University Hospital ranged from 3.63 to 3.71 and 3.64 to 3.68 for Riley.

The nursing staff at Indiana is particularly worthy of their high scores. Ninety percent of the nurses here have bachelor's degrees, and most unit directors have a master's degree in nursing. Several nursing staff members have been cited for outstanding clinical and other nursing leadership roles.

Patient satisfaction with the hospital facilities and with its doctors and nurses partially explains why this is Indiana's primary referral center. Providing tertiary care for residents of the entire state, University Hospital and James Whitcomb Riley Hospital for Children are the cornerstone of the Indiana University Medical Center. In addition, over 9 percent of those seeking care at the medical center come from outside the state. The center serves as the teaching hospital for the university, whose medical complex includes schools of medicine, dentistry, and nursing; a division of allied health sciences; some 90 specialty clinics; and five separate hospitals.

Patients are often referred to University Hospital for critical care or complicated diagnoses. Two-thirds of the patients are admitted with two or more diagnoses of different medical problems in addition to the primary diagnosis. The hospital is a leader in cancer-care, cardiac care, treatment for hypertension, neurosurgery, and rheumatology.

The cancer-care programs offer diagnosis and treatment of more than 200 types of cancer. Adult and pediatric patients benefit from the expertise of physicians who have special interests in childhood malignancies including Wilms' tumor, colorectal, gynecologic, hematologic, lung, urologic tumors, neuroblastoma, Hodgkin's disease, and sarcomas.

The cardiac care program focuses on the prevention, treatment, and care of all cardiovascular disease. It is divided into adult and children's services. Adult outpatient services are provided at the Krannert Institute for Cardiological Diagnosis and Ambulatory Care. All services are supported by 19 adult and 18 pediatric cardiac-care unit beds and a specially educated nursing staff.

Riley is the only children's hospital in Indiana and thus serves as a specialty referral center for infants, children, and adolescents of Indiana and adjacent states. Riley provides services generally not available in hospitals throughout the state for the management of unusual, complex, or therapeutic problems. Children's needs are the focus throughout, as exemplified in many family-centered programs. Educational programs and services are provided to parents in an effort to help them better understand and cope with their child's disease. Some of the special facilities include a new Pediatric Intensive Care Unit and an eight-bed Pediatric Burn Center, the only one of its type in Indiana.

Riley is one of the nation's major centers for children's cardiovascular surgery. It offers a comprehensive range of care for children suffering from cancer, leukemia, and problems in a variety of other areas, such as arthritis, gastroenterology, infectious diseases, and ophthalmology. The advanced Newborn Surgical Intensive Care Unit serves as a comprehensive referral center for critically ill newborns from hospitals throughout the state. The Mobile Newborn Intensive Care Unit provides specialized emergency treatment during transportation. Riley's newborn hotline, an around-the-clock telephone consultation service, offers expert advice on the problems of the high-risk mother and newborn infant.

The kidney programs at Indiana are designed to handle all forms of congenital and acquired renal disease. The comprehensive adult program includes special services for hypertension, metabolic stone disease, renal failure and end-stage renal disease, and hypertensive manifestations of systemic problems, such as collagen vascular disease and diabetes. The program is well known for its innovative home dialysis services as well as more complex hospital-based dialysis programs. The pediatric program handles all forms of childhood kidney disease and emphasizes home dialysis. The Renal Transplant Program performed over 80 transplants in 1985 and is supported by a 20-bed special-care unit.

The Eating Disorders Program is designed to assist adults and children in dealing with psychologically based eating disorders. Treatment for anorexia nervosa and bulimia includes physical stabilization and weight restoration and attempts to remedy the psychological problems that cause these disorders. Using a combination of therapies, the treatment takes two to three months and is used on both an inpatient and outpatient basis. For children, family therapy plays an important role.

The Endocrinology/Metabolism Program includes four major centers. The Hypertension Center treats all types of hypertension, including adrenal, essential, malignant, renovascular, and other secondary forms. The multidisciplinary team of experts develops a strategic plan for each patient that incorporates treatment and patient control over drugs and diet. The Diabetes Center serves adults and children with disorders of glucose metabolism such as diabetes insipidus, diabetes mellitus, and hypoglycemia. The Metabolic Bone Disease Center helps patients who are at risk of osteomalacia, osteoporosis, or Paget's disease of bone. The Children's Endocrine Center is staffed by pediatric endocrinologists who diagnose and treat dysfunction of the endocrine glands in infants, children, and adolescents. Patients with growth failures benefit from team management of pediatric specialists.

Ophthalmologists at Indiana have been performing corneal transplants for the past twenty-five years. The Lions Club of Indiana established here the only accredited eye bank in the state. Patient-care services in all areas of ophthalmology are also provided, including a special pediatric program, the only eye diagnosis and care program in Indiana devoted exclusively to children.

The Arthritis Center has over 70 physicians and scientists and the resources to handle the entire spectrum of degenerative connective tissue diseases. The center is one of the few programs in the United States that offers comprehensive clinical services in rheumatology management. A variety of services treat, rehabilitate, and educate patients in the treatment of amyloidosis, juvenile rheumatoid arthritis, osteoarthritis, rheumatoid arthritis, and scleroderma, among many other conditions.

Every county in Indiana sends patients here, which is why over 600,000 people are treated annually in all the clinics and hospitals that encompass Indiana University Medical Center. Also, Indiana is one of the largest medical schools in the country.

## Specialties

Specialties at University Hospital include Cardiac Transplants, Cardiology and Cardiac Care, Dentistry, Dermatology, Endocrinology, Family Practice, Gastroenterology, Gerontology, Hematology, Internal Medicine, Infectious Diseases, Medical Genetics, Neonatology, Nephrology, Neurology, Obstetrics/Gynecology, Oncology, Ophthalmology, Orthopedics, Otolaryngology, Plastic Surgery, Psychiatry, Renal Transplants, Rheumatology, Surgery, and Urology.

Specialized services are available for allergies, arthritis, bone marrow transplants, corneal transplants, eating disorders, epilepsy, nuclear medicine, renal dialysis, sleep studies, speech therapy, sports medicine, and ultrasound.

Specialized pediatric services at Riley include treatment for arthritis, bone marrow transplants, burns, cancer, cardiology, cerebral palsy, clubfoot, corneal transplants, diabetes, eating disorders, epilepsy, genetic testing, growth anomalies, hemophilia, intensive care, kidney transplants, muscular dystrophy, myelomeningocele, and psychiatry. Special programs include adolescent medicine, the Infant Nurture School Age, the Parent Care Unit, and the Teen Unit.

---

**STATISTICAL PROFILE**

Number of Beds: 620
Bed Occupancy Rate: 81%
Average Number of Patients: 503
Average Patient Stay: 9 days
Annual Admissions: 18,000
Births: 1,127
Outpatient Clinic Visits: 160,000
Emergency Room/Trauma Center Visits: The Emergency Room is a
   self-contained unit, not part of the Medical Center.

Hospital Personnel:
   Physicians: 600
   Residents: 593
   Registered Nurses: 1,200
   Total Staff: 3,400

---

# Well-known Specialists

Dr. John P. Donahue, urology; specialist in adrenal disease, cancer of the genitourinary tract, and renovascular hypertension.

Dr. Mark L. Dyken, neurology; specialist in cerebral vascular disease, strokes, and diagnostic problems in neurology, coauthor of *Cerebrovascular Diseases*, a physician's reference.

Dr. Clarence E. Ehrlich, obstetrics/gynecology; specialist in cancers of the cervix and uterine, ovarian, and endometrial cancer.

Dr. Lawrence Einhorn, internal medicine and hematology; specialist in genitourinary tumors.

Dr. Harvey Feigenbaum, internal medicine and cardiovascular disease; specialist in cardiology and echocardiography.

Dr. Charles Fisch, internal medicine; specialist in cardiac arrhythmias.

Dr. Morris Green, pediatrics; specialist in child development and psychological aspects of child health.

Dr. Jay Grosfeld, general and pediatric surgery, neonatal surgery, pediatric surgical oncology, and pediatric trauma.

Dr. C. Conrad Johnston, internal medicine and endocrinology; specialist in metabolic bone disease and osteoporosis.

Dr. Richard E. Lindseth, orthopedic surgery; specialist in myelomeningocele, pediatric spine deformities, knee and foot disorders, and congenital scoliosis.

Dr. Richard L. Schreiner, pediatrics and neonatal-perinatal medicine; specialist in perinatal aspiration syndromes.

Dr. August Watanabe, internal medicine and cardiovascular diseases; specialist in cardiovascular pharmacology.

## Research

In 1986 research funding at the Indiana University Medical Center totaled $21 million. The various schools at the university support 429 research projects. Research institutes include Cardiology, Psychiatric Research, the Regenstrief Institute of Health, and the Walther Oncology Center. Among the major areas of investigation are cardiology, dermatology, oncology, pediatrics, and rheumatology.

Well known for its advances in cardiology, Indiana University was the founding institution for echocardiology. Another aspect of cardiology research here is testing TPA (tissue plasminogen activator), a drug that dissolves blood clots.

Between 50 and 60 protocols in pediatrics are being studied at the medical center; Indiana is particularly strong in pediatric pulmonary and pediatric trauma research.

Oncology studies investigate gynecologic, pelvic, and testicular cancers. Research on cancer drugs and treatments is partially sponsored by the National Cancer Institute.

## Admission Policy

Indiana is a true referral hospital; almost all its patients are referred by their physicians. The hospital accepts only limited self-referrals, athough patients can make appointments in some of the clinics.

There is no financial requirement for admission because this is a state hospital. About $5 million worth of indigent care is provided per year.

**ROOM CHARGES** (per diem)

|  | Riley | University Hospital |
|---|---|---|
| Private: | $273 | $231 |
| Semiprivate: | $265 | $226 |
| Ward: | $278 |  |
| ICU: Newborn | $445 | $591 |
| Pediatric | $665 | $445 |
| Cardiac | $665 | $445–$591 |

**AVERAGE COST PER PATIENT STAY:**    $6,864

**MAILING ADDRESS**               **TELEPHONE**
1100 West Michigan Street    317-274-5000
Indianapolis, IN 46223

# University of Iowa Hospitals and Clinics

**IOWA CITY, IOWA**

---

Americans living in rural areas have often found it difficult to obtain quality medical care beyond the primary level. Today the continuing crisis in the farm economy and the attendant drop in farm population—over a half-million people left rural areas between 1980 and 1985 alone—have joined forces with the recent changes in Medicare payment dispersal to play havoc with the economic stability of hospitals throughout the Farm Belt. As their occupancy rates fall, hospitals are being forced to restructure. As a consequence, the services offered by the major, heavily subsidized academic medical centers are bound to grow in importance.

University of Iowa Hospitals and Clinics have long been the primary providers of secondary- and tertiary-care services in this region. Opened in 1870 as a clinical training area for the medical school, the first University Hospital was built in 1898; by 1914 it had 250 beds and a growing reputation. Today it is the largest university-owned teaching hospital in the United States, employing over 1,000 doctors in more than 100 specialties. While there are only 150,000 people in Iowa City and nearby Cedar Rapids combined, Iowa Hospitals and Clinics register just over 400,000 patient visits per year. Most come from Iowa (all 99 counties) and from Illinois, although there are patients from almost every other state and from 20 or more foreign countries annually. For while the rich black soil of the Iowa cornfields may actually be visible from some of the buildings, what they practice here isn't farmland medicine, but state-of-the-art medicine with facilities including nuclear magnetic resonance imaging scanners, lasers, laser linear accelerators, and the lithotriptor.

Several of the tertiary-care services at Iowa have achieved national recognition, including their transplantation programs. Since 1969 over 1,000 kidney transplants have been performed; about 80 are done each year. Heart and liver transplant programs were begun only recently, but Iowa should become a regional referral center for these procedures over the next few years; the hospital is already performing most of the region's pancreas transplants (over 20 a year). In bone marrow transplantation, Iowa is one of the nation's leaders. Over 200 such transplants have been done here, just over 40 a year on the average, and the program has gained special attention because of the doctors' success with unrelated donors and recipients.

Iowa's Department of Otolaryngology is nationally known for its work with cochlear implants. Over 30 have been performed here, and many other patients have been evaluated for this procedure.

Every major medical specialty and subspecialty is practiced at Iowa, and most of the departments sponsor programs that serve the entire state. Ophthalmology, for example, runs a statewide screening program for glaucoma and is also the leading referral center for cornea transplants (over 100 are done each year). Internal Medicine sponsors the Renal Dialysis Network, which through ten hospitals around the state provides initial diagnostic evaluation for patients with renal disease as well as preparation for home dialysis or possible transplantation.

One of the most active departments in terms of statewide programs is Pediatrics. Children with cancer from all parts of Iowa are given an examination and initial treatment; most are then returned to their home communities for continued therapy. In 1976 Iowa's pediatric hematologists initiated the Statewide Children's Hemophilia Program, which has helped identify and treat some 200 patients. Physicians here are also active in the perinatal and neonatal fields; the Neonatal Intensive Care Unit is a 43-bassinet center treating some 700 critically ill infants from all parts of Iowa and western Illinois annually. Genetics provides a complete range of diagnostic, therapeutic, and educational services in pediatrics through 15 regional clinics.

Iowa is also the home of the state's most comprehensive and sophisticated Burn Center, where an average of 160 patients—most of the major burn victims in the state—are treated each year. The Emergency Treatment Center is Iowa's only comprehensive emergency treatment center. At the Iowa Psychiatric Hospital, which has 58 adult and 12 children's beds, more than 900 inpatients and 1,700 outpatients are treated annually, making it the largest such facility in the state.

These hospitals and clinics are also the site of the largest cancer treatment center in the state, and one of the largest in the Midwest. Almost 5,000 cancer patients are helped here each year, more than 2,000 of them new cases. Many patients are referred to Iowa because of the availability of several advanced therapies (including intraoperative radiation) and hard-to-find technological marvels such as a laser linear accelerator.

## Specialties

Iowa's clinical services are organized through 16 departments: Anesthesiology, Dermatology, Family Practice, Hospital Dentistry, Internal Medicine, Neurology, Obstetrics/Gynecology, Ophthalmology, Orthopedics, Otolaryngology–Head and Neck Surgery, Pathology, Pediatrics, Psychiatry, Radiology, Surgery, and Urology. These departments encompass a total of 110 specialties and subspecialties. Each clinical service has its own inpatient and outpatient sections and special diagnostic areas where applicable.

Clinics include Allergy-Immunology, Alzheimer's/Dementia, Arthritis,

Cardiovascular, Hematology/Oncology, Iowa Lions Cornea Center, Muscular Dystrophy, Pain, Pediatric Cardiology, Sleep Disorders, and Sports Medicine.

---

**STATISTICAL PROFILE**

Number of Beds: 922
Bed Occupancy Rate: 80%
Average Number of Patients: 720
Average Patient Stay: 7.1 days
Annual Admissions: 37,081
Births: 2,461
Outpatient Clinic Visits: 368,032
Emergency Room/Trauma Center Visits: 17,490

Hospital Personnel:
　Physicians and Dentists: 455 (on staff)
　Residents (Physicians and Dentists): 602
　Registered Nurses: 1,335
　Total Staff: 6,832

---

# Well-known Specialists

Dr. Francois Abboud, internal medicine.
Dr. Douglas M. Behrendt, cardiothoracic surgery.
Dr. Reginald R. Cooper, orthopedics.
Dr. Robert J. Corry, surgery; specialist in transplantation.
Dr. Antonio Damasio, neurology; specialist in Alzheimer's disease.
Dr. Charles E. Driscoll, family practice.
Dr. Edmund A. Franken, radiology.
Dr. Bruce Gantz, director of the cochlear implant program.
Dr. Roger D. Gingrich, director of bone marrow transplantation.
Dr. Richard G. Lynch, pathology.
Dr. Brian F. McCabe, otolaryngology; specialist in head and neck surgery.
Dr. Allyn L. Mark, director of cardiology.
Dr. John C. Montgomery, hospital dentistry.
Dr. Frank Morriss, pediatrics.
Dr. Roy M. Pitkin, obstetrics/gynecology.

Dr. John S. Strauss, dermatology.
Dr. John H. Tinker, anesthesiology.
Dr. John C. VanGilder, neurosurgery.
Dr. Thomas Weingeist, ophthalmology.
Dr. Richard D. Williams, urology.
Dr. George Winokur, psychiatry.

# Research

The size and scope of Iowa's medical research programs have helped this institution achieve its strong recognition. With over $48 million in research grants in 1985–86, the University of Iowa ranks among the top institutions in terms of support. It houses one of the NIH's specially funded Clinical Research Centers, where a large number of highly specialized trials are conducted, including studies in cystic fibrosis, diabetes, glaucoma, hyperactivity in children, and hypertension.

Given the university's location, there's a good deal of research devoted to problems peculiar to rural America. The Division of Agricultural Medicine, for example, has demonstrated that farmers who raise hogs in confinement experience a much higher rate of infections and respiratory problems; physicians and scientists are now trying to discover ways of teaching farmers alternative methods.

Every department at Iowa has several major research projects in progress at all times. Generally speaking, however, the strongest research programs reflect the hospital's best-known services, cochlear implants and organ transplantation. There are also separately designated research centers for Alzheimer's disease, cancer (especially bone marrow transplantation), cardiovascular problems including arteriosclerosis and ischemic heart disease, diabetes, and digestive diseases. A long-range study into the childhood origins of heart disease, which was begun in 1970, has resulted in the establishment of national standards for childhood blood pressures.

# Admission Policy

Most patients are referred to Iowa by community physicians, however, referrals are not necessary. Anyone can call the hospital and make an appointment with the appropriate department or clinic.

No proof of insurance is required. Each year the hospital provides $35 million worth of indigent care, of which about $25 million is reimbursed by the state of Iowa.

**ROOM CHARGES (per diem)**
Private: (Not available. Most rooms are semiprivate, 2 beds.)
Semiprivate: $159–$504
ICU: $416 (burn unit)–$834 (transplants)

**AVERAGE COST PER PATIENT STAY:**    $6,041 (without physician's fee)

**MAILING ADDRESS**        **TELEPHONE**
650 Newton Road          319-356-1616
Iowa City, IA 52242

# The Menninger Foundation
**TOPEKA, KANSAS**

"No greater illusion prevails than that mental illness is usually hopeless or has at best a bad outlook," wrote Dr. Karl Menninger. "Precisely the reverse is true. Most of its victims recover."

The Menninger Foundation was established in 1925 when Dr. Charles Menninger and his two sons, Dr. Karl and Dr. Will, bought twenty acres of land on the outskirts of Topeka and remodeled an existing farmhouse to serve as a 13-bed psychiatric hospital. Although it was not the first psychiatric hospital in the United States, it was the first to use a "total environment" approach, involving a family atmosphere, physical exercise, and a multidisciplinary team of doctors. "Often called 'The Mayo Clinic of psychiatric hospitals,' The Menninger Foundation is regarded as one of the major psychiatric treatment and teaching facilities in the world," reported the *New York Times* in a November 13, 1975, article. More than 130,000 patients have been seen at The Menninger Foundation over the past sixty-one years.

The Menninger Foundation is a national center for the diagnosis and treatment of severe mental illness, a major source for the education of mental-health professionals, a research center for the development of basic knowledge about human behavior, and a pioneer in the prevention of mental illness, particularly in business and industry.

Management consultants Booz, Allen & Hamilton recently reported that professionals and lay public alike regarded The Menninger Foundation as an institution of high quality and innovation. They also noted that no other institution offers the breadth of services available here in treatment, education, research, and prevention of mental illness. Inpatient and outpatient clinical services include hospitals for adults and children offering comprehensive psychiatric evaluation, diagnosis, and consultation as well as psychoeducational evaluation, neurological evaluation, neurosurgery, and neuropsychological testing.

The Children's Hospital treats patients aged five to seventeen in a hospital setting with a staff-to-patient ratio of two to one and a separate school with individualized instruction (class size is limited to five students). Children between the ages of two and five who suffer emotional difficulties or learning disabilities are treated in the Preschool Day Treatment Center. The Menninger Youth Program provides group homes and services for dependent and neglected children in 33 communities in six states and the District of Columbia, with additional homes in the planning stage.

Workshops for divorcing couples and stepfamilies present methods parents can use to help their children deal with the emotional trauma of divorce. Practical issues—including property settlement, child custody and visitation, and spousal and child support—are also addressed.

A Rehabilitation Program provides disability management services and comprehensive vocational assessments of disabled people and injured workers. The program also serves as a job resource center for disabled people and employers.

Employee assistance programs provide on-the-job help for workers with concerns about marital, family, emotional, job stress, alcohol, and drug abuse issues.

The Menninger Foundation is an internationally recognized training center for mental-health professionals. More than 170 active faculty members work with students in many disciplines. "We like to think [our students] have learned what limits to place on their expectations. . . . But their hope should remain unextinguished and unextinguishable. They should believe steadfastly that there is no patient for whom something helpful cannot be done," wrote Dr. Karl Menninger in *The Vital Balance*.

The Karl Menninger School of Psychiatry and Mental Health Sciences trains physicians in general and child psychiatry. The school offers postdoctoral training in clinical psychology, postmaster's training in psychiatric social work, and training for practicing mental-health professionals focusing on marriage, family counseling, and other specialties. The Topeka Institute for Psychoanalysis provides training in psychoanalysis.

In the past sixty-one years The Menninger Foundation has demonstrated that timely and skillful therapeutic intervention in the lives of troubled patients, in an atmosphere of optimistic expectation and caring, can lead to improved health.

## Specialties

Psychiatric and neurological services for both children and adults include comprehensive diagnosis, individualized treatment plans, a team concept of treatment, family involvement through the treatment process, and consultative services provided by a multidisciplinary staff.

Special programs include alcohol and drug abuse treatment; psychosocial services for cancer patients and their families; career assessment evaluation for clergy; eating disorders treatment; emergency admission treatment; family therapy, marriage counseling, and sex therapy; forensic consultation and evaluation; headache management and treatment; hypnosis and hypnotherapy; remedial groups for neurologically impaired patients and their families; premenstrual syndrome evaluation and treatment; individual and group psychotherapy; and speech and hearing evaluation and therapy.

**STATISTICAL PROFILE**

|  | Menninger Hospital | Children's Hospital |
|---|---|---|
| Number of Beds: | 166 | 69 |
| Bed Occupancy Rate: | 91% | 94% |
| Average Number of Patients: | 150 | 65 |
| Average Patient Stay: | 125 days | 125 days |
| Annual Admissions: | 471 | 51 |

Outpatient Clinic Visits: 138,257

Hospital Personnel:
There are more than 1,100 full- and part-time employees. The clinical staff includes more than 240 psychiatrists, psychoanalysts, psychologists, psychiatric social workers, internists, neurologists and neurosurgeons, dieticians, nurses, and activity therapists, as well as theologians, special educators, audiologists, and speech pathologists.

# Well-known Specialists

Dr. C. Alton Barnhill, eating disorders.
Dr. Robert W. Conroy, alcoholism and drug abuse.
Dr. Steven L. Fahrion, Ph.D., biofeedback.
Dr. Glen O. Gabbard, borderline personality disorders.
Dr. Joseph M. Hyland, psychosocial effects of cancer.
Dr. Erwin T. Janssen, child and adolescent psychiatry.
Stephen A. Jones, M.S.W., marriage and family therapy.
Dr. Stephen E. Katz, depression and psychopharmacotherapy.
Dr. William Kearns, geriatric psychiatry.
Dr. Eric Kulick, schizophrenia.
Dr. William S. Logan, forensic psychiatry.
Dr. Roy Menninger, stress.
Dr. W. Walter Menninger, chronic mental illness.
Dr. Jack L. Ross, psychoanalysis.
Dr. John B. Runnels, neurology and neurosurgery.
Dr. Joseph D. Sargent, psychosomatic medicine, including headache treatment.
Dr. William S. Simpson, sex therapy.
Dr. William H. Smith, Ph.D., hypnosis.
Dr. Glenn Swogger, Jr., preventive psychiatry.

# Research

Research programs at The Menninger Foundation emphasize the multidisciplinary study of mental illness to contribute to the understanding of its causes, prevention, and treatment. Research funding amounts to almost $2 million; about 48 percent is funded by The Menninger Foundation and the rest by various groups, including the American Psychoanalytic Association, the Department of Health and Human Services (specifically the National Institute of Mental Health and the National Heart, Lung, and Blood Institute, which funds research of nondrug treatment for hypertension), the U.S. Department of Education, and pharmaceutical companies.

Some areas in which research is currently being conducted at the foundation include biofeedback as a method for controlling migraine headaches, hypertension, and other psychosomatic illnesses; postoperative counseling for cancer patients; child-rearing and child-care practices; genetics, to explore whether behavior can be passed from one generation to another; hospital treatment evaluation and follow-up studies; the nature of mental illness, specifically schizophrenia; and prediction of suicide potential.

# Admission Policy

The Menninger Hospitals accept applicants who desire and need hospitalization. Referral may come through psychiatrists, other mental-health professionals, or the patient or family.

The Admissions Office requests that applicants call or write the office to discuss their problems and treatment needs; the therapist currently treating the applicant should communicate with the foundation by phone or letter, and the person who is financially responsible for treatment should contact the Admissions Office to discuss treatment costs.

Members of the family should accompany the applicant and participate in the admission process, which usually takes from two to four days (during which time the family members generally stay in a local motel).

The process begins with a preadmission consultation to clarify the patient's desire for treatment and the appropriateness of treatment at the foundation. It is during this consultation that the final decision regarding admission is made.

**ROOM CHARGES (per diem)**
The fee for room, meals, nursing care, medication, social work, activity therapists, hospital supplies, and use of facilities is $350 a day. The fee for the hospital psychiatrist is first day, $95; second day, $70; each additional day, $55. (Fees are charged for a five-day week.)

Charges at prevailing rates will be made for other services including initial clinical examination by a clinical social worker; psychological testing; laboratory charges; X ray, electroencephalogram, and EKG; and services of the internist and neurologist. Laboratory charges are approximately $225, and psychological testing is about $525. Individual psychotherapy is $85 per hour.

Services of specialists within the community are billed by the specialist and are not part of the foundation's statements.

It is the policy of The Menninger Foundation that the first month's charge for hospital services and medical services is payable upon admission. A minimum admission deposit of $1,500 is required. The foundation provides over $1 million per year in indigent care.

**AVERAGE COST PER PATIENT STAY:**   $48,890

**MAILING ADDRESS**  **TELEPHONE**
P.O. Box 829        913-273-7500
Topeka, KS 66601

# The Ochsner Clinic and Hospital

**NEW ORLEANS, LOUISIANA**

---

We received some idea of how highly regarded the Ochsner Clinic is when doctors kept referring to it in the same context as The Mayo Clinic and the Cleveland Clinic. While not nearly as large or as famous as those two institutions, Ochsner does see about 160,000 people a year, and almost half of them come from outside the New Orleans area; 10,000 are from Latin America. Ochsner's regional reputation is so strong that over the last few years its administrators have initiated a twenty-four-hour emergency helicopter transport service that serves a 200-mile radius. They've opened six neighborhood clinics in New Orleans that have over 65,000 patient encounters a year, and in 1986 they opened two facilities in Baton Rouge.

People come to the Ochsner Clinic for a thorough diagnostic evaluation, officially called a Clinic Check, or for one of the specific medical services described in the following paragraphs. The Clinic Check normally takes about a week and costs anywhere from $600 for males under forty-five to $1,200 for females over forty-five. The Pediatric Clinic Check usually requires three or four days and its costs vary greatly. If a patient's condition warrants hospitalization, a clinic physician will admit him or her to the Ochsner Foundation Hospital, which is adjacent to the clinic. Or patients may choose to return to their referring physicians for admission to a hometown hospital.

Patient satisfaction is high for hospital services here. Market research by the hospital indicates that overall measures of satisfaction consistently average 90 percent. In addition, more than half of all discharged patients have recommended Ochsner to at least one person in need of hospitalization. Elaborate quality-assurance programs are a source of great pride to Ochsner. Unlike most other hospitals, Ochsner was willing to reveal some of the results of its quality-assurance programs, including the fact that its hospital-acquired infection rate has been consistently and significantly lower than the national average, 3 percent versus 5 percent.

The high quality of patient care is matched by Ochsner's commitment to obtaining the latest tools of medical technology. Ochsner was one of the first facilities in the region to acquire a lithotriptor and the first in New Orleans to build a Magnetic Resonance Imaging Center.

Cardiac surgery is recognized as a major strength here. About 400 bypass operations are performed here annually, and the hospital has recently become a regional center for heart transplants, with a minimum of 12 per year being planned. Pediatric cardiac surgery is also a specialty.

The Ochsner Kidney Transplant Center is the largest in Louisiana and has a success rate of over 90 percent. It provides services for Louisiana, adjoining states, and many Latin American countries. A new immune monitoring panel of tests is used for posttransplant immunosuppression management.

The Department of Colon and Rectal Surgery, one of the first independent departments established in this specialty in the United States, provides a full range of surgical procedures, including diagnostic and operative colonoscopy. Minor surgical procedures and several kinds of therapy are offered on an outpatient basis. Areas of special interest in gastroenterology include absorptive disorders, diagnostic and therapeutic endoscopy, inflammatory bowel disease, diseases of the liver, and motor disorders of the gastrointestinal tract. Outpatient and inpatient services are available for hypertensive diseases. Treatment emphasizes life-style modification as well as pharmacological therapy. Ochsner is involved in clinical trials of new drugs for hypertension, which are available to patients.

Special care areas in the hospital include the Coronary Care Unit and the Intensive Care Unit. The Neonatal Intensive Care Unit and the Pediatric Intensive Care Unit are regional referral centers.

The Department of Psychiatry has a special unit limited to adolescent and young women. It offers long-term therapy dealing with emotional and psychological stress that may be manifested as anorexia, behavioral problems, depression, or other conditions that are best addressed in an all-female psychiatric inpatient setting. A stress treatment unit offers care to older adolescents and adults with stress-related illnesses. Patients may be referred to the unit by their own physician, a professional agency, or a psychologist.

The Patient/Family Education Department and the Ochsner Cancer Institute cosponsor the Ochsner Cancer Education Program, which provides free educational forums to help cancer patients and their families anticipate and cope with the variety of problems of living with the disease.

Ochsner's tradition of fine medical care dates back almost half a century. Founded in 1941 by five surgeons, the Ochsner Clinic was named after one of them—Dr. Alton Ochsner, a world-renowned surgeon and teacher as well as the first physician to draw a connection between cigarette smoking and lung cancer. In 1944 the partners of the Ochsner Clinic established the nonprofit Alton Ochsner Medical Foundation. Today the Ochsner Clinic is a private partnership of physicians and surgeons who practice in over 50 specialties and subspecialties. Its professional staff also serve as the attending medical staff of the adjoining Ochsner Foundation Hospital.

According to *The New Orleans Citibusiness*, "Unlike many not-for-profit hospitals which contract with several so-called 'doctor corporations' for services such as emergency room service, only one 'doctor corporation' exists at Ochsner. . . . Of the 200 physicians, 108 are partners, the others are 'employee physicians' who generally become partners during their fourth year of work at Ochsner."

The Ochsner Medical Foundation also sponsors one of the nation's largest non-university-affiliated graduate medical education programs for approximately 200 new physicians per year. Postgraduate medical education programs at Ochsner take from two to seven years to complete and usually involve specialization.

The School of Allied Health Sciences offers 12 full programs leading to careers including health-care administration, dietetic internship, extracorporeal technology, nuclear medicine technology, radiological technology, respiratory therapy, and diagnostic ultrasound technology.

## Specialties

Allergy and Clinical Immunology, Anesthesiology, Cardiac Surgery, Cardiology, Colon and Rectal Surgery, Dermatology, Emergency Medical Services, Endocrinology, Gastroenterology, Hand and Microvascular Surgery, Hematology and Oncology, Hypertensive Diseases, Infectious Diseases, Internal Medicine, Neonatology, Nephrology, Neurology, Neurosurgery, Nuclear Medicine, Obstetrics/Gynecology, Occupational Medicine, Ophthalmology, Oral Surgery, Organ Transplant, Orthopedic Surgery, Otorhinolaryngology, Pathology, Pediatric Surgery, Pediatrics, Plastic and Reconstructive Surgery, Psychiatry, Psychology, Pulmonary Diseases, Radiation Therapy, Radiology, Rehabilitation and Physical Medicine, Rheumatology, Spinal Surgery, Sports Medicine, Surgery, and Urology.

In addition to physician services, diagnosis and treatment of children with learning disorders, psychological testing and social work services, speech and hearing tests, and patient instruction on arthritis, cardiac rehabilitation, diet, hypertension problems, smoking elimination, weight control, and other health issues are available.

---

**STATISTICAL PROFILE**

Number of Beds: 483
Bed Occupancy Rate: 70%
Average Number of Patients: 333
Average Patient Stay: 7 days
Annual Admissions: 17,200
Births: 775
Outpatient Clinic Visits: 144,500
Emergency Room Visits: 24,320

Hospital Personnel:
  Physicians: 225
  Residents: 220
  Registered Nurses: 525
  Total Staff: 2,550

# Well-known Specialists

Dr. William Brannan, urology.
Dr. Edward D. Frohlich, hypertensive diseases.
Dr. J. Byron Gathright, colorectal surgery.
Dr. Jay P. Goldsmith, neonatology.
Dr. Franz H. Messerli, hypertensive diseases.
Dr. Noel L. Mills, cardiac surgery.
Dr. John L. Ochsner, cardiac surgery; head of the heart transplant team.
Dr. George A. Pankey, infectious diseases.
Dr. John E. Ray, colorectal surgery.
Dr. Frank A. Riddick, Jr., endocrinology and metabolic diseases.
Dr. George T. Schneider, obstetrics/gynecology.

# Research

The research budget at Ochsner is less than that of many of the other hospitals in this book, but of its approximately $3.2 million, almost $2.2 million is internally funded by the Alton Ochsner Medical Foundation, and the foundation research program is growing.

Ochsner's major areas of research center on cancer and cardiovascular disease (particularly hypertension). A new initiative in cancer research has focused on the molecular biology of cancer and ongenes and immunological methods for diagnosis and treatment using monoclonal antibody technology and lymphokine therapy. A nationally recognized program on hypertension includes studies of the atrial natriuretic hormone, a material synthesized in the heart that causes water and salt loss and may play an important role in hypertension and congestive heart failure.

Other studies investigate AIDS, bone marrow transplantation, thrombolytic therapy of coronary artery disease, esophageal motility, septic shock, gastrointestinal blood flow during shock, transplantation surgery and immunology, and the cellular biology of vasoactive peptides.

# Admission Policy

The Ochsner Clinic provides service on an appointment basis only. Patients are encouraged to make an appointment with any clinic doctor they wish to see. Patients are taken in order of their appointments unless laboratory testing procedures require a change in schedule.

Appointments with any clinic physician or department (except Audiology, Cardiology, Obstretrics/Gynecology, Oral Surgery, Otorhinolaryngology, Pediatrics, Psychiatry, and Speech Therapy, which schedule appointments separately) can be made by telephoning the Appointment Desk at 504-838-4111. For the other departments call the clinic's general number: 504-838-4000.

There is a financial requirement for admission to the hospital. Patients must provide proof of insurance coverage or make a cash deposit estimated on the basis of the reason they are entering the hospital and the expected length of stay provided by the physician. Patients may also be asked to make a deposit for amounts not covered by insurance.

The Brent House, an on-campus 200-room hotel, is available for patients and their families.

---

**ROOM CHARGES (per diem)**
The average daily cost of hospital care in this area of Louisiana is about $600, considerably less than the $800- to $1,000-a-day figures for cities such as New York or San Francisco.
  Private: $245
  Semiprivate: $210
  ICU: $630
  Room Charges at Brent House: $57–$65 per night

**AVERAGE COST PER PATIENT STAY:**   $7,050

**MAILING ADDRESS**          **TELEPHONE**
1516 Jefferson Highway    Hospital: 504-838-3000
New Orleans, LA 70121    Clinic: 504-838-4000

---

# Johns Hopkins Medical Institutions
## BALTIMORE, MARYLAND

Staffed by physicians from a world-renowned medical school, the Johns Hopkins Medical Institutions provide care in almost every area of modern medicine, including bone marrow and organ transplantation (cornea, heart and lung, kidney, liver, and pancreas). While every department is highly regarded, several—cardiology, neurology, neurosurgery, oncology, ophthalmology, pediatrics, and urology, for example—have international reputations, so patients are referred here from around the world. Almost half of Hopkins's patients are from outside the Baltimore area, and in recent years patients from almost 60 countries have been referred here.

At the center of Hopkins's renown in the medical community is one of the world's largest and most respected medical research programs, whose clinical impact is especially strong, as a few recent examples will illustrate. Physicians and scientists at Hopkins have developed a test for predicting bone marrow rejection, a sinus surgery never before performed in the United States, a prenatal hemophilia and Huntington's disease test, an objective test to diagnose nerve injury, a shunt proven successful in patients with liver disorder, a drug treatment to replace surgery for many infants with hydrocephalus, new devices in the treatment of thigh-bone fractures, a new type of surgery for children with severe genetic disorders, and a program changing the treatment for alcoholism.

The discoveries of Adrenalin, Dramamine, Mercurochrome, and vitamin D all happened here, as did the development of cardiopulmonary resuscitation. During the 1970s the Nobel Prize–winning discovery of restriction enzymes, which gave birth to the genetic engineering industry, also took place at Hopkins.

It would, however, be a mistake to conclude that research is the predominant activity at Hopkins. The melding of research and patient care at Hopkins is part of a tradition dating back to 1889, when the hospital first opened; it was followed four years later by the medical school. Both were the outright gifts of Johns Hopkins, a Quaker merchant. Along with several other hospitals and medical schools at that time, Hopkins helped to usher in the era of modern medical training by bringing students from the classroom to the hospital.

Only a handful of hospitals can match Hopkins in terms of the number of services offered; fewer still can equal its reputation for excellence in so many areas.

A recent addition to Hopkins's services is the Neuroscience Critical Care Unit, one of the few to offer patients with life-threatening brain diseases, including Guillain-Barré syndrome, a combination of specialists—neurologists, neurosurgeons, and anesthesiologists—and the most modern equipment in a single unit. Patients who have undergone or will undergo neurosurgery are also treated here. About 800 patients a year are expected to benefit from this unit.

Alcoholism is a major focus at Johns Hopkins, which has initiated a program that could become a national model for diagnosing alcoholism early enough for successful treatment. The program teaches physicians to recognize early stages of alcoholism, plan treatment, and motivate patients to comply with treatment.

At the Center for Aging, which includes the Mason F. Lord Chronic Hospital at the Francis Scott Key Medical Center, the goal is to integrate research, inpatient care, home health services, professional training, and nursing to meet the psychological and social as well as medical needs of the elderly. The Center for the Study of Dementia, which trains health professionals, also extends its education to patients' families through regular support group meetings and counseling sessions. Geriatric psychiatry programs include Alzheimer's disease, Huntington's disease, and neuropsychiatry.

The Children's Center houses a pioneering adolescent pregnancy project and a major program to consolidate health services for high-risk young people. (Urban youths aged fifteen to twenty-four are the only group in the United States with increasing death rates.)

Hopkins is the Pediatric Trauma Center for Maryland, and a large number of patients with head injuries are treated here annually. Other special interests in pediatric neurosurgery are hydrocephalus and brain tumors. Parents may room-in with children during hospitalization. Child Life workers are also available to provide age-appropriate education and recreation.

The Wilmer Eye Institute was created in 1925 within the framework of the Johns Hopkins Medical Institutions. Wilmer is an international leader in the study and investigation of the causes and treatment of eye disease. It provides diagnostic and evaluative services to patients with all forms of ophthalmic problems. The institute has pioneered the use of lasers for aging macular degeneration, diabetic retinopathy, and glaucoma. Areas of expertise include studies of retinitis pigmentosa, intraocular lenses for cataract surgery, perfection of techniques for removing damaged vitreous gel, corneal transplantation, and eye muscle and orbital surgery. Last year the 100 physicians and scientists at Wilmer published over 500 scientific journal articles and 15 books. There are 55,000 office visits and 4,500 surgical operations at Wilmer each year; patients are referred here from all over the world.

The Chronic Pain Treatment Program emphasizes the treatment of chronic pain of benign origin. Techniques include behavioral therapy, drug withdrawal, implantable stimulators, active rehabilitation, and surgery.

The Oncology Center was designated by the NIH as one of about 20 Comprehensive Cancer Centers when it opened in 1976. It provides advanced diagnostic and treatment services for patients with a variety of disorders, with special emphasis on the management of aplastic anemia, brain tumors, breast cancer, Hodgkin's disease, leukemia, primary liver cancer, carcinoma of the lung, lymphoma, multiple myeloma, and ovarian and testis cancer. Over 5,000 patients come here each year, including many children.

The Department of Gynecology and Obstetrics provides a broad range of services, from routine obstetrics and reproductive health counseling to high-risk obstetric care, in vitro fertilization, and treatment of all forms of gynecologic disorders. The department's Prenatal Birth Defect Center provides multidisciplinary genetic consultation to patients at risk for bearing children with birth defects.

Today the Johns Hopkins Medical Institutions are composed of The Johns Hopkins Hospital, The Johns Hopkins University School of Medicine, the School of Public Health, and the School of Nursing. The institutions consist of 37 buildings situated on a 44-acre complex in Baltimore.

## Specialties

Hopkins's directory of referrals lists 226 clinical services, covering just about every medical specialty and subspecialty. Major divisions include Allergy and Immunology, Anesthesiology, Cardiology, Dermatology, Endocrinology, Gastroenterology, Gynecology and Obstetrics, Laboratory Medicine, Medicine, Neurology, Neurosurgery, Oncology, Ophthalmology, Orthopedic Surgery, Otolaryngology, Pathology, Pediatrics, Psychiatry and Behavioral Sciences, Radiology and Radiological Science, Rehabilitation Medicine, Rheumatology, Surgery, and Urology.

In addition to standard adult emergency services, Hopkins provides emergency specialty services in eye, oral and maxillofacial, otolaryngological, pediatric, psychiatric, renal, and respiratory care. Helicopter transport service is also available.

A selected list of clinics and services includes Adolescent Medicine, the Adolescent Pregnancy Program, Adult Seizures, Affective Disorders, Allergy, Anxiety, Behavioral Medicine, Birth Defects, Burn Treatment, Breast Reconstruction, Cardiac Arrhythmia, the Cornea and Anterior Segment Surgery Center, Dementia Research, the Dermatology Ambulatory Care Unit, Diabetes, Eating Disorders, Emergency Services, the Endocrine Clinic, Epilepsy, Eye Consultation, Facial Nerve, Facial Rehabilitation, the Fertility Control Center, the Foot Clinic, Fractures, Genetics, Glaucoma, Gynecological Oncology, the Hand Clinic, Head and Neck Trauma, Head Injuries, Hearing and Speech, Hematology, High Risk Obstetrical, Immunodeficiency, Infectious Diseases, In Vitro Fertilization, the Lipid Clinic, Low Vision, Male Infertility, Medical Genetics, Movement Disorder, Multiple Sclerosis, the Neuromuscular Clinic, Occupational Medicine, Ocular Oncology, Oncology (Pediatrics), Ophthalmologic Surgery, Orthopedics, Pain Treatment, Plastic Surgery, Prenatal Birth Defects, Prenatal Diagnostics, Preventive Cardiology, Psychogeriatrics, Retinal Consultation, Retinal Degenerations, the Sarcoidosis Consultation Service, Schizophrenia, Scoliosis,

Sexual Behavior Consultation, Sleep Disorders, the Spine Clinic, Surgical Diagnostics and Consultation, Swallowing, Thyroid, Urology, Urological Oncology, and Voice Disorders.

Supplementing the alcoholism program are community services, a daytime recovery unit, emergency services, walk-in services/day hospital, inpatient services, and an outpatient clinic.

---

**STATISTICAL PROFILE**

Number of Beds: 1,087
Bed Occupancy Rate: 81%
Average Number of Patients: 880
Average Patient Stay: 8 days
Annual Admissions: 35,864
Births: 3,016
Outpatient Clinic Visits: 453,964
Emergency Room/Trauma Center Visits: 95,756

Hospital Personnel:
    Physicians: 1,611; 714 full-time
    Residents: 503
    Registered Nurses: 1,504

---

## Well-known Specialists

Dr. Fred Berlin, authority on sex offenders and their treatment.

Dr. John L. Cameron, surgery; specialist in gastrointestinal surgery, biliary tract, liver, and pancreatic diseases.

Dr. Susan Folstein, researcher in Huntington's disease.

Dr. John Freeman, pediatric neurology; specialist in epilepsy and restoring children with seizure disorders to drug-free life.

Dr. Robert Jeffs, pediatric urology.

Dr. Steven Kopits, orthopedic surgery; specialist in surgically correcting deformities in dwarfs.

Dr. Paul McHugh, psychiatry; specialist in major eating disorders, such as anorexia nervosa and bulimia.

Dr. John Money, Ph.D., authority on human sexuality and gender identity problems.

Dr. Frank Oski, chief of pediatrics, author of *Don't Drink Your Milk* and the *Yearbook of Pediatrics*.

Dr. Arnall Patz, ophthalmology; specialist in eye problems related to diabetes, pioneer in the use of lasers in treating eye problems, director of the Wilmer Eye Institute.

Dr. Peter Rabins, psychiatry; specialist in Alzheimer's disease, author of *The 36 Hour Day*.

Dr. Walter Stark, ophthalmology; specialist in intraocular lens implants, researcher in cataracts and cornea transplants.

Dr. Patrick Walsh, urology; perfecter of surgery to remove the prostate while preventing impotence.

## Research

Federal funding for the research program at the Hopkins medical school and its related institutions totals over $90 million, while private corporations and foundations provide another $25 million, giving Hopkins one of the three largest medical research programs in the country. This money goes to over 1,000 projects, more than 900 of them clinical investigations.

Virtually every area of medicine is covered. Among the largest specialties are oncology ($8.2 million), ophthalmology ($8.0 million), psychiatry ($7.0 million), and neurology ($4.5 million). Intense investigation is taking place in AIDS, bone marrow and organ transplantation, Down's syndrome, hypertension, liver cancer, movement disorders, and stroke. Hopkins is also one of only a few NIH-funded institutions doing special research in Alzheimer's disease.

Two federally sponsored Clinical Research Centers are located here. For adults, coronary heart disease, Huntington's disease, lung cancer, and sickle-cell anemia are just a few of the diseases under investigation; for children, there are programs in endocrinology, genetic diseases, nephrology (chronic renal failure), and neurology.

## Admission Policy

Most of the patients at Hopkins have been referred by their physicians or by one of the local hospitals, but anyone can make an appointment at the clinics (phone 301-955-JHMI) and if hospitalization is required will be admitted by a Hopkins physician.

All patients admitted to Hopkins are interviewed to determine financial responsibility. It is the policy of the hospital to establish with each patient, or the individual assuming responsibility for the patient's bill, a reasonable arrangement for payment. Patients without insurance are expected to deposit, on admission, a sum based on their estimated charges. The deposit may be reduced or waived depending on the patient's financial situation and the urgency of need for medical care.

In recent years Hopkins has absorbed over $15 million in bad debts annually and provided about $6 million in free care. The hospital has rendered more charity care to the poor of the city than any other private or public institution in Baltimore.

Elective admissions are postponed until estimated charges are paid or insurance coverage is obtained. It is also the policy of Hopkins that uninsured foreign nationals must pay 100 percent of their estimated hospital bill before admission.

---

**ROOM CHARGES (per diem)**
Private: $260–$300 depending on unit
          $595 in oncology unit
Semiprivate: $5 less than private rooms
ICU: $355–$565
          $865 for transplant, coronary, neuro, and critical care

**MAILING ADDRESS**          **TELEPHONE**
600 North Wolfe Street     301-955-5000
Baltimore, MD 21205

---

# The Warren Grant Magnuson Clinical Center of The National Institutes of Health

**BETHESDA, MARYLAND**

The Warren Grant Magnuson Clinical Center is the research hospital of The National Institutes of Health. The clinical center accepts a limited number of patients for study and therapy. All patients consent to participate in research studies and are treated for free. Unlike most hospitals the clinical center does not offer general diagnostic and treatment services. Admission is very selective: patients are chosen solely because they have an illness or disease that is under study by one or more of the institutes.

One of the unique features of the clinical center is the proximity of the laboratory to the patient here; the two are often merely the width of a hospital hallway apart. Traffic across this short distance is decidedly two way. Advances realized in the laboratory are brought to the patient's bedside, and new avenues of investigation are often opened by the health-care team's observations of patients. An amusing consequence of this interaction occurred in 1986 when a long-time patient of the clinical center claimed partial credit for the 1985 Nobel Prize in medicine awarded to Drs. Michael S. Brown and Joseph L. Goldstein, both of whom cared for him while they trained here.

Studies at the NIH often make national headlines—for instance, in December 1985 an article in the *New England Journal of Medicine* reported the results of the work by Dr. Steven Rosenberg and his colleagues on interleukin-2 treatment for cancer tumors. Twenty-five patients with advanced tumors of various types, from skin cancer to lung cancer, were treated with the drug in conjunction with the patient's own blood components. In 11 cases, the tumors shrank by 50 percent and, in one patient, they disappeared entirely. Rosenberg has called this process "adoptive immunotherapy."

Rosenberg's work is only one of dozens of studies that are always under way at the clinical center. Transfusion medicine, clinical pathology, and a major department of nuclear medicine equipped with its own cyclotron and PET scanners are only three areas of investigation.

The NIH is divided into 12 research institutes. Those with clinical research programs are Aging; Alcohol Abuse and Alcoholism; Allergy and Infectious Diseases; Arthritis and Musculoskeletal and Skin Diseases: Cancer; Child Health and Human Development; Dental Research; Diabetes and Digestive and Kidney Diseases; the Eye; Heart, Lung, and Blood; Mental

Health; and Neurological and Communicative Disorders and Stroke. Within these institutes almost every branch of medicine is covered.

Nearly all the institutes maintain their own laboratory and clinical research programs. Well over 2,600 research projects are in progress at all times on the NIH's Bethesda site, making it one of the largest research sites in the world. Over the years the NIH has supported the work of 70 Nobel Prize winners. Four of these scientists have been or are currently at work at NIH— Dr. Christian B. Anfinsen, Dr. Julius Axelrod, Dr. D. Carleton Gajdusek, and Dr. Marshall W. Nirenberg.

Physicians from each of the institutes offer medical care at the clinical center. Nursing care and other support services are provided by staff members. In addition, numerous guest scientists from this country and abroad collaborate in NIH activities. The clinical center also offers training in research medicine for young physicians, medical students, and nursing students. Bench scientists in some 1,100 laboratories work side by side with clinicians caring for patients. The clinical center contains 540 beds.

The NIH is the principal medical research arm of the federal government and one of the six health agencies of the Public Health Service, a component of the U.S. Department of Health and Human Services. The NIH supports research in universities, medical schools, hospitals, and research institutions; conducts research in its own labs and clinics; supports training for promising young researchers; identifies research findings; promotes effective ways to communicate biomedical information; and develops policies relating to the conduct and support of biomedical research. Of the total national investment in health research and development of about $6.2 billion, the NIH supports more than 40 percent, and provides more than two-thirds of the federal funds for this purpose.

The principal laboratories, clinics, offices, animal quarters, and other specialized facilities of the NIH are located on a 306-acre campuslike setting in suburban Bethesda, Maryland, about ten miles from downtown Washington, DC.

Also part of the NIH is the National Library of Medicine, the world's largest reference center devoted to a single subject. Currently the library's collection includes 2.5 million items. As one of its services the library produces and publishes the *Index Medicus*, an indispensable reference journal for investigators and practitioners throughout the world.

A new 13-story Ambulatory Care Research Facility provides space for the hospital's rapidly expanding outpatient program. The facility handles an estimated 145,000 outpatient visits each year.

## Specialties

Patients, upon referral by their physicians, are admitted to clinical studies conducted by the various institutes. Some of the specific diseases studied here include AIDS, Alzheimer's disease, Cushing's syndrome, hypertension, and many genetic disorders.

Physicians can obtain a booklet describing the diseases currently under study by writing to Clinical Center Communications, NIH, Building 10, Room 1C255, Bethesda, MD 20892. (Telephone: 301-496-2563.) Specific trials change frequently so this booklet is published yearly.

---

**STATISTICAL PROFILE**

Number of Beds: 540
Bed Occupancy Rate: 64%
Average Number of Patients: 318
Annual Admissions: 7,500
Outpatient Clinic Visits: 145,000

Hospital Personnel:
Physicians: 1,000
Registered Nurses: 700
Total Staff: 5,000, of which 20 percent hold doctoral degrees

---

## Well-known Specialists

Dr. Duane F. Alexander, director of National Institute of Child Health and Human Development.
Dr. John L. Decker, director of the Clinical Center.
Dr. Vincent T. Devita, Jr., director of the National Cancer Institute.
Dr. Anthony S. Fauci, director of the National Institute of Allergy and Infectious Diseases.
Dr. Murray Goldstein, director of the National Institute of Neurological and Communicative Disorders and Stroke.
Dr. Frederick Goodwin, director of the National Institute of Mental Health.
Dr. Enoch Gordis, director of the National Institute on Alcohol Abuse and Alcoholism.
Dr. Carl Kupfer, director of the National Eye Institute.
Dr. Claude J. M. Lenfant, director of the National Heart, Lung, and Blood Institute.
Dr. Harald A. Löe, director of the National Institute of Dental Research.
Dr. Lawrence E. Shulman, director of the National Institute of Arthritis and Musculoskeletal and Skin Diseases.
Dr. T. Franklin Williams, director of the National Institute on Aging.

# Admission Policy

Patients can be considered for admission to the clinical center only upon referral from their physician or dentist. Admissions are limited to those patients who have an illness being investigated at one or more of the institutes. The number of beds available for a particular study and the length of the waiting list of qualified patients are also important in determining admission.

Patients may leave the clinical center at any time they wish. However, when they are admitted, the general plan of the study is explained, the importance of the patients' role is outlined, and their cooperation for the duration of the study is enlisted. When participation in a study is completed and their condition permits, patients are returned to the care of their own physicians. Periodic follow-up examinations may be conducted, or treatments may be given for months or years afterward.

About 8,500 such inpatients are admitted each year from throughout the United States. The clinical center also admits about 300 "normal volunteers" annually. These healthy people (about 15 percent of the patient population) provide an index of normal body functions against which to measure the abnormal. Normal volunteers come under varied sponsorship such as that of colleges, civic organizations, and religious groups.

The clinical center welcomes calls from physicians and dentists regarding referrals. The Patient Referral Service can be reached at 301-496-4891.

---

**ROOM CHARGES** (per diem)
There are no charges for services because patients are volunteering to be part of specific research groups funded by the federal government.

**MAILING ADDRESS**      **TELEPHONE**
9000 Rockville Pike      301-496-4114 (Director's Office)
Building 10
Bethesda, MD 20205

# Beth Israel Hospital

**BOSTON, MASSACHUSETTS**

If a hospital is to be judged on the quality of its nursing program, then Beth Israel will certainly be rated one of the best in the country. Its nursing department has been cited as a model for nursing practice by the *New York Times*, the *Boston Globe*, and many professional journals. Nurses at Beth Israel have averaged more than 30 publications a year since 1980 and four times that many presentations. Beth Israel was selected by the American Academy of Nursing as one of 41 magnet hospitals in the United States and was asked to participate in three national studies examining nursing care, which were sponsored by the Division of Nursing Health and Human Services, the National Commission on Nursing, and the Institute of Medicine. In addition, nurses from more than 20 countries and 20 states have requested either a field placement or observation experience at Beth Israel during the last five years, and some have returned for second visits.

The primary-care nursing program at Beth Israel, developed in 1974, has one of the longest and most successful histories in the country and has served as a model for many other hospitals. Each patient is assigned a registered nurse, who is responsible for developing a coordinated individual plan of care. The primary nurse accepts twenty-four-hour accountability for maintaining continuity of care from admission to discharge or transfer and provides direct nursing care to primary patients and other assigned patients while on duty. The primary nurse leaves clear directions to other staff when not on duty. This hospitalwide system allows nurses to give more personalized care and helps ensure that competent care is maintained throughout hospitalization.

Beth Israel offers a full range of adult inpatient, outpatient, walk-in, and emergency services and extensive programs in teaching and research.

Inpatient medical services cover cardiology, medicine, neurosurgery, neuromedicine, obstetrics/gynecology, orthopedics, psychiatry, surgery, and medical and surgical intensive care units.

Beth Israel's Berenson Emergency Unit is part of the Longwood Area Trauma Center, which handles the most difficult emergencies from the Greater Boston region and beyond. The unit treats more than 35,000 patients a year.

Beth Israel maintains an innovative general medicine center for ambulatory care (BI Healthcare Associates) and outpatient specialty units. The Home Care Program provides more than 7,000 visits to homebound, chronically ill patients by nurse practitioners, physicians, or social workers acting as a team.

Beth Israel is one of the major teaching facilities for Harvard Medical

School, and most of its physicians hold faculty appointments at the school. There are over 320 interns and residents each year in medicine, pathology, surgery, and other medical specialties. Nearly 150 postgraduate fellows continue in training for subspecialties, practice, research, and teaching. Beth Israel has led the country in providing innovative training programs in geriatrics and primary-care medicine.

Nursing students from five area schools; social work students from two colleges; and dietary intern students in medical technology, pharmacy, physical and occupational therapy, respiratory therapy, and radiological technology all receive part of their clinical education at Beth Israel.

Nursing research is an integral part of the professional practice model of the Division of Nursing. Nurse researchers with doctoral degrees conduct studies and publish their findings.

Biomedical research at Beth Israel is conducted in all areas of adult medicine, including cardiology, computer sciences, dermatology, endocrinology, gastroenterology, hematology, infectious disease, nephrology, neurology, nutrition, obstetrics, oncology, orthopedics, psychiatry, pulmonary diseases, rheumatology, surgery, and other fields related to clinical medicine and its underlying scientific basis.

Beth Israel was established in 1916 by the Boston Jewish community to meet the needs of the growing immigrant population. The hospital moved to its current location in 1928, when its affiliation with Harvard Medical School began.

In 1972 Beth Israel was the first hospital in the nation to issue a written statement on the rights of patients, including the rights to be treated with privacy, personal dignity, and respect and to receive full and detailed information about their cases. The statement is distributed to each patient admitted and to each new employee. It has served as a model for similar statements issued by other hospitals and enacted as legislation in various states.

## Specialties

Cardiology, Gastroenterology, General Surgery, Gerontology, Infertility, Nephrology, Neurology, Neurosurgery, Obstetrics/Gynecology, Oncology, Orthopedics, and Radiation Therapy.

Beth Israel offers many preventive, informational, and health-promotion programs, such as smoking cessation, weight loss, and treatment of stress-related illnesses, including allergies, chronic illness, high blood pressure, and hypertension, through behavioral medicine techniques. The Men's Program for the Treatment of Sexual Dysfunction offers a comprehensive approach to impotence.

The Beth Israel Dental Unit is a private group practice covering all areas

---

**STATISTICAL PROFILE**

Number of Beds: 460
Bed Occupancy Rate: 93%
Average Number of Patients: 413
Average Patient Stay: 6.5 days
Annual Admissions: 25,293
Births: 4,592
Outpatient Clinic Visits: 181,113
Emergency Room/Trauma Center Visits: 35,735

Hospital Personnel:
  Physicians: 262
  Residents: 192
  Registered Nurses: 967
  Total Staff: 4,071

---

from routine checkups to oral surgery. The Walk-In Center provides prompt medical care for minor emergencies.

# Well-known Specialists

Dr. Kenneth A. Arndt, author of the standard textbook on diagnosis and treatment of skin disorders, pioneer in the use of lasers to treat port wine stains, chief of dermatology.

Dr. Eugene Braunwald, author of the standard textbook on heart disease, editor in chief of the standard text *Harrison's Principles of Internal Medicine*, physician in chief.

Dr. Clyde Crumpacker, virology; specialist in infectious diseases such as AIDS and herpes.

Dr. Emanuel A. Friedman, creator of the Friedman curve, the widely used scientific description of the labor process, chief of obstetrics/gynecology.

Dr. Albert Galaburda, specialist in the relation between brain structure and dyslexia.

Dr. Robert Goldwyn, author of numerous books, including *Beyond Appearance: Reflections of a Plastic Surgeon*, chief of plastic surgery.

Dr. William Grossman, author of the standard textbook on cardiac catheterization, chief of cardiology.

Dr. John Hedley-Whyte, U.S. representative to the international standards committee on anesthesiology, chief of anesthesiology.

Dr. Steven Locke, psychiatry; specialist in the relation between stress and illness, author of several books, including *The Healer Within*.

Dr. Mitchell T. Rabkin, president of Beth Israel and professor of medicine at Harvard Medical School, author of the landmark Beth Israel "Statement on the Rights of Patients," leader in development of innovative systems of health care, such as primary nursing practice and a hospital-based ambulatory care center.

Dr. John Rowe, specialist in research on aging, chief of gerontology.

Dr. Lowell Schnipper, president of the Massachusetts Division of the American Cancer Society, chief of oncology.

Dr. William Silen, specialist in gastrointestinal surgery, editor of Cope's *Acute Abdomen*, chief of surgery.

Dr. Augustus A. White, III, specialist in back pain, author of the best-selling *Your Aching Back*, chief of orthopedic surgery.

Dr. Paul Zoll, cardiology; developer of the cardiac pacemaker.

## Research

Since the Harvard Medical School annually receives almost $60 million in research funding from NIH, it's not surprising that Beth Israel, its major teaching affiliate, is nationally recognized as an important center for clinical research. In 1986, the hospital itself received $17 million in research grants ($4 million of it from nonfederal sources) to support major programs in the study of AIDS, Alzheimer's disease, and epilepsy, among other things. At the NIH-funded Clinical Research Center there are special projects in chronic renal disease and hypertension, as well as extensive programs in the fields of endocrinology, gerontology, and hematology.

Several research projects here have received widespread media coverage, including the development of a method to deliver insulin nasally, the use of lasers with balloon catheters in treating cardiovascular disease, and the beginnings of several new techniques to help eliminate coronary bypass operations. In cancer research, one of the most dramatic breakthroughs of recent years came toward the end of 1986 when doctors at Beth Israel announced that they had developed a new blood test, using magnetic resonance imaging, to detect all forms of cancer. In a study of 330 people the test had an accuracy rate of well over 90 percent. Since early cancer detection has long been regarded as crucial to survival, this new test could become the most significant diagnostic tool of cancer specialists.

## Admission Policy

Patients can be admitted to Beth Israel without a physician's referral through the emergency room or clinic.

There is no financial requirement for admittance.

**ROOM CHARGES (per diem)**
Private: $409
Semiprivate: $380
ICU: $975

**AVERAGE COST PER PATIENT STAY:**    $800 per inpatient day

**MAILING ADDRESS**        **TELEPHONE**
330 Brookline Avenue    617-735-2000
Boston, MA 02215

# Brigham and Women's Hospital
## BOSTON, MASSACHUSETTS

Although the people of Boston are engulfed by history on almost every street corner and surrounded by the monuments of centuries' old traditions of academic excellence, they seem certain that their city belongs to the future—and with good reason. The youthful population, ubiquitous construction sites, and visible high-tech industries are all unmistakable signs that, in the coming decades, Boston will again be in the forefront of American cities.

This blending of past accomplishments with future hopes gives Boston a distinctive atmosphere, one that pervades just about every endeavor, including its extraordinary health-care system. Through the area's network of first-rate hospitals, one can trace the history of modern medicine and also see clearly the contours of scientific marvels still being developed. Perhaps the best example of this is Brigham and Women's Hospital, a world-famous tertiary-care center, a teaching affiliate of the Harvard Medical School, and one of Boston's most popular hospitals.

The Brigham, as it is often called, is located in a new, dramatically styled 16-story tower. Although the hospital opened officially in this facility in 1980, it was actually the result of a merger of three of Boston's oldest and most prestigious hospitals: the Peter Bent Brigham Hospital, the Robert B. Brigham Hospital, and the Boston Hospital for Women.

For decades the Boston Hospital for Women set the standard in obstetrics and gynecology, while doctors at Peter Bent Brigham achieved international recognition for initiating what became modern neurosurgery, for developing the artificial kidney machine, and for performing the first successful kidney transplant in 1954.

Today, some 1,200 kidney transplants later, the new Brigham and Women's Hospital remains a major center for all renal problems as well as for every facet of obstetrics and gynecology. In fact, nearly 10,000 babies are born here annually, placing the hospital sixth in the nation and first in New England in this category. About 2,000 babies spend some time in the Neonatal Intensive Care Unit, which is regarded as one of the best in the nation. The Brigham also has an active in vitro fertilization program and a special menopause unit, which attracts patients from all over New England.

The Department of Rheumatology and Immunology is one of the nation's oldest and largest. Its staff includes more than 30 physicians, as well as physical therapists, occupational therapists, psychologists, and nurses with special training in arthritis problems. About 400 young people are seen annually in the pediatric rheumatology unit, while the lupus clinic follows more than 300 patients and sees over 200 new ones each year.

These specialties alone would make the Brigham stand out, even among Boston's many fine hospitals. But if you consider the other services offered here, it's clear why this hospital is an invaluable regional resource. In orthopedic surgery, for example, doctors perform over 900 joint replacement operations a year, and the hospital serves as a regional referral center for disorders of the hand and upper extremity. In cardiothoracic surgery the hospital is considered a major transplant center (19 heart transplants were done here in 1985) and one of the leading facilities for bypass surgery (more than 800 were performed in 1985). The Brigham is internationally known for its cardiac care and cardiovascular services; it offers acute coronary care, angioplasty, and treatment of heart rhythm disturbances. The expertise of the radiation therapy department attracts thousands of patients from all over the United States as well as from Europe; close to 20,000 treatments for leukemia, tumors, and genetic disorders are performed each year. The Brigham also houses New England's only bone marrow transplant unit for adults and one of the few Level I Trauma Centers and burn centers in the region.

Not surprisingly, the Brigham has a high occupancy rate (86 percent), and an excellent reputation with the general public. To help secure this position in a crowded hospital market and in the midst of overall declining patient admissions, the administration recently linked itself to New England's largest health maintenance organization, the Harvard Community Health Plan. With well over 200,000 members, this group will help to solidify the Brigham patient base while attracting new members by promising access to one of the nation's leading hospitals.

---

**STATISTICAL PROFILE**

Number of Beds: 720
Bed Occupancy Rate: 86%
Average Number of Patients: 655
Average Patient Stay: 6.8 days
Annual Admissions: 32,154
Births: 9,844
Outpatient Clinic Visits: 224,441
Emergency Room/Trauma Center Visits: 37,780

Hospital Personnel:
  Physicians: 1,410
  Residents: 239 (Fellows: 216)
  Registered Nurses: 1,042
  Total Staff: 5,847

## Specialties

Asthma and Allergic Diseases, Bone Marrow Transplantation, Cardiology and Cardiothoracic Surgery (including heart transplantation), Gynecologic Cancer; Kidney Dialysis and Transplantation, Microsurgery, Neurology, Neurosurgery, High-Risk Obstetrics and Newborn Medicine, Orthopedic Surgery, Psychiatry, Radiation Therapy and Diagnostic Imaging, Rehabilitative Medicine, Rheumatology and Immunology, and Trauma.

There are special services for victims of lupus, multiple sclerosis, and stroke, as well as an occupational medical service, a pain treatment unit, and a thyroid diagnostic service.

## Well-known Specialists

Dr. K. Frank Austen, chairman of the rheumatology and immunology department.

Dr. Eugene Braunwald, cardiology; chairman of the Department of Medicine, head of the research team investigating a new drug to unclog blocked arteries.

Dr. C. Norman Coleman, director of the Joint Center for Radiation Therapy.

Dr. John Collins, director of cardiothoracic surgery.

Dr. Robert Demling, director of the burn/trauma unit.

Dr. Michael Epstein, neonatology.

Dr. Bernard Lown, cardiology; specialist in heart rhythm abnormalities, head of a special BWH cardiovascular group that bears his name.

Dr. Kenneth J. Ryan, chairman of the obstetrics and gynecology department.

Dr. Dennis J. Selkoe, neurology; specialist in research in and treatment of Alzheimer's disease.

Dr. Clement B. Sledge, chairman of the orthopedic surgery department.

Dr. Nicholas R. Tilney, kidney transplant surgery.

Dr. Howard Weiner, neurology; specialist in multiple sclerosis.

## Research

With grants totaling over $50 million a year, the Brigham's research program is one of the larger and more respected in the country. In 1985 the Brigham ranked first in the nation among independent hospitals in total grants from the NIH—$40 million. Also in 1985 the hospital took over nine floors in a new Biosciences Research Building (Harvard Medical School has four floors), further expanding the scope and potential impact of its research. The special Center for Neurologic Diseases, for example, now occupies an entire floor of the new facility, where researchers are studying the causes of three degenerative diseases of the central nervous system: Alzheimer's disease, ALS, and multiple sclerosis.

While physicians and scientists here conduct investigations in almost every area of medical science, many of the best-known programs are in fields where the hospital is especially strong clinically. In women's health problems, osteoporosis and menopausal hot flashes are being investigated. In rheumatology, doctors are studying ways of improving the functional capability and relieving the pain of rheumatoid arthritis patients who don't respond to conventional therapy; radiation synovectomy has helped some patients avoid surgery. Other researchers are working on new drug therapies for arthritis, including the use of cyclosporine, the immune suppressant developed for organ transplant patients.

The Brigham is also an NIH-sponsored Clinical Research Center, where studies in arrhythmias, cancer (interleukin-2 trials), juvenile diabetes, and metabolic bone disease, among other ailments, are conducted. Other major grants come from the American Heart Association and the American Cancer Society.

## Admission Policy

Given the nature of the illnesses treated at the Brigham and the hospital's affiliation with the Harvard Community Health Plan, most patients come through physician referrals. But patients can also be admitted through the emergency room as well as through some of the many ambulatory services. In addition, appointments with Brigham physicians can be made through the Patient Communications Office at 617-732-6636.

Prospective nonemergency patients are expected to have insurance coverage or prove their ability to pay. The Brigham does, however, have a long-standing record as the state's most generous private hospital, providing over $8 million annually in charity care.

---

**ROOM CHARGES (per diem)**
Private: $370
Semiprivate: $340
Nursery: $120
ICU: $835–$999
Neonatal Intensive Care: $650–$800

**MAILING ADDRESS**   **TELEPHONE**
75 Francis Street   617-732-5500
Boston, MA 02115

# Dana-Farber Cancer Institute
## BOSTON, MASSACHUSETTS

At the Dana-Farber Cancer Institute scientists work closely with physicians, carrying on a swift bench-to-bedside transfer of medical discoveries. This partnership has helped produce a remarkable record of achievements against many childhood and adult cancers that a generation ago claimed the lives of most of their victims. For example, in the United States, childhood leukemia has risen from a cure rate of less than 5 percent in 1960 to 50 percent overall and up to 80 percent in some forms of the disease. Osteogenic sarcoma, a bone cancer for which the cure rate was less than 15 percent, is now over 60 percent curable. Wilms' tumor, the second most common childhood tumor, has risen from roughly 40 percent to over 85 percent curable. Hodgkin's disease, a lymphoma that strikes children and adults, was approximately 40 percent curable in 1960 and is now approaching an 80 percent cure rate. Diffuse histiocytic lymphoma, a major form of adult lymphoma, has risen from 30 percent to 60 percent curable. Disseminated testicular cancer has gone from 10 percent to over 80 percent curable. Specialists at the institute have also made vital contributions to the treatment of childhood lymphoma and soft tissue sarcoma, as well as breast, head and neck, lung, and ovarian cancers.

Quality of life is the focus of many of the institute's most innovative treatment programs. Dana-Farber has introduced limb-saving techniques for osteogenic sarcoma, developed breast-preserving procedures using lumpectomies and radiotherapy for women with breast cancer, and pioneered research in drugs to combat nausea among chemotherapy patients.

The institute began in 1947 as the Children's Cancer Research Foundation, one of the world's first research and treatment centers devoted exclusively to pediatric cancer. Its programs in patient care, clinical investigation, and basic research grew to such an extent that in 1969 the institute expanded to provide services to anyone with cancer, regardless of age. As one of a network of about 20 federally designated regional Comprehensive Cancer Centers, Dana-Farber conducts basic and clinical research and provides pediatric and adult patient care, training and education of future cancer specialists, and outreach programs to disseminate up-to-date cancer treatment information to laypeople and to affiliated community hospitals and physicians throughout northern New England.

Any major surgery required by patients of the institute is performed at Beth Israel Hospital (see page 131), Brigham and Women's Hospital (see page 136), or the New England Deaconess Hospital. Pediatric patients are treated at The Children's Hospital.

Dana-Farber is a teaching affiliate of Harvard Medical School and maintains alliances with the other Harvard teaching hospitals. Institute professional staff hold appointments at Harvard Medical School or one of the other Harvard faculties. An oncology fellowship program is provided annually for young pediatricians and internists.

The institute is named for Dr. Sidney Farber, whose pioneering work with chemotherapy in 1947 enabled him to produce the first complete remissions in children with acute leukemia, and for the Charles A. Dana Foundation, which has helped support the institute for more than two decades.

In addition to focusing on the treatment of cancers with surgery, radiotherapy, and/or chemotherapy and providing the necessary support services, Dr. Farber recognized the importance of social and psychological factors affecting cancer patients and the need to maintain the best possible quality of life for them. This philosophy became known as "total patient care" and is still adhered to today.

According to Dr. Emil Frei III, director and physician in chief at Dana-Farber, programs in bone marrow transplants and the use of new drugs in combination chemotherapy and immunotherapy augur well for the future.

Working within the limits of chemotherapy, institute investigators have continued to develop innovative approaches to the treatment of cancer, most recently head and neck cancer. Combination chemotherapy administered before surgery or radiation can shrink these tumors to the point where they can be treated much more effectively with follow-up surgery, radiation, or a combination of the two. As a result, some previously inoperable tumors may now be curable. This approach has been extended to some patients with a specific type of lung cancer as well.

The institute's Division of Biostatistics and Epidemiology is considered one of the world's outstanding statistical centers for multi-institutional cancer clinical tests. It is the statistical center for the Eastern Cooperative Oncology Group, one of the leading cancer clinical cooperative groups in the United States. More than 200 treatment centers throughout the world, participating in approximately 100 studies, send their clinical data to the division for analysis.

The institute's Communication Office operates the Cancer Information Service to provide cancer patients and their families, health professionals, and the public with up-to-date information on the detection, diagnosis, and treatment of cancer. Its toll-free number serving Massachusetts, Maine, New Hampshire, and Vermont is 800-422-6237.

## Specialties

Biostatistics and Epidemiology, Blood Component Laboratory, Cancer Control, Cancer Genetics, Cancer Pharmacology, Cell Growth and Regulation, Gynecologic Oncology, Immunogenetics, Medical Oncology, Medicine, Oncodiagnostic Radiology and Nuclear Medicine, Pediatric Oncology, Radiotherapy, Respiratory Therapy, Social Work, Surgical Oncology, Tumor Immunology, and Tumor Virology.

Laboratories include Eukaryotic Transcription, Gene Regulation, Immunopathology, Membrane Immunochemistry, Molecular Biology, Molecular Carcinogenesis, Molecular Genetics, Molecular Immunobiology, Molecular Immunochemistry, Molecular Immunology, Neoplastic Disease Mechanisms, Structural Molecular Biology, and Tumor Virus Genetics. Other labs include Biochemical Pharmacology, Clinical Pharmacology, and Infectious Diseases.

---

**STATISTICAL PROFILE**

Number of Beds: 57
Bed Occupancy Rate: 80%
Average Number of Patients: 46
Average Patient Stay: 7–8 days
Annual Admissions: 2,200
Outpatient Clinic Visits: 25,437

Hospital Personnel:
    Physicians: 92
    Fellows: 35
    Registered Nurses: 88
    Total Staff: 1,113

---

## Well-known Specialists

A spokesperson for Dana-Farber requested that we ask prospective patients not to phone the doctors listed below. Instead, the public is advised to call one of the clinic numbers listed under "Admission Policy."

Dr. Steven J. Burakoff, chief of pediatric oncology.
Dr. George P. Canellos, chief of medical oncology.
Dr. Emil Frei III, chief of medicine.

## Research

At Dana-Farber more than 300 physicians and scientists in nearly 30 separate divisions and laboratories are addressing two central questions concerning cancer: What causes normal cells to transform into malignant or destructive cells? What is the best way to destroy each type of cancer cell?

In basic research geneticists and cell biologists are exploring the types of damage to human DNA that may trigger gene-activated eruption of cancerous cells. Virologists are investigating the roles of infectious viral invaders in restructuring the host cells. And immunologists are attempting to train the body's immune defense system to seek and destroy foreign matter without harming the host organs.

In clinical research chemotherapy programs developed for children with acute leukemia are being used with increasing success in the treatment of adults. Other chemotherapy protocols initiated at Dana-Farber are increasingly accepted as the best treatment of some forms of malignant lymphoma. In addition, the institute is pioneering the use of monoclonal antibodies in cancer diagnosis, prognosis, and treatment, most prominently in bone marrow transplantation.

## Admission Policy

Patients may be referred to Dana-Farber by their primary physicians, or they may inquire directly about admittance to consultation or treatment programs. For further information call the appropriate number.

Adult: 617-732-3476
Breast Evaluation Center: 617-732-3666
Head and Neck Clinic: 617-732-3090
Lung Cancer Clinic: 617-732-3468
Pediatric: 617-732-3315
Sarcoma Clinic: 617-732-3339

---

**ROOM CHARGES** (per diem)
Private and Semiprivate: $405

**MAILING ADDRESS**      **TELEPHONE**
44 Binney Street      617-732-3000
Boston, MA 02115

---

# Lahey Clinic Medical Center
## BURLINGTON, MASSACHUSETTS

Like those at the Mayo and Cleveland clinics, physicians at the Lahey Clinic Medical Center work on salary, not on a fee-for-service basis, and treat patients through the team approach of consultation and coordinated care. This approach has wide-reaching effects. The clinic is staffed and governed by full-time physicians whose control over quality the clinic believes is much more effectual than in other hospital organizations. The Lahey Clinic's quality-assurance program is unusually impressive, as exemplified in two reviews by the Joint Commission of Accreditation of Hospitals, undertaken when the new clinic facility opened in 1980. The clinic passed both reviews with no contingencies, no criticism, no areas to be corrected. This is very unusual and indicates that the Lahey Clinic offers the highest level of patient care.

Another evidence of the quality of care at Lahey is sheer numbers. The bed occupancy rate here is 95 percent, far higher than most hospitals, including the hospitals in this book. More than 70 percent of all nurses at Lahey have a bachelor's degree. The quality of nursing care is unusually high here, in part because the clinic primarily hires registered nurses with experience along with a small number of new graduates with bachelor's degrees. In their outpatient clinics, physicians at Lahey see between 1,400 and 1,700 patients a day.

The clinic is located in Burlington, twelve miles north of Boston, and is a not-for-profit institution concerned with providing coordinated diagnosis and treatment in nearly every medical specialty and subspecialty. It is a center of expertise in areas such as brain surgery, diagnostic imaging, management of hypertension, treatment of kidney disorders, laser surgery, pancreatic autotransplants, and use of radiation therapy for cancer.

Lahey's medical specialists focus on problems as diverse as cancer, cardiovascular disease, and gastrointestinal, neurological, and pulmonary disorders. More specifically, in the treatment of cancer, the clinic has developed specialized procedures, including the rotational therapy technique and special techniques for protecting normal tissue during treatment. In gastroenterology the clinic treats the full range of digestive disorders, with particular experience in inflammatory bowel disorders, diseases of the pancreas, motor disorders of the esophagus, and hyperalimentation.

The clinic has expertise in the full range of general surgical procedures, particularly those of the biliary tract, liver, pancreas, and thyroid, and performs pioneering work in renal vascular bypass surgery, surgical treatment of secondary hypertension and restoration of kidney function, clinical evaluation of YAG laser irradiation of bladder cancer cells as an alternative to removal of the bladder, and reconstructive surgery of the upper and lower urinary tract.

Diagnostic specialists use CAT scanning, digital subtraction angiography, ultrasound, and other sophisticated technology to detect and define disease. Magnetic resonance imaging is a major resource in the Department of Diagnostic Radiology.

As a means of minimizing hospitalization and reducing the cost of health care, the Lahey Clinic stresses the development and use of techniques of testing and treatment on an ambulatory basis. For this reason it has long undertaken diagnostic tests related to an approaching hospital stay on an outpatient basis, days in advance of hospital admission. With clinical departments and self-contained ambulatory surgery facilities, the clinic is designed to accommodate a large outpatient population. Physicians for the clinical departments have their offices and examining rooms within the medical center's Charles A. Dana Ambulatory Care Center. The Mary and Arthur Clapman Hospital provides inpatient care.

In 1980 Lahey established the Lahey Clinic Blue Cross and Blue Shield Health Maintenance Plan, a prepaid health plan that serves more than 20,000 members in 40 cities and towns in eastern Massachusetts. Health-plan members receive care from the same physicians as other Lahey Clinic patients. (At present enrollment is through employer group contracts only.)

Tel-Med is a library of telephone tapes on more than 250 health topics presented as a public service by the Lahey Clinic/Blue Cross and Blue Shield Health Maintenance Plan. The three- to seven-minute tapes, which can be listened to in privacy over the telephone, provide basic information on a variety of health-care issues and problems. Brochures listing the tapes available from the clinic's Department of Public Relations can be obtained by calling 617-273-8733.

Lahey's social services department provides professionally trained social workers and continuing care nurses to hospitalized patients and their families. This staff helps in planning for discharge home or to another facility and in counseling for emotional or social problems related to illness or hospitalization.

In addition to its central focus on patient care, the Lahey Clinic is strongly committed to research and education. The Department of Research concentrates on developing new instrumentation and refining surgical and medical techniques while coordinating research projects undertaken by physicians throughout the medical staff. Special interests include biomedical research, biomedical statistics, cancer immunology, and regional cancer chemotherapy. The clinic's Eleanor Naylor Dana Laser Research Laboratory is one of its special facilities for testing and refining new applications of laser technology.

The training of physicians at Lahey follows the tradition of the team approach. At any given time approximately 45 physicians are serving here in residency and fellowship programs in ten specialties. In addition, physicians from throughout the United States and abroad attend the clinic's continuing education program.

The Lahey Clinic was established in 1923 as a small, private clinic operated by Dr. Frank H. Lahey, a prominent Boston surgeon, in his apartment in the city. Although the initial staff consisted of only four physicians, the clinic at that time was an exception to the prevailing concept of Boston medical practice, which emphasized physicians practicing on a solo basis and treating difficult cases in the medical schools. Today the Lahey Clinic's team approach by physicians of differing specialties is followed by many major health-care institutions.

Sixty percent of Lahey Clinic patients come from Greater Boston. Twenty-five percent come from outside Massachusetts. Seventeen percent are from Massachusetts, and approximately 2 percent come from outside the United States.

**STATISTICAL PROFILE**

Number of Beds: 200
Bed Occupancy Rate: 95%
Average Number of Patients: 190
Average Patient Stay: 7.2 days
Annual Admissions: 8,631
Outpatient Clinic Visits: 350,000
Emergency Room/Trauma Center Visits: 40,000

Hospital Personnel:
  Physicians: 171
  Residents: 55
  Registered Nurses: 581
  Total Staff: 1,700

# Specialties

Allergy and Dermatology, Anesthesiology, Cardiology, Colon and Rectal Surgery, Diagnostic Radiology, Emergency Medicine, Endocrinology, Gastroenterology, Gynecology, Hematology, Infectious Diseases, Internal Medicine, Nephrology, Neurology, Neurosurgery, Oncology, Ophthalmology, Orthopedic Surgery, Otolaryngology/Head and Neck Surgery, Pediatric and Adolescent Medicine, Plastic Surgery, Psychiatry and Behavioral Medicine, Pulmonary Medicine, Radiotherapy, General Surgery, Rheumatology, and Urology.

Multispecialty clinics include the Breast Cancer Clinic, the Head and Neck Tumor Clinic, the Pain Management Program, the Raynaud's Clinic, the Center for Renal Stone Disease, and the Sports Medicine Clinic.

## Well-known Specialists

Dr. John W. Braasch, surgery; specialist in biliary, liver, and pancreatic surgery.

Dr. Eugene P. Clerkin, internal medicine; specialist in endocrinology and hypertension.

Dr. F. Henry Ellis, thoracic surgery; specialist in esophageal surgery.

Dr. Charles A. Fager, neurosurgery; specialist in cranial, nerve, and spinal surgery.

Dr. John A. Libertino, urology; pioneer in renal artery surgery and laser treatment of bladder cancer.

Dr. Samuel Moschella, allergy and dermatology; specialist in skin cancer and leprosy.

Dr. F. Warren Nugent, gastroenterology; specialist in Crohn's disease.

Dr. Stanley Shapshay, otolaryngology/head and neck surgery; pioneer in using lasers to treat head and neck tumors.

Dr. Malcolm C. Veidenheimer, specialist in mucosal proctectomy for ulcerative colitis and familial polyposis, chairman of the Department of General Surgery.

Dr. Leonard Zinman, urology; specialist in reconstructive surgery of the upper and lower urinary tracts.

## Admission Policy

Anyone with a health concern can come to the Lahey Clinic for diagnosis and treatment. Appointments may be made either by the patient directly or through referral by a physician. Individuals can make appointments for themselves by calling the Appointment Office at 617-273-8000.

Appointment coordinators are specially trained to match patients with physicians based on their health-care needs and preferences. Prospective patients may also request appointments with specific physicians. Physicians referring patients can do so most easily by calling the Physician Referral Office at 617-273-8899.

A patient can be admitted as an inpatient only by a member of the Lahey Clinic medical staff. Patients are required, at the time of admission, to indicate their method of payment, which may include private insurance, Medicare, Medicaid, or welfare.

**ROOM CHARGES** (per diem)

Single-bedded: $300 (The Lahey Clinic hospital has only single-bedded or single-occupancy rooms; for billing purposes these are considered the equivalent to semiprivate rooms in other hospitals and, in reimbursement terms, are not considered "private" rooms.)

ICU: $700

**MAILING ADDRESS**
41 Mall Road
Box 541
Burlington, MA 01805

**TELEPHONE**
617-273-5100

# McLean Hospital
## BELMONT, MASSACHUSETTS

Located on a 240-acre campus in Belmont, just outside Boston, McLean Hospital has the look of a small New England college. Yet in this bucolic setting important work is carried on at this private, nonprofit psychiatric hospital affiliated with Massachusetts General Hospital (see page 154) and the Harvard Medical School. Each day it treats up to 328 people in its inpatient services and almost twice as many in its outpatient and aftercare programs.

The quality of care at McLean is a result, in part, of its staff-to-patient ratio, which is among the highest of any teaching institution. Counting only mental-health professionals engaged in direct patient care, McLean has a ratio of two clinical staff members to every patient. This does not take into account other professionals on staff who are directly involved with patients, such as teachers at the two schools for patients, clergy, research assistants, and research psychiatrists.

The third oldest psychiatric hospital in the United States and the first to open in Massachusetts, McLean was founded in 1811 as part of Massachusetts General Hospital, and it actually opened before Mass General.

Over the years the age mix of patients treated at McLean has shifted dramatically. In the early 1950s, for example, the average age of half of McLean's patients was seventy-seven. During the 1960s adolescent admissions tripled, and they have remained high ever since. While McLean does treat all ages, from one to eighty, its patients today are predominantly under age forty.

McLean meets the needs of the mentally ill through over 25 specialty programs plus several generic units, an accredited high school, and a medical clinic. Inpatient, outpatient, and community residential services are available. The Evaluative Service Unit continually monitors the effectiveness of treatment programs.

Every patient is approached with the expectation that no matter what the diagnosis and the severity of the emotional illness, he or she can be treated. Therapies range from traditional psychoanalysis to such newer techniques as behavior and family therapy, but the goal is always to return patients to their communities as quickly as possible.

The Community Residential and Treatment Services for emotionally disabled people encourage patients to function independently. The services include around-the-clock staffed programs, independent apartments, and specialty programs for adolescents and the elderly. Collectively, these services have almost 100 beds and can serve an additional 60 individuals in partial hospitalization programs. Community Residential Services have been specially designed to provide the highest level of clinical care possible at the lowest cost to the consumer. The programs include six staffed community residences, five on hospital grounds and one in Boston. There are also three cooperative apartment programs providing more independent living in Belmont. All these programs serve as transitional steps between hospital and community for some residents and as alternatives to hospitalization for others.

McLean has always educated psychiatric professionals. Today over 400 students annually train at McLean for careers in nursing, social work, psychology, psychiatry, and other human service professions. An even larger number of practicing professionals come to McLean for continuing education programs that cover subjects as diverse as neurochemistry and couples therapy. In addition, the staff at McLean frequently serve as faculty for programs offered by the American Psychiatric Association and other national professional societies. Through contractual arrangements the staff also work with people in schools, prisons, and other community settings.

When McLean first admitted patients, in 1818, the goal was to treat all the mentally ill, rich and poor alike. But overwhelming community needs proved too much to handle, so around 1840, as state hospitals opened and assumed some of the burden, McLean began concentrating on offering high-quality care to patients who could pay for treatment.

As the social status of patients changed, more commodious patient quarters resulted, as did the flat refusal of patients to engage in "manual industries," such as farm and kitchen work, which had been a traditional part of therapeutic programs. It was not until the 1960s, when insurance for psychiatric care became more widely available, that McLean patients again began reflecting a breadth of socioeconomic groups. It was then also that McLean opened its Outpatient Clinic expressly for people unable to afford private psychiatric care.

In 1983 McLean rejected a proposal from Hospital Corporation of America to purchase the hospital and turn it into a for-profit institution. In a report from the Faculty Advisory Committee to the dean of Harvard Medical School, the reasons for this opposition were clearly defined: "the operation of hospitals, and particularly teaching hospitals, should not be influenced by the motivation for profit."

At the time of the proposed purchase, many concerns were raised by the faculty regarding control over patient care, clinical research, the academicity of McLean, and even its long-term survival if linked with a for-profit chain. In discussing the report, Dean Tosteson of Harvard said he believed that stronger cooperative arrangements between for-profit companies and private universities could benefit both sectors, and that rejection of the HCA proposal did not mean it would be impossible to construct an arrangement with an investor-owned hospital/company that would be acceptable to Harvard Medical School.

The passionate debates that this proposal aroused at McLean were in sharp contrast to the faculty's ready acceptance of a unique alliance between McLean Hospital and American Medical International, Inc. (AMI), founder of the investor-owned hospital industry, in February 1986. Out of this partnership grew McLean Hospital Services, Inc., a for-profit company owned jointly by McLean Hospital and AMI. The joint venture unites the resources of this private psychiatric hospital and an international health-care organization, while respecting the autonomy of both partners and the integrity of McLean's long-standing affiliations with Massachusetts General Hospital and Harvard Medical School.

Today McLean markets high-quality psychiatric treatment programs and services in diverse settings throughout the United States. Initial efforts have focused on psychiatric services in acute-care hospitals, community residential and treatment services, and employee assistance programs.

## Specialties

Modes of treatment include individual, couples, family, group, and behavior therapy; chemotherapy, rehabilitation therapies; psychological testing; medical, pediatric, and neurological evaluation/care: and detoxification and other therapies related to chemical dependency.

Inpatient services include the following programs: the Adolescent and Family Treatment and Study Center; the Alcohol and Drug Abuse Treatment Center; the Behavior Therapy Unit; the Hall-Mercer Children's Center; the Depression Treatment Unit; Clinical Evaluation Units; Generic Units;

---

**STATISTICAL PROFILE**

Number of Beds: 328
Bed Occupancy Rate: 91%
Average Number of Patients: 293
Median Patient Stay: 42 days, adults; 77 days, children
Annual Admissions: 3,500 (more than half in outpatient clinics and
   community residences)

Hospital Personnel:
  Psychiatrists: 146
  Psychologists: 71
  Nursing Staff: 480
  Social Workers: 63
  Rehabilitation Professionals: 42
  Principal Research Investigators: 108
    Total: 680
  Regular Full-Time and Part-Time Employees: 1,426

the Neuropsychiatry Unit; the Proctor House Older Adult Service; and the Short-Term Pavilion Unit.

Outpatient services include the Adult Outpatient Clinic, the Affective Disease Program, the Hall-Mercer Children's Center Outpatient Service, the Tardive Dyskinesia Program, the Appleton Family Program, the Geriatric Outpatient Clinic, and the Appleton Outpatient Evening Clinic.

## Well-known Specialists

Dr. Ross J. Baldessarini, bipolar disorder.
Dr. Edward D. Bird, Huntington's disease.
Dr. Bruce Cohen, M.D., Ph.D., schizophrenia.
Dr. Jonathan O. Cole, depression.
Dr. John G. Gunderson, personality disorders.
Dr. Philip G. Levendusky, Ph.D., eating disorders.
Dr. Joseph F. Lipinski, bipolar disorder.
Dr. Benjamin Liptzin, geriatric psychiatry.
Dr. Nancy K. Mello, Ph.D., alcoholism.
Dr. Jack H. Mendelson, substance abuse.
Dr. Silvio Onesti, childhood disorders.
Dr. Harrison G. Pope, Jr., eating disorders.
Dr. Alan F. Schatzberg, depression.
Dr. Edward R. Shapiro, adolescent disorders.
Dr. Roger Weiss, substance abuse.
Dr. Bryan T. Woods, neuropsychiatry.

## Research

McLean ranks first among all U.S. private psychiatric hospitals in the size of its research program. In 1985 McLean received over $8.4 million in grants. (In 1980 an NIH publication cited McLean as number one among U.S. psychiatric hospitals in receipt of Public Health Services–supported research funds, and twelfth among all U.S. institutions classified as hospitals.)

Mailman Research Center, opened in 1977, is one of the world's most comprehensive facilities for basic scientific research into mental illness. Scientists at Mailman are working in close collaboration with psychiatrists carrying on clinical studies, thereby integrating physiological and psychological approaches to psychiatric research.

With over 100 principal investigators on staff, studies include basic research on brain systems, architecture, and neurochemistry and clinical and/or laboratory investigations of diseases such as Alzheimer's, anorexia nervosa and bulimia, depressive disorders, Huntington's, and schizophrenia; the effects of commonly abused drugs, such as alcohol, cocaine, and marijuana;

and the actions of antipsychotic and other psychoactive drugs. During 1985 McLean investigators published (or had in press) well over 200 research reports in national and international journals.

## Admission Policy

Generally, admissions to McLean are scheduled in advance by telephone. While a family member or prospective patient often makes the first contact and provides information on the patient's history and current condition, admissions are arranged with the recommendation of a qualified health professional—except in the hospital's drug and alcohol dependency units, where patients may refer themselves. For prospective patients not working with a health professional, the admissions staff can arrange private interviews.

Also, before admission, families are asked to call the hospital's Patient Accounts Office to discuss financial arrangements. Over 90 percent of patients here are insured for varying degrees of treatment costs. While limited in its ability to offer free care, the hospital provides about $500,000 of such care annually.

---

**ROOM CHARGES (per diem)**
Daily rates vary among programs, depending on the level of care and service provided. Continuous-care rooms with twenty-four-hour staff support average $400 per day for adults and $608 per day for children. Community residential and treatment services range between $19 and $123 per day. Apartments are available at $900 per month. Outpatient services are $34 per visit for adults and $55 per visit for children.

Current rate cards are available upon request, and some of the services may be reimbursable by third parties, including Medicare. In fact, recent figures show that 95 percent of the patients admitted to the inpatient service were covered for varying degrees of the costs involved by some form of insurance.

**MAILING ADDRESS**      **TELEPHONE**
115 Mill Street          617-855-2000
Belmont, MA 02178

---

# Massachusetts General Hospital

**BOSTON, MASSACHUSETTS**

Although the Boston metropolitan area ranks only tenth in population and twenty-seventh in per capita income in the country, most people realize that its status in health care is unquestionably at the top. Only two or three cities in the United States can approach Boston in terms of the availability of high-quality medical care. Boston offers not only a high number of physicians in relation to the population (471 per 100,000; as compared with New York's 370, Los Angeles's 243, or Houston's 207), but also three of the best-known medical schools and more than ten fine teaching hospitals (New England Deaconess, University, and Carney, for example). A measure of the quality of hospital care here was shown in a recent federal government report listing Boston City Hospital, the local municipally funded facility, as having the lowest mortality rate among Medicare patients in the entire state of Massachusetts.

With so many fine medical facilities clustered together in such a small area, it's difficult to believe that one institution could emerge as the dominant hospital of the region. But in the minds of many doctors and hospital administrators, Massachusetts General is not only Boston's most important hospital but also one of the best in the country. Mass General, as it is called, delivers primary care to hundreds of thousands of Bostonians while also serving as one of the major tertiary-care centers of New England. It is by far the largest of the Harvard-affiliated hospitals, and it is also the oldest and most influential.

Chartered in 1811 and first opened in 1821, Mass General was probably the single most important American setting for the evolution of modern medicine. The use of an anesthetic (ether) during surgery, for example, was first publicly demonstrated here in 1846; and in 1886 the first description of appendicitis and the recommendation of a surgical treatment were made here. In 1926 physicians at Mass General were instrumental in finding the causes of lead poisoning and developing a treatment for it; they also discovered a surgical cure for hyperparathyroidism, a common endocrine disorder, in 1929 and did pioneering work in nuclear medicine as early as 1937.

Following World War II, Mass General's reputation as an important research institution continued to grow, especially after one of its physicians shared the Nobel Prize in 1953 for discovering coenzyme A and describing its role in metabolism. During the 1960s two important breakthroughs—the first successful replantation of a human arm and the discovery of a way to make practical the freezing of blood—brought Mass General enormous national media attention. And Mass General's importance as a research hospital has only increased, as has its national and international influence.

**154**

Today people come to Mass General from around the world. About 1,000 patients a year are from foreign countries, and more than 5,000 are from outside Massachusetts. Many have been referred by their physicians because the medical staff at Mass General has developed an excellent reputation for diagnosing difficult cases.

Most people who travel to Mass General, however, come for one of the many specialized care services in areas such as arthritis, dermatology, diabetes, neurosurgery, thyroid disease, and recently developed laser treatments for dermatologic birth defects and for kidney stones. In addition, patients are flown into the specially designed and equipped Redstone Burn Center from around the entire Northeast. Mass General is also the leading center in New England for organ transplantation and carries out bone, heart, kidney, liver, and pancreas transplants. Cardiac surgery is a major specialty, with over 1,200 open-heart procedures performed each year. Orthopedic surgery too is a very active department, with about 410 artificial joint replacements done each year, along with arthroscopic procedures of the elbow, knee, and shoulder.

These complex medical services and the research programs are the principal reasons for Mass General's widespread fame, but to the people of Greater Boston it is the easy access to doctors in a host of fields that makes this hospital vital. In fact, the only medical specialty not practiced here is obstetrics (although there is a very active neonatal intensive care unit run by the Pediatrics Department). Ophthalmology and otolaryngology are, strictly speaking, offered at a separate hospital, the world-famous Massachusetts Ear and Eye Infirmary. This 16-story, 174-bed facility is a major teaching hospital of the Harvard Medical School. It has its own impressive research program ($15 million from NIH alone), and treats almost 150,000 patients a year, more than half on an outpatient basis. Because Mass General and Mass Eye and Ear are actually adjacent to each other, they are usually viewed as contiguous institutions.

What follows is a brief rundown of Mass General's major services, starting with the most important, cancer.

Physicians at Mass General were concerned with the treatment of cancer patients long before they opened their first so-called Tumor Clinic in 1925. Today the hospital's cancer center is the largest facility for oncological treatment and research in New England. Over 3,500 new patients come here every year, and more than 11,000 are treated annually, mainly on an outpatient basis. About 120 physicians from a variety of departments—including the special Pediatric Hematology Oncology Unit—are involved in treating patients with the most up-to-date therapies and advanced technology, including a cyclotron, one of two in the country for cancer treatment.

Mass General is also equipped with four linear accelerators, which move streams of electrons at a very high speed to produce X rays in the order of millions of electron volts. Used to focus a single high dose of radiation on a tumor, the linear accelerator is only one of several forms of radiation treatment available here. When last tabulated in 1983, the Mass General Radiation Service ranked second in the nation in the number of procedures performed (over 46,000). Standard forms of chemotherapy are also available.

Long-term rehabilitation medicine is provided at Spaulding Rehabilitation Hospital, the largest facility of its kind in the world. Spaulding's 127 physicians sustain 16 comprehensive programs to prepare patients to return to families and communities at their highest level of independence. Renowned for its ability to provide intensive rehabilitation while managing complex medical problems, Spaulding treats over 2,800 inpatients and 2,600 outpatients each year.

The Vincent Memorial Hospital specializes in the treatment of gynecologic cancer and other women's diseases. Here a group of internists, gynecologists, and psychiatric professionals have formed the Women's Health Associates, a unique primary-care and clinical research program providing comprehensive health care to women. Each new patient receives a complete physical and gynecologic exam, which includes consideration of daily habits that can undermine or support good health. In addition, Vincent offers the latest techniques for treating infertility, including a computerized pump that releases a carefully calculated amount of hormone into the bloodstreams of infertile women to help them conceive.

Former patients of Mass General are overwhelmingly positive about the treatment they received here. A large portion of the patients have been here before and chose to return—this despite the fact that many of the buildings are out of date, the rooms small and not luxurious.

Like so many other old and prestigious hospitals, Mass General is in the midst of a major rebuilding program that will result in a total replacement of facilities holding more than half the beds. Two new inpatient towers are scheduled for completion around 1991.

## Specialties

Allergy and Immunology, Anesthesiology, Cardiac Surgery, Cardiology, Dermatology, Endocrinology, Gastroenterology, Genetics, Gerontology, Gynecology, Hypertension, Infectious Diseases, Neonatology, Nephrology, Neurology, Neurosurgery, Obstetrics, Oncology and Hematology, Oral and Maxillofacial Surgery, Organ Transplantation, Orthopedic Surgery, Pathology, Pediatrics, Pediatric Surgery, Plastic and Reconstructive Surgery, Psychiatry, Pulmonary Medicine, Radiation Medicine, Rehabilitation Medicine, Replantation of Limbs, Rheumatology, Thoracic Surgery, Urology, and Vascular Surgery.

Just about every department has offices in the Ambulatory Care Center, where over 550,000 patients a year are treated in more than 70 specialized outpatient clinics. Here's a brief alphabetical listing of some of them: Adolescent Gynecology, Allergy, Arthritis/Rheumatology, the Cancer Center Unit (includes nine clinics), Cardiac Ambulatory Care, Child Psychiatry,

Cystic Fibrosis, Diabetes, Eating Disorders, Huntington's Disease, Infectious Disease (the Traveler's Advice Center), Infertility, Learning Disorders, Movement Disorders, Muscular Dystrophy, Neurovisual Disorders, Occupational Health, the Pain Group, Plastic and Reconstructive Surgery, Psychiatry (Acute and General), Radiation Medicine, Reproductive Endocrinology, Scoliosis (Adult and Child), Sleep Disorders, and the Thyroid Unit.

---

**STATISTICAL PROFILE**

Number of Beds: 1,082
Bed Occupancy Rate: 85%
Average Number of Patients: 921
Average Patient Stay: 9.2 days
Annual Admissions: 32,168
Outpatient Clinic Visits: 574,669
Emergency Room/Trauma Center Visits: 70,236

Hospital Personnel:
    Physicians: approximately 1,400
    Residents and Interns: 405
    Registered Nurses: 1,020
    Total Staff: 8,413

---

# Well-known Specialists

This list represents only a fraction of the well-known specialists practicing at Mass General.

Dr. W. Gerald Austen, cardiac surgery; introducer of the intraaortic balloon pump in 1968, chief of general surgical services.
Dr. Mortimer J. Buckley, Austen's partner in introducing the pump, chief of cardiac surgery.
Dr. William F. Crowley, specialist in infertility, chief of the Reproductive Endocrine Unit.
Dr. Roman W. DeSanctis, director of clinical cardiology.
Dr. Patricia K. Donahoe, director of pediatric surgery.
Dr. Thomas B. Fitzpatrick, dermatologist in chief.
Dr. Arlan F. Fuller, gynecology; specialist in gynecologic cancer.
Dr. Hermes C. Grillo, thoracic surgery.
Dr. William H. Harris, orthopedic surgery.
Dr. Adolph M. Hutter, cardiology.
Dr. Kurt J. Isselbacher, gastroenterology.
Dr. Henry J. Mankin, chief of orthopedic surgery.

Dr. Joseph B. Martin, chief of neurology.

Dr. Martin C. Mihm, dermatology; specialist in melanoma.

Dr. Robert G. Ojenlann, neurosurgery.

Dr. Herman D. Suit, chief of radiation medicine.

Dr. I. David Todres, director of the Neonatal and Pediatric Intensive Care units.

Dr. Earle W. Wilkins, thoracic surgery.

Dr. William C. Wood, director of the Cancer Center.

Dr. Peter M. Yurchak, cardiology.

Dr. Nicholas T. Zervas, chief of neurosurgery.

# Research

Over $60 million a year in research funds are available to physicians and scientists at Mass General, making it the single largest research hospital in the nation. A recent publication listing all the research projects being conducted here runs over 900 pages and covers just about every area of medicine and biochemistry; it includes topics in bioengineering, epidemiology, and preventive medicine as well as the standard clinical areas, especially cancer, cardiology, neurology, neurosurgery, and burns, one of the hospital's most important specialties.

The success of Mass General's research program has helped keep funding at a high level. Over the last ten years physicians and scientists here have been involved in the development of magnetic resonance imaging, in creating the first artificial skin, and in cultivating skin for patients with severe and extensive burns. Several important discoveries were made here involving HTLV-III, the AIDS virus, by a team of physician-researchers headed by virologist Martin Hirsch. Mass General continues to be in the forefront of AIDS research and has recently begun clinical trials of two promising types of drugs to halt the spread of this disease.

Less dramatic discoveries, many of which have immediate clinical value, are made seemingly every month. Recently physicians here developed a new experimental treatment for lung cancer using interleukin-2, devised a test for very early diagnosis of ectopic pregnancies, and found ways to strengthen hip replacements and to reduce serious blood clots after this kind of surgery.

Important ongoing research projects include the search to expand use of lasers in medicine (Mass General has the most extensive such program in the nation), and studies for understanding and preventing mental retardation, which take place in the Joseph Kennedy, Jr., Memorial Research Laboratories for Mental Retardation.

Some of the topics of investigation at Mass General's NIH-funded Clinical Research Center are Cushing's disease, depression, diabetes, infertility, osteoporosis, and Paget's disease. A special Center Without Walls for the study and treatment of Huntington's disease is based partly in this unit.

# Admission Policy

Although this is one of America's best-known hospitals, a place where famous people such as John Wayne, Henry Kissinger, and Yelena Bonner are treated, Mass General treats far more people whose names are not household words. Patients can be referred by their doctors to a specialist on staff, or they can inquire about doctors through a special patient referral number: 617-726-3400. Patients calling this number will most likely be directed to a doctor in the Wang Ambulatory Care Center. Of course, those needing immediate help will be treated—and if need be admitted—through the Emergency Ward or the Medical Walk-in Unit; in fact, a surprising 40 percent of all admissions enter the hospital this way.

The hospital strives to keep its doors open to people from all walks of society. In fact, in recent years Mass General has annually provided more than $20 million worth of charity and bad debt medical care.

---

**ROOM CHARGES (per diem)**
Private: $342–$457
Semiprivate: $204–$382
ICU: $583–$999

**AVERAGE COST PER PATIENT STAY:**   $7,831

**MAILING ADDRESS**     **TELEPHONE**
32 Fruit Street     617-726-2000
Boston, MA 02114

# New England Medical Center

**BOSTON, MASSACHUSETTS**

Even with all the competition in Greater Boston, New England Medical Center stands out—for many reasons. First, the medical center, the primary teaching hospital of Tufts University School of Medicine, provides excellent services that are enhanced by its numerous and varied research projects and educational programs.

One example is the Division of Clinical Decision Making, the only unit in the world that ties the principles of logical decision analysis to the care of individual patients. It is concerned with identifying strategies of patient care that minimize unnecessary tests and procedures, increase patients' participation in decisions affecting their care, and decrease the cost of medical care. The division uses computers and other related tools, and the microcomputer programs developed here are the standard for medical decision making throughout the country.

Another example is the Pratt Diagnostic Clinic. A nationally recognized specialty referral center, the clinic provides second opinions and expert diagnostic evaluations for difficult medical problems. The Pratt has helped make New England Medical Center one of the leading diagnostic centers in the country.

In terms of medical services, the New England Medical Center offers comprehensive inpatient and outpatient care for both adults and children. It provides all levels of health care—from the most basic health maintenance and primary care to the most complex, such as brain surgery, cancer treatment, heart bypass surgery, organ transplants, and stroke management.

New England Medical Center began with the establishment of the Boston Dispensary, created in 1796 by a group of Boston citizens to ensure that the poor of the city had access to health care. Over the years other institutions have become part of the medical center: The Floating Hospital for Infants and Children (1894), Pratt Diagnostic Clinic (1930), New England Center Hospital (1948), and the Rehabilitation Institute (1958).

The Floating Hospital for Infants and Children provides both inpatient and outpatient care for newborns to teenagers. Its state-of-the-art facility includes a neonatal intensive care unit, a special-care nursery, and a pediatric psychiatric unit. Among other things, the Floating Hospital is a regional and national center for diagnosis, evaluation, and treatment of children with rheumatic diseases, including juvenile rheumatoid arthritis, rheumatic fever, systemic lupus erythematosus, and spondylitis. The Pediatric Cardiac Catheterization Laboratory is one of the most advanced units in the country, providing highly complex diagnostic and treatment capabilities. The Kiwanis Pediatric Trauma Institute—which was one of the first regional trauma centers combining transportation, treatment, and rehabilitation exclusively for children—is located at the Floating Hospital. The hospital's aggressive protocol for the treatment of pediatric leukemia and its multidisciplinary approach have also distinguished it as a cancer center.

The Rehabilitation Institute at the medical center maintains a position of leadership in patient care, education, and research. Patients come to the institute from New England and beyond. In addition to offering services to disabled adults, the institute is a national leader in pediatric rehabilitation and a source of primary and consultative care for physically disabled children. It provides care for a wide range of disabilities, including cancer, cardiopulmonary disorders, progressive degenerative diseases, limb deficiencies, musculoskeletal diseases such as arthritis, neuromuscular diseases such as stroke and spinal cord injuries, chronic pain and other behavioral disorders, and peripheral vascular diseases. The Lung Tumor Evaluation Center specializes in the diagnosis and treatment of lung tumors and other abnormalities of the chest.

The Stroke Service is a multidisciplinary center that provides extensive inpatient and outpatient diagnostic evaluation, management, and treatment for adults with cerebrovascular diseases. The service works in close collaboration with the medical center's surgical and rehabilitative programs.

The Breast Health Center provides comprehensive diagnostic, therapeutic, and educational services for women with benign and malignant breast problems. A team of specialists from obstetrics/gynecology, oncology, pathology, plastic surgery, radiology, therapeutic radiology, and surgery provides multidisciplinary expertise in one location. Test results, diagnosis, and assessment of treatment options are usually available during the initial visit.

The New England Medical Center is a founding member of both the Boston Center for Liver Transplantation and the Boston Center for Heart Transplantation. The medical center was the first Boston hospital to perform both heart and liver transplants.

The Cardiovascular Center offers a full complement of diagnostic facilities for the evaluation and treatment of cardiac disease. Available technologies include cardiac catheterization, clinical electrophysiology, Doppler echocardiography, stress testing, and more.

The Gastroenterology Department provides inclusive diagnostic and treatment services for adults and children with problems such as liver disease and peptic ulcers.

The Fertility Center is a full-service clinical program for couples who have been unable to conceive; available therapies include artificial insemination, in vitro fertilization, laser surgery, microsurgery, and ovulation induction.

The Department of Psychiatry offers comprehensive evaluation, consultation, and treatment for adults, adolescents, and children with disturbances and disorders related to behavior, emotions, learning, and thought processes. Specialized expertise is available in anxiety, depression, eating and weight problems, intractable pain, clinical psychopharmacology, psychosis, psycho-therapy, and sleeping and memory disorders.

Among the medical center's ambulatory care services are the Day Surgery Center, the Frances Stern Nutrition Center, and the Sports Medicine Center.

## Specialties

New England Medical Center's areas of expertise include Cardiology, Cardiothoracic Surgery, Gastroenterology, Gynecologic Oncology, Infectious Diseases, Neonatology, Neurology, Neurosurgery, Oncology, Pediatric Rheumatology, Psychiatry, and Vascular Surgery.

Clinic services cover a full range of medical problems, such as allergy, arthritis, bed-wetting, cerebral palsy, cleft palate, cystic fibrosis, diabetes, dizziness, glaucoma, headache, hypertension, lupus, pain, retina disorders, scoliosis, stroke, Tourette's syndrome, and tropical diseases.

---

**STATISTICAL PROFILE**

Number of Beds: 469
Bed Occupancy Rate: 90%
Average Patient Stay: 9.3 days
Annual Admissions: 15,000
Outpatient Clinic Visits: 260,000
Emergency Room/Trauma Center Visits: 26,000

Hospital Personnel:
    Physicians: 350
    Residents: 400
    Registered Nurses: 725
    Total Staff: 4,000

---

## Well-known Specialists

Dr. Louis Caplan, specialist in the central nervous system, particularly strokes, neurologist in chief.
Dr. Weiner Chasin, otolaryngology.
Dr. Richard Cleveland, cardiothoracic surgery; pioneer in using lasers in open-heart surgery.
Dr. Jane Desforges, hematology.
Dr. Sidney Gellis, pediatrics; specialist in genetic counseling.
Dr. Herbert Levine, cardiology.

Dr. Carol Nadelson, psychiatry; first woman president of the American Psychiatric Association.

Dr. David Parkinson, oncology; researcher on interleukin-2 in the treatment of some forms of cancer.

Dr. Jane Green Schaller, pediatrics; specialist in pediatric rheumatology.

Dr. Bernard Schwartz, ophthalmology.

Dr. Robert Schwartz, hematology/oncology.

Dr. R. Michael Scott, pediatric neurosurgery.

Dr. Sheldon Wolff, specialist in fever and infectious diseases, physician in chief, cochairman of the national task force on AIDS organized by the National Academy of Sciences and the Institute of Medicine.


# Research

Several major research projects are currently under way at New England Medical Center, one of six institutions designated by the NIH to begin treating cancer patients with interleukin-2. Researchers at the National Cancer Institute, where the therapy was developed, report that the treatment successfully activated the immune system to kill cancer cells in ten out of 25 patients with advanced forms of cancer. Although the results are only preliminary, and the treatment is highly toxic and costly, it is shrinking tumors and suppressing cancer activity in some patients with renal cancer, melanomas, and colorectal cancers, none of which responds well to chemotherapy.

A new treatment for patients with malignant glioma, a form of deep-seated brain tumor that is virtually always fatal, is being developed by a team of medical center clinicians. Treatment involves delivering radioactive iridium-192 through catheters directly to the tumor. A computer program has been developed to help determine the proper amount of radioactive seeds, based on the volume of the remaining tumor.

Another research team is perfecting techniques to remove plaque from coronary arteries. Doctors are developing a fiber-optic system that will allow surgeons to "vaporize" blockages with lasers threaded through the arteries.

The NIH awarded the medical center, in conjunction with St. Margaret's and Brigham and Women's hospitals, a $1.7-million grant for a clinical study on treating premature infants with respiratory problems with high-frequency ventilation. These infants are placed on mechanical ventilators set at very high breathing rates. High-frequency ventilation requires less air pressure and air volume, so there is less risk of lung damage.

These studies and new techniques are only a fraction of the broad spectrum of research conducted in both the laboratory and clinical settings of the medical center. Many other studies are done through the federally funded Clinical Research Center here.

## Admission Policy

Patients can be admitted to the New England Medical Center through the clinics or emergency room, referred by their physician, or self-referred.

The medical center accepts all major forms of insurance. There is no financial requirement to be admitted to the hospital, and financial assistance is available. Last year the medical center provided $9 million of "uncompensated" care to indigent patients.

---

**ROOM CHARGES (per diem)**
Private: $407
Semiprivate: $373
ICU: $995

**AVERAGE COST PER PATIENT STAY:**   $1,009 per day for inpatients; $182 per visit for outpatients (includes ancillary lab charges)

**MAILING ADDRESS**      **TELEPHONE**
750 Washington Street    617-956-5000
Boston, MA 02111

---

# Harper-Grace Hospitals

## DETROIT, MICHIGAN

The largest health-care center in Michigan is The Detroit Medical Center, and predominant in the center is Harper-Grace Hospitals, which includes Harper Hospital, a 900-plus-bed referral hospital; and Grace Hospital, a 400-bed community-oriented facility.

The Detroit Medical Center hospitals are the only ones in Detroit that have full university affiliations, and give research a primary concern. Heads of most medical departments at the hospitals are also chairmen of departments at the School of Medicine of Wayne State University.

The hospitals are a central part of the Meyer L. Prentis Comprehensive Cancer Center of metropolitan Detroit, one of 20 such NIH-funded centers in the country. To expand and improve Harper's cancer radiation facilities, the world's first superconducting cyclotron built for medical purposes is to be installed in 1987. It will be especially useful in combating cancers of the bladder, bones, cervix, head and neck (especially salivary glands), prostate, and soft tissue. Opening at about the same time will be a magnetic resonance imaging center. It will yield more exact and accurate diagnosis of heart defects, the extent of cancerous growths, nerve degeneration from multiple sclerosis, brain damage from strokes, spinal disc problems, and a host of other illnesses. It will be valuable for examining pregnant women because it uses no ionizing radiation.

The diagnosis and treatment of heart disease is another of Harper's major specialties. Harper has been a leader in heart surgery since 1952, when its doctors invented the world's first heart machine, a device used to keep blood circulating during open-heart surgery. About 800 open-heart operations are performed at Harper annually, more than in any other hospital in Michigan. A recent study of the outcome of heart surgery showed that Harper is one of the safest specialty centers in the country to have such operations. Harper's heart specialists, like its cancer specialists, participate in research on newly developed medicines and techniques.

Another major specialty at Harper is the treatment of vision disorders at the Kresge Eye Institute, which treats more than 40,000 visually impaired people a year. Eye specialists perform about 12 operations and many more diagnostic procedures a day. It was at Harper that the first radial keratotomy operation to correct nearsightedness was performed in the United States. Among current developments the institute is perfecting a test for the very early detection of glaucoma. Operations to remove cataracts and implant artificial lenses are now routine, as is a rare operation to correct glaucoma, remove cataracts, and implant artificial lenses all in one procedure. The institute has its own instrument laboratory, a facility that designs and makes special implements for research projects.

Harper is also noted for other specialties, including the reattachment of fingers, hands, arms, and legs that have been cut off in accidents, and the care of victims of head injuries.

Grace Hospital, while basically geared to serving its community, has also developed some outstanding programs. It is the national headquarters for a group known as ROMP (Recovery of Male Potency). The organization uses a program of instruction coupled with surgery that was pioneered at Grace and has been so successful that chapters have been launched in other cities.

A Grace Hospital doctor has pioneered the use of a laser to reverse vasectomies. This procedure is faster, less expensive, and easier on the patient than the usual surgical operation. Several of the men who have undergone it have already become fathers.

Grace Hospital has one of Detroit's leading obstetric services, providing a variety of delivery methods, ranging from conventional childbirth followed by several days of hospitalization to the newer techniques using a family birthing unit and eliminating any overnight hospital stay. For babies born with medical problems the hospital has a neonatal intensive care unit.

There are few medical problems for which Grace and Harper cannot provide expert help. In addition to those already discussed, there are spe-

## STATISTICAL PROFILE

|  | Harper Hospital | Grace Hospital |
|---|---|---|
| Number of Beds: | 917 licensed; 737 active | 402 licensed |
| Bed Occupancy Rate: | 80% | 80% |
| Average Number of Patients: | 720 | 320 |
| Average Patient Stay: | 10.7 days | 6.6 days |
| Annual Admissions: | 22,000 | 13,000 |
| Births: | 0 | 2,500 |
| Outpatient Clinic Visits: | 91,000 | 38,000 |
| Emergency Room/ Trauma Center Visits: | 16,000 | 19,000 |
| | | |
| Hospital Personnel: | | |
| Physicians: | 1,200 (same staff for both hospitals) | |
| Residents: | 145 | 35 |
| Total Staff: | 3,300 | 1,400 |

cialized programs for the treatment of anorexia, breast cancer, deformities, diabetes, dizziness and loss of equilibrium, drug and alcohol addiction, high blood pressure, chronic pain, psychiatric problems, sports injuries, strokes, and other illnesses.

Grace is also developing a specialized service for the assessment and treatment of physical and mental illnesses afflicting the elderly.

## Specialties

Anesthesiology, Cardiovascular Disease, Dermatology, Endocrinology and Metabolism, Family Practice, Gastroenterology, General Surgery, Hand Surgery, Hematology, Infectious Diseases, Internal Medicine, Nephrology, Neurology, Neurosurgery, Obstetrics and Gynecology, Oncology, Ophthalmology, Orthopedic Surgery, Otolaryngology, Pathology, Plastic Surgery, Psychiatry, Pulmonary Disease, Radiology, Rheumatology, Thoracic and Cardiovascular Surgery, and Urology.

## Well-known Specialists

Dr. Lawrence H. Baker, chief of oncology.
Dr. Ramon Berguer, chief of vascular surgery.
Dr. Lawrence R. Crane, researcher in AIDS, chief of infectious diseases.
Dr. George Grunberger, diabetes.
Dr. Robert S. Jampel, chief of ophthalmology.
Dr. George M. Kazzi, vice chief of obstetrics and gynecology.
Dr. Robert P. Lisak, researcher and clinician in neuromuscular disease, chief of neurology.
Dr. Elliot D. Luby, chief of psychiatry.
Dr. Gordon Luk, chief of gastroenterology.
Dr. William E. Powers, chief of radiation therapy.
Dr. Vainutis K. Vaitkevicius, cancer researcher and clinician, chief of medicine.
Dr. Joshua Wynne, chief of cardiology.

## Admission Policy

Patients are admitted to Harper or Grace by their own physicians or through an emergency room. Patients who have no doctor or want a specialist can call the hospital-operated doctors' appointment desk service at 313-745-9626. The service will recommend several specialists and, if desired, arrange the initial appointment.

Through The Detroit Medical Center, patients can be transported to the hospitals via helicopter. The helicopter, Sky Team, carries a flight physician and nurse and serves a wide area of Michigan, Ohio, and Indiana. Arrangements for transportation can be made by calling 800-362-1717.

The hospitals accept most insurance coverages, and arrangements are made for people who lack coverage. In 1985 the hospitals provided about $12.5 million of free care.

---

## HARPER

**ROOM CHARGES (per diem)**
Private: $412
Semiprivate: $400
ICU: $1,120

**AVERAGE COST PER PATIENT STAY:**   $10,336

| **MAILING ADDRESS** | **TELEPHONE** |
|---|---|
| 3990 John R Street | 313-745-8040 |
| Detroit, MI 48201 | |

## GRACE

**ROOM CHARGES (per diem)**
Private: $393
Semiprivate: $383
Ward: $377
ICU: $985

**AVERAGE COST PER PATIENT STAY:**   $5,710

| **MAILING ADDRESS** | **TELEPHONE** |
|---|---|
| 18700 Meyers Road | 313-966-3135 |
| Detroit, MI 48235 | |

# Henry Ford Hospital

## DETROIT, MICHIGAN

For over seventy years Henry Ford Hospital (HFH) has been as vitally important to the people of Detroit as the motor company bearing the same name. The first Henry Ford founded this hospital at just about the time he shocked the young automobile industry by offering workers $5 a day—twice the going rate—to assemble his Model Ts. When the 48-bed hospital opened in 1915, it became a symbol of Ford's commitment to the people who were building a powerful industry and a great city.

In recent years urban decay, racial problems, and a rapidly shifting global economy have all conspired to victimize the city of Detroit and to humble the automobile industry. For the 4 million people who live and work in the Detroit metropolitan area today, however, there are unmistakable signs of hope for the future; many of them, like HFH, are still linked to the days of past glory.

Today HFH is a 940-bed specialty referral center and teaching hospital where over 500 doctors pool their talents in a group practice similar to those of the Mayo and Cleveland clinics. There are now eight buildings on the Detroit campus, including a regional trauma center and an ambulatory care center, as well as research and educational facilities. Patients come from 30 states and even from overseas to obtain sophisticated medical care in over 40 specialties. Almost every piece of modern medical technology can be found here, including the most up-to-date magnetic resonance imaging equipment, lasers for various types of surgery and treatments (including a newly developed one for early diagnosis and treatment of lung cancer), and the lithotriptor for destroying kidney stones.

Although HFH has been transformed from one small facility to a nationally recognized health-care system, it remains an essential resource for the people of Detroit and its suburbs. Over 5,000 physicians throughout southeast Michigan use HFH as a referral center for their most critically ill patients. Each year more than 35,000 patients are admitted to the hospital and 1.6 million are seen in the clinic here and in 14 outpatient centers the hospital has set up in areas surrounding the city. Opened in the early and mid-1970s, these medical centers are staffed with HFH specialists who have access to many of the same testing facilities as the main hospital; a mobile CAT scan, ambulatory surgery, and twenty-four-hour emergency care are offered at the centers in Dearborn, West Bloomfield, and Sterling Heights. The other centers are located in Ann Arbor, Canton, Plymouth, Rochester, Royal Oak, St. Clair Shores, Southfield, Sterling Heights (two sites), Taylor, Troy, and Warren.

The hospital runs a health education program and provides community training in cardiopulmonary resuscitation. It is a major educational resource for the allied health professions, offering 25 programs to over 450 students. A school of nursing, a graduate program for residents in other area hospitals, and a continuing education program enrolling 2,000 doctors a year are all indicative of HFH's crucial role in keeping Detroit's medical population well trained and well informed.

While HFH is large, and some people complain about the inconveniences sheer size can cause, patient responses to surveys about their care are, on the whole, positive. One important reason for this is the presence of 1,000 registered nurses, an extraordinary number in a hospital with fewer than 1,000 beds. Still, we would be less than candid if we didn't convey our impression that the people who run the hospital are not overly concerned about negative comments from patients. They are much more interested in discussing the medical services offered. Even the following brief description will tell you why.

The Bone and Joint Specialty Center is the only such center in Michigan and offers treatment for conditions such as arthritis, bone cancer, osteoporosis, and scoliosis. The Bone and Mineral Division is one of ten in the United States where histological structure of the bone is studied. More than 1,000 new patients with metabolic diseases pertaining to the skeletal system, kidney stones, and parathyroid glands are seen annually at this regional referral center.

The hospital also serves as a regional center for the diagnosis and treatment of kidney disease and is one of the largest hemodialysis centers in Michigan. In addition, it is one of the state's major kidney transplant facilities; in 1986, 569 kidney transplants were performed.

The neurology department's noninvasive cerebral blood flow system, one of only about 50 in the United States, is used to study illnesses such as hydrocephalus, epilepsy, migraine, and stroke that involve the rate of blood flow to the brain. Specialists here in neurosurgery are well recognized for innovations in the development of brain mapping, microneurosurgical techniques, and advances in surgical treatment of disorders of the brain and spinal cord.

The hospital has a history in cardiovascular medicine and surgery. The heart transplant team, under the direction of Dr. Donald J. Magilligan, has an almost unparalleled success rate of 96.7 percent, compared with the national one-year survival rate of 80 percent. Heart surgeons here are pioneering the use of ultrafiltration during open-heart surgery to remove excess body fluid. Current offerings include angioplasty and balloon valvuloplasty as alternatives to open-heart surgery for some patients, heart transplants, electrophysiology, and implantable defibrillators for diagnosis and treatment of arrhythmias. In vascular surgery HFH is recognized for work in replacing diseased arteries with prostheses.

The oncology department is a coordinated, cooperative effort by more than 30 specialists in a number of fields. Research projects include cloning of human tumors, immunization of tumor patients with healthy human-donor tissue, development of monoclonal antibodies to fight cancer, new drug development, and the study of heredity's role in cancer.

Orthopedics and Sports Medicine is staffed by surgeons with extensive training in subspecialties including pediatric orthopedics. The hospital's Center for Athletic Medicine, which addresses the health needs of competitive and recreational athletes, is one of only a few such comprehensive diagnostic, treatment, and preventive centers to be housed within a hospital complex.

Other special programs at HFH include the Chemical/Alcohol Dependency Program, a planned hospice program for the terminally ill, and a future transplantation center to include heart-lung, liver, and pancreas transplants.

## Specialties

Allergy, Anesthesiology, Chemical/Alcohol Dependency, Dermatology, Diagnostic Radiology, Emergency Medicine, Endocrinology, Geriatrics, Gynecology/Obstetrics, Infectious Diseases, Internal Medicine, Neurological Surgery, Neurology, Ophthalmology, Otolaryngology, Pediatrics, Psychiatry, Pulmonary Medicine, Rheumatology, Surgery, Therapeutic Radiology, and Urology.

Specialty "centers of excellence" include bone and mineral disease, cardiovascular medicine and cardiac surgery, nephrology, neurosurgery and neurology, oncology, orthopedics and sports medicine, and sleep disorders,

---

**STATISTICAL PROFILE**

Number of Beds: 940
Bed Occupancy Rate: 87.2%
Average Number of Patients: 803
Average Patient Stay: 8.2 days
Annual Admissions: 35,055
Births: 2,356
Outpatient Clinic Visits: 1,649,473 (includes all 14 outpatient
   centers)
Emergency Room/Trauma Center Visits: 180,059

Hospital Personnel:
   Physicians: 550
   Residents: 434
   Registered Nurses: 1,000
   Total Staff: 6,500

including sleep apnea. In addition, HFH offers special programs such as those for genetic counseling, handicapped children, kidney stones, lung cancer, and other areas benefiting from the multispecialty approach to care.

## Well-known Specialists

Dr. James Ausman, one of the few surgeons in the world who performs a back-of-the-brain "bypass" for stroke victims, a pioneer in microsurgical procedures on the brain and spinal cord, chairman of neurosurgery.

Dr. Calvin B. Ernst, specialist in vascular malformation, vascular prosthesis, and visceral ischemia, division head of vascular surgery.

Dr. Sidney Goldstein, specialist in heart disease research, codirector of the Henry Ford Heart and Vascular Institute.

Dr. Michael Kleerekoper, specialist in the treatment of osteoporosis, head of the Bone and Mineral Division.

Dr. Donald J. Magilligan, specialist in heart bypass surgery, cardiac valve replacement, and ultrafiltration techniques, codirector of the Henry Ford Heart and Vascular Institute.

Dr. Thomas Roth, specialist in sleep disorders, including jet lag, narcolepsy, and sleep apnea.

Dr. K. M. A. Welch, specialist in stroke and migraine, chairman of neurology.

Dr. Fred Whitehouse, specialist in the diagnosis and treatment of metabolic disorders, including diabetes.

## Research

More than 200 basic and clinical research projects, with $10 million annual funding, are under way at HFH. Major research areas include blood clotting, bone loss, cancer, genetics, heart disease, hypertension, sleep disorders, and stroke.

The NIH has designated the hospital's Department of Neurology as one of 12 Stroke Centers in the country and has awarded it a three-year grant of more than $2 million. The funds will support research into the causes and treatment of stroke.

In 1980 HFH was selected as one of only three medical centers nationwide to test Eli Lilly and Co.'s genetically engineered "human" insulin for diabetics. It was thus one of the first facilities to offer the approved product to patients who are allergic to animal insulin.

One of the Bone Division's major clinical studies, supported by a million-dollar, five-year grant from the NIH, is investigating postmenopausal women who have osteoporosis. Only HFH and the Mayo Clinic have received federal grants to study the safety and effectiveness of sodium fluoride in preventing further fractures in patients with the disease.

Sleep research at HFH's Sleep Research and Disorders Center has resulted in findings involving jet lag and sleep-inducing medication. The center was one of the first in the United States accredited by the Association of Sleep Disorders Centers.

## Admission Policy

Most appointments can be made directly by calling the nearest HFH facility and asking for the appointment desk of the specialty clinic desired. If the specialty is not available at the nearest HFH center, patients are given information about the closest site where it is available.

Callers will be asked for brief information, including their HFH medical record number. Anyone ever seen at an HFH facility has a permanent medical record number, which gives physicians at all HFH locations access to the patient's complete medical history.

Family physicians can also make referrals to HFH. They will then be kept informed of their patients' status and care at HFH. Physicians may call the Referring Physician Offices at Consult Line: 800-662-8242 (Michigan) or 800-521-7946 (out of state); calls are accepted twenty-four hours a day.

The hospital contributes more than $10 million per year in uncompensated health care for the indigent, the poor, and those without adequate health insurance.

---

**ROOM CHARGES (per diem)**
Private: $400–$420
Semiprivate: $380–$390
ICU: $1,075 (average)

| **MAILING ADDRESS** | **TELEPHONE** |
|---|---|
| 2799 West Grand Boulevard | 313-876-2600 |
| Detroit, MI 48202 | |

# University of Michigan Medical Center

**ANN ARBOR, MICHIGAN**

The University of Michigan (UM) Medical Center is not alone in issuing statements in its annual report pledging to "renew and improve upon the humanness with which we provide health care." But this is one hospital that translated its rhetorical commitment into action. Nowhere is this more apparent than in the construction of a new building complex that opened in February 1986. Before ground was even broken, the UM Medical Center conducted a patient-and-visitor survey of over 3,000 individuals on everything from color preferences to the advantages of wall-mounted televisions versus arm modules connected to the bed. (Results of this survey are now being requested and copied by hospitals around the country.)

The brand-new patient rooms at the UM Medical Center were designed and built in accordance with the findings from this extensive survey. For example, windows in all rooms were lowered to make it easier for bedridden patients to see outside. Bathrooms with showers are in every patient room, and there is a nurse call button in every shower stall. Every room also has a bulletin board so that patients can display cards and personal mementos. These details may seem small, but in many ways they reflect the kind of personal attention that exemplifies the special care patients can expect to receive here, both in its rooms and, more importantly, in its high-quality health care.

The UM Medical Center is a comprehensive treatment, research, and education center providing health-care services to over 500,000 people a year in 112 outpatient clinics. The medical center offers a full range of medical and surgical services as well as diagnostic and treatment facilities, laboratories, and pharmacies.

Many of the services combine the most up-to-date equipment with academic achievement. For example, the latest techniques for detecting and treating diseases of the skin can be found here, in one of the nation's oldest academic dermatology departments. Laser surgery for warts and other skin abnormalities, high-intensity ultraviolet light therapy for psoriasis, microsurgery for skin cancer (including Mohs surgery), and promising new drugs for hair regeneration are some of the treatment methods being practiced and refined here.

The UM Medical Center is one of the leading transplant centers in the United States. Specialty services include a transplant team performing heart, kidney, liver, and pancreas transplants. Bone marrow, heart-lung, and an artificial heart program are anticipated. Accompanying the transplant program is the nation's first Transplant Policy Center to study and collect information on how organ transplants affect individuals, their families, and society.

The departments of neurology, neurosurgery, and psychiatry offer among the best programs in the state. The Department of Neurology provides diagnostic and therapeutic services for patients with cancer affecting the nervous system, movement disorders, neuromuscular diseases, and seizure disorders and dementia, and also has many research projects under way in these areas.

The Section of Neurosurgery has recently established a new program in surgical management of pain and movement disorders, the only one in the state. At the hospital and in satellite clinics, chronic pain management is treated through a combination of exercise, medication regimens, nerve blocks, and nerve stimulations.

The Department of Psychiatry offers programs in anxiety disorders, grief survival, and substance abuse; it also has programs for children with borderline personality disorders. The Adolescent Psychiatry Service focuses on depression, eating disorders, personality disorders, and suicide.

Approximately 450 newborns were treated at Holden Perinatal Hospital last year; 315 of them were premature. Holden provides care for newborns who need intensive care or surgery or who have a life-threatening disease. Pediatrics is another well-known specialty of the UM Medical Center, which treats over 6,000 children a year as inpatients. Pediatric specialties include birth defects, cardiology, cystic fibrosis, endocrinology, hematology/oncology, surgery, and many others.

The UM Medical Center is one of the world's leading centers for the study of rheumatic diseases and diabetes. In addition, the medical center has been a pioneer in nuclear medicine and in the intraoperative use of ultrasound in neurosurgery, the use of angioplasty during emergency treatment of heart attacks, and the use of TPA (tissue plasminogen activator), a drug that dissolves blood clots and helps keep heart attacks from damaging the heart.

The Spinal Cord Injury Center here is designated by the National Institute for Handicapped Research. It provides care from the accident site through hospitalization, rehabilitation, and follow-up.

Among other services available are the Nurse-Midwifery Program for both obstetrics and well-woman care, the Breast Care Center and the Breast Cancer Detection Center, the Sleep Disorders Center, an in vitro fertilization program, a comprehensive hearing center, and the Osteoporosis Test Center. MedSport is a center for the treatment of sports injuries and the prevention of injuries and disease through proper training and life-style habits. Treatment for melanoma patients is conducted at the newly established Multidisciplinary Melanoma Clinic. Emergency services include a full trauma center support, a replantation and microvascular reconstruction team on twenty-four-hour call, a nationally recognized burn unit, and the Survival Flight helicopter and emergency jet service.

Patients at the UM Medical Center not only receive counseling but have access to dozens of educational books and films. For example, The Pediatric Burn Coloring Book helps children and parents get through the trauma of severe burns. A videotape helps teenagers with curvature of the spine understand their treatment and adjust to being in a cast for a year. A UM Medical Center videotape shows patients how to exercise while bedridden in the hospital or at home. Patient education programs are conducted in the hospital, and home-care programs, such as the Breast Cancer Support Group, are offered through ambulatory services. Special programs also help educate diabetics.

The medical center comprises the UM Hospitals and the UM Medical School. The hospitals include University Hospital (adult, acute care); Ambulatory Care Services, including the A. Alfred Tubman Health Care Center; C. S. Mott Children's Hospital; Women's Hospital; Holden Perinatal Hospital; Adult Psychiatric Hospital; Child and Adolescent Psychiatric Hospital; W. K. Kellogg Eye Center; and Turner Geriatric Services.

---

**STATISTICAL PROFILE (all UM hospitals)**

Number of Beds: 888
Bed Occupancy Rate: 82%
Average Number of Patients: 727
Average Patient Stay: 8.8 days
Annual Admissions: 30,106
Births: 1,657
Outpatient Clinic Visits: 430,906
Emergency Room/Trauma Center Visits: 33,378

Hospital Personnel:
  Physicians: 765
  Residents: 687
  Total Staff: 5,231

---

## Specialties

Anesthesiology, Burns, Cardiology, Clinical Research, Critical Care Medicine, Dentistry, Dermatology, Endocrinology and Metabolism, Emergency Services, Gastroenterology, General Medicine, Geriatrics, Gynecology, Hematology, Infectious Diseases, Internal Medicine, Neonatology, Nephrology, Neurology, Neurosurgery, Nuclear Medicine, Obstetrics, Ophthalmology, Orthopedics, Otorhinolaryngology, Pathology, Pediatrics, Physical Medicine and Rehabilitation, Physical Therapy, Plastic Surgery, Psychiatry,

Pulmonary Medicine, Radiation Therapy, Radiology, Rheumatology, Surgery, Thoracic Surgery, and Urology.

Specialty clinics include Allergy, Ambulatory Care Services, Asthma, Cardiac Rehabilitation, Cleft Palate, Hyperlipidemia, Hypertension, Immunization, Nutrition, Occupational Therapy, Osteoporosis Testing, Pain Management, Retina Service, Thyroid, and many others.

## Well-known Specialists

Dr. Kenneth L. Casey, neurology; specialist in pain management.

Dr. Luis Diaz, dermatology; specialist in skin immunology disorders.

Dr. Preston V. Dilts, Jr., gynecology and obstetrics; specialist in maternal-fetal medicine.

Dr. Kenneth Foon, hematology/oncology; specialist in using interferon to treat hairy cell leukemia.

Dr. E. Richard Harrell, Jr., dermatology; specialist in fungal infections.

Dr. Alan Lichter, radiation therapy.

Dr. Roger F. Meyer, ophthalmology; specialist in the cornea.

Dr. George W. Morley, specialist in gynecologic cancer.

Dr. Mark Orringer, thoracic surgery; specialist in esophageal surgery.

Dr. Eric Topol, cardiology.

## Research

More than $50 million supports research at UM Medical Center, which ranks sixteenth in NIH funding. An NIH-supported Clinical Research Center is located in University Hospital. And a unit of the Howard Hughes Medical Research Institute has been established here with a core group in molecular genetics.

About 15 percent of the clinical activity of the medical center is in oncology. The UM Cancer Center has more than 200 scientists conducting research funded by more than $18 million.

The medical center is one of the world's leading testing centers for antihypertension drugs and the study of rheumatic diseases. It also established one of the first research and teaching centers for diabetes.

The Department of Psychiatry's Diagnostic Research Unit has developed a number of protocols investigating the neurobiology of childhood disorders such as autism and depression and children at risk of alcoholism.

In the Section of Pediatric Surgery, research activities focus on parenteral nutrition, body fluid compartment changes during total parenteral nutrition, and metabolic changes in postoperative newborns.

The Section of Neurosurgery focuses on cerebrovascular diseases, cerebral ischemia, and the edema process. These investigations are particularly relevant to stroke patients and those experiencing progressive neurological deficits after arterial occlusion.

The Department of Neurology conducts studies of brain tumors, dementia, Huntington's disease, and stroke, among many others.

The Clinical Research Center received funding for studies of childhood obesity and zinc metabolism, and two studies of treatments for kidney cancers are funded by the National Cancer Institute.

The Department of Dermatology is in the forefront of research into the mechanisms and treatment of psoriasis and has developed a new biopsy technique for the diagnosis and treatment of hair loss. In addition, a quick and inexpensive test for herpes simplex was recently proven effective by UM dermatologists.

## Admission Policy

Patients can usually be admitted to the UM Medical Center without a doctor's referral, through the emergency room or a clinic. Appointments for clinic services should be made through the outpatient service, or the patient can come to the Pediatric or Adult Walk-in Service or Emergency Department.

There is no financial requirement for emergent, life- or limb-threatening cases.

---

**ROOM CHARGES (per diem)**
Private: $492
Semiprivate: $487
ICU: $1,020–$1,670

**AVERAGE COST PER PATIENT STAY:**   $7,303

**MAILING ADDRESS**                  **TELEPHONE**
1500 East Medical Center Drive       313-936-4000
Ann Arbor, MI 48109

---

# The Mayo Clinic and Hospitals
## ROCHESTER, MINNESOTA

The Mayo Clinic is one of the few medical institutions in the United States whose status can legitimately be called legendary.

So widespread is the fame of the Mayo Clinic that every year some 280,000 people come here for evaluation and treatment; 60,000 of them travel over 500 miles to do so. They come from every state and from dozens of foreign countries. According to a recent survey by the clinic, 85 percent of the patients interviewed said they were "extremely or very satisfied" with their treatment, and 92 percent said they would return to Mayo if they needed medical attention.

Begun in the late 1880s as the family practice of Dr. William Worall Mayo and his two physician sons, the Mayo Clinic evolved into the first so-called group practice, whereby doctors pool their knowledge and skills in treating all kinds of illness. By the turn of the century, the medical achievements (especially in surgery) of the Mayos and their growing number of associates had created a reputation for the Mayo Clinic that spread far beyond the surrounding area. In 1915 the success of the clinic was further demonstrated when the Mayo family donated $1.5 million to found the now world-famous Mayo Graduate School of Medicine.

Mayo's reputation for excellence continued to grow in the decades that followed. Well-known statesmen, socialites, athletes, and movie stars came here with the hope of finding treatment for ailments other doctors proclaimed incurable. A few novels and movies in the 1940s and 1950s helped popularize the notion that Mayo doctors had answers that others didn't. Then again, those hopes, both the real and the fictional, were not without foundation. In 1922, for example, doctors at Mayo first used iodine to treat goiters successfully; in 1933 the first blood bank was established here, and just after World War II two Mayo doctors discovered the drug cortisone and won the Nobel Prize.

Today more than 800 physicians and scientists are continuing the Mayo tradition. The core of the Mayo approach is still group practice. Most cases are studied by several specialists who review the patient's records and tests with the primary physician and jointly decide on diagnosis and treatment.

In almost every specialization the clinic staff has achieved a high degree of recognition. Mayo is, for example, the federally designated Comprehensive Cancer Center for this region. Every year an average of 27,000 cancer patients come here for treatment; about 6,000 are new patients, making Mayo the largest cancer practice for new patients in the country. More than 100 physicians from throughout the clinic are involved in treatment of and research in cancers including colorectal, gastroenterological, neurological,

**179**

and pulmonary. There are also separate pediatric and rehabilitation oncology units. In addition to the standard therapeutic options, patients can participate in an extensive clinical trials program in therapies still in the experimental stage.

The Mayo Clinic is also a major center for kidney and liver transplantation. Over 1,000 kidney transplants have been performed here since the program began in 1963, and over 80 percent have been successful. Liver transplantation was begun here only in 1985, but Mayo is already considered one of the leading places for this difficult operation. Under the leadership of Dr. Ruud Krom, whom the clinic recruited from the Netherlands, more than 75 transplants have taken place with a one-year success rate of 85 percent.

Other kinds of transplantation are also available at Mayo. Cornea transplants have been performed here since 1950, and today about 100 a year are done with a success rate approaching 95 percent. Bone marrow transplantation, on the other hand, was only started in 1982; as of March 1986, 50 percent of the transplants have been successful. Finally, while bone grafts from bone banks have been done for many years, only recently have doctors been using long bones from donors to replace bones destroyed by tumors (15 such operations were done here in 1985).

As the list of medical specialties available here makes clear, there is very little the Mayo Clinic and its two hospitals don't offer. And what they do here, they do on a scale significantly larger than almost any other medical facility in the world. Since every new patient is required to take Mayo's comprehensive examination, the clinic will, on an average working day, do more than 2,000 X rays, 850 blood tests, and 650 electrocardiograms, while analyzing 500 lab tests and administering 140 CAT scans. About 20 percent of Mayo's patients require hospitalization, and most need surgery of some kind. Every year over 55,000 surgical procedures (including more than 2,000 artificial joint replacements and almost 1,000 coronary bypass operations) are performed in the two major hospitals that have been affiliated with the Mayo Clinic for years. Neurosurgery is a specialty in which Mayo has one of the largest practices in the world.

Only a handful of medical centers can provide more than 1,800 hospital beds and 81 operating rooms, the combined totals at Rochester Methodist and Saint Mary's, both of which officially became part of the Mayo Foundation in May 1986. Saint Mary's was actually the first tiny hospital used by the Mayos before the turn of the century. Today it is a five-building medical complex staffed by almost 3,600 highly trained professional and support staff, some of whom are members of the religious order that founded the hospital a century ago. This order, the Sisters of St. Francis, still sponsors the hospital.

Rochester Methodist, first opened in 1954, was recently cited by the American Nursing Association as a superior place for nurses to work because of its concern for the quality of nursing care. One result of this attention to attracting and training highly skilled nurses is that both hospitals in the Mayo Foundation are given excellent ratings in their surveys of former patients, each consistently receiving responses of over 95 percent "satisfied" or "very satisfied."

Mayo is a large, complex organization dispensing medical services in the precise, almost military fashion that allows it to handle the many people who come here every year. Still, there can be no doubt that most patients here sense they are in the hands of caring people whose medical knowledge is second to none.

One measure of that knowledge is the extensive educational programs conducted by Mayo and budgeted at over $40 million. Each year about 800 residents and more than 150 research fellows are in training programs in the Mayo Graduate School of Medicine, where more than 60 specialties are taught by clinic staff members. There are also continuing medical education programs for practicing physicians. At the Mayo Medical School, which opened in 1972 and which accepts only 40 students a year out of 1,600 applicants, the teaching staff is also made up exclusively of physicians from the clinic. In addition, about 250 students from other medical schools come here each year for intensive, short-term training. Finally, the Mayo School of Health Related Sciences trains about 200 students a year in 12 allied health programs, including physical therapy, laboratory technology, and nurse anesthesia.

Reaching out, to the medical community at large as well as to the farm community of the upper Midwest, has been a central part of Mayo's development. In 1985 the boundaries of Mayo's influence were expanded when it announced that two satellite clinics would open in Jacksonville, Florida, and Scottsdale, Arizona, in 1986 and 1987. The Jacksonville Clinic has been almost overwhelmed by demand since it opened in October 1986.

## Specialties

Adolescent Chemical Dependency, Alcohol and Drug Dependence, Allergic Diseases, Anesthesiology, Cardiovascular Diseases, Cardiovascular Surgery, Child and Adolescent Psychiatry, Colon and Rectal Surgery, Community and Area Medicine, Critical Care, Dentistry, Dermatology, Dialysis, Emergency Medicine, Endocrinology, Family Medicine, Gastroenterology, Gastrointestinal Surgery, General Surgery, Gynecologic Surgery, Gynecology, Hematology, Hemophilia, Immunology, Infectious Diseases, Internal Medicine, Medical Genetics, Neonatology, Nephrology, Neurologic Surgery, Neurology, Neuro-Oncology, Obstetrics, Oncology, Ophthalmology, Oral Surgery, Orthopedics, Otolaryngology, Outpatient Surgery, Pediatrics (including Pediatric Allergy, Cardiology, Endocrinology, Gastroenterology, Infectious Diseases, Learning Disabilities, Nephrology, Oncology, and Rheumatology), Perinatology, Plastic Surgery, Physical Medicine and Rehabilitation, Preventive Medicine, Psychiatry and Psychology, Radiology, Reproductive Endocrinology, Rheumatology, Sleep Disorders, Surgical Oncology, Thoracic Diseases, Thoracic Surgery, Transplantation Surgery, Urology, and Vascular Surgery.

---

**STATISTICAL PROFILE**

|  | Saint Mary's | Rochester Methodist |
|---|---|---|
| Number of Beds: | 1,065 | 788 |
| Bed Occupancy Rate: | 77% | 65% |
| Average Number of Patients: | 780 | 520 |
| Average Patient Stay: | 9 days | 7.6 days |
| Annual Admissions: | 31,800 | 24,909 |
| Births: | 0 | 2,063 |
| Emergency Room/ Trauma Center Visits: | 29,015 | 18,219 |

Hospital Personnel (both hospitals):
Nursing Staff:
1,600 (Saint Mary's)
1,100 (Rochester Methodist)
Total Staff: 5,753

Hospital Personnel (Mayo Clinic):
Physicians and Medical Scientists: 850
Residents: 800–850
Paramedical Personnel: 5,800

---

# Well-known Specialists

Dr. Thomas Bunch, rheumatology.
Dr. Robert Frye, cardiology.
Dr. William Furlow, urology; specialist in impotence and incontinence.
Dr. Clark H. Hoagland, hematology; head of the bone marrow transplant unit.
Dr. Keith Kelly, gastroenterological surgery.
Dr. Patrick Kelly, neurosurgery; specialist in brain tumors.
Dr. Ruud Krom, head of the liver transplant team.
Dr. Robert Kyle, oncology; specialist in myeloma.
Dr. Edward Laws, neurosurgery.
Dr. Charles Moertel, oncology; specialist in colon cancer.
Dr. J. Desmond O'Duffy, rheumatology.
Dr. W. Spencer Payne, thoracic surgery.

Dr. Mark Pittelkow, dermatology; specialist in skin growth for burn victims.
Dr. Douglas Pritchard, orthopedic surgery.
Dr. Charles Reed, chairman of the allergic diseases department.
Dr. David Utz, urology; specialist in prostate cancer.
Dr. Jack Whisnant, neurology; specialist in cerebrovascular disorders.
Dr. John Woods, plastic surgery.

## Research

Some observers say that much of the Mayo Clinic's success is based on good old common sense, especially of the kind found on midwestern farms. But the special brand of medicine practiced here is actually based on intense teamwork among a tightly knit group of first-rate physicians who are supported by an extensive research program.

Because so much of its energy is given to patient care, most people don't think of Mayo as one of the nation's leading research institutions. But in fact about 100 physicians and 800 staff employees work full-time in research here; in addition, just about every doctor on the staff is involved in some form of research. In 1985 alone Mayo Clinic physicians and scientists published more than 2,800 articles in medical journals and books.

Current research programs, supported by a budget of almost $60 million, span the entire gamut of medicine. The largest amount of money is spent on a broad array of basic and clinical research projects in cancer. Other areas under investigation include artificial joints, diabetes, fertility and sterility, heart disease (including arrhythmias), intestinal disorders, myasthenia gravis, osteoporosis, and strokes. Mayo is a designated Clinical Research Center funded by the NIH.

There is also a good deal of research devoted to implementing and improving new medical techniques. The clinic played a key role in developing the mechanical heart-lung bypass machine and, in 1973, was the first medical center in the country to use CAT scanning. More recently researchers at Mayo have developed a nonsurgical means for removing gallstones and a new laser therapy for lung tumors.

A Mayo surgeon has developed a method of neurosurgery that uses both lasers and computers. Called computer-assisted stereotactic neurosurgery, it enables doctors to operate deep in the brain with precise accuracy and vaporize tumors once considered inoperable. It will also help in the treatment of motor function ailments such as epilepsy, multiple sclerosis, and Parkinson's disease.

## Admission Policy

The Mayo Clinic is open to everyone, and no physician's referral is necessary (in fact only about 20 percent of all patients are referred here by outside doctors). Anyone can make an appointment by calling the Appointment Information Desk at 507-284-2111.

Although several thousand people come here every year without making advance appointments, this is not advisable, especially between May and October, when the majority of patients arrive.

There is no official financial prerequisite for admission. Between $16 and $18 million per year of indigent care is provided.

Hotels, motels, and rooming houses are all plentiful in Rochester, with prices ranging from $75 to $80 a night for a deluxe hotel room to as little as $10 for a room in a private house. The clinic will send a hotel/motel guide upon request.

---

**ROOM CHARGES (per diem)**
Private: $173
Semiprivate: $170
Ward: $155
ICU: $385–$475

**AVERAGE COST PER PATIENT STAY**
Approximately $403 per day (not including charges for Mayo Clinic services provided in the hospital, such as lab tests or physical therapy)
Cost of a Comprehensive Examination (2–4 days) for a generally healthy person: $600–$800
Cost of Transplant:
  Kidney: $20,000–$25,000
  Liver: $105,000–$120,000

**MAILING ADDRESS**         **TELEPHONE**
220 First Street, S.W.     507-284-2511
Rochester, MN 55901

---

# The University of Minnesota Hospitals and Clinics

**MINNEAPOLIS, MINNESOTA**

Hospital consultants consider the Twin Cities area one of the most competitive hospital markets in the country. There are 27 hospitals here, many of them offering excellent care, and a few (Hennepin County Medical Center and St. Paul–Ramsey Medical Center, for example) that have national reputations in several fields. Only one, however, offers the variety and depth of service that one looks for in a truly extraordinary medical center.

Although it is only up the road, quite literally, from the world-famous Mayo Clinic (see page 179), The University of Minnesota Hospitals and Clinics (UMHC) has maintained its place as a leading regional referral center and arguably the most influential medical institution in the state. More than half of UMHC's patients come from outside the Twin Cities, and almost one-quarter come from other states and foreign countries. Best known to the general public for its outstanding work in organ transplantation, UMHC is also highly regarded in medical circles for programs including those in nephrology, neurology, neurosurgery, oncology, ophthalmology, pediatrics, and psychiatry.

Founded in 1911 as the Elliot Memorial Hospital (125 beds, 25 doctors), UMHC was one of the first university-affiliated hospitals in the country. Today it is a modern medical complex comprising six buildings, almost 600 beds, nearly 400 doctors, 1,400 nurses, and just about every piece of sophisticated medical technology, including a nuclear magnetic resonance imaging unit, a lithotriptor, all types of lasers, and a hyperthermia machine that treats deep-seated malignant tumors.

In the spring of 1986 UMHC opened a new 450-bed hospital to replace its older principal facility. Within the new hospital is the Variety Club Children's Hospital, a fully equipped facility with six patient units exclusively for pediatric care. Everything about the new building represents the latest thinking in hospital design, including rooms with views of the Mississippi River and an internal transport system that sends medicines, lab specimens, medical records, and such at a rate six times faster than the old system. There's also a state-of-the-art air filtration system that purifies the air and removes spores to a degree rare in any hospital (the air in the lobby, for example, is kept 99.97 percent pure).

Organ transplantation is a central concern of UMHC; in fact, this is one of the world's largest transplantation centers. In 1985 surgeons performed 181 kidney transplants, 26 liver transplants, 25 segmental pancreas transplants, and 14 heart transplants. In 1986 the hospital acquired the services of Dr. Stuart Jamieson, a former member of Dr. Norman Shumway's heart

**185**

transplant team at Stanford and one of the very few surgeons experienced in heart-lung transplantation. With Dr. John Najarian, a specialist in kidney transplantation, and other well-known surgeons here, Jamieson places Minnesota in the top echelon of transplantation work.

The University of Minnesota medical community sees itself as an integral part of Minnesota's health-care system. Over half the state's physicians as well as thousands of allied health personnel receive their training here. Through the special Rural Physician Associate Program, hundreds of third-year medical students have spent a year with practicing physicians in the state's remote rural areas; almost 60 percent of them return to rural family practice after training is completed. Through a wide variety of outreach programs the staff here provides both service and education to health professionals and allied health personnel throughout Minnesota and the upper Midwest. Programs range from one-day seminars for nurses to month-long tutorials for physicians.

A variety of services for the community and full range of clinics and specialty centers are available to anyone; some of these are described in the following paragraphs. A comprehensive pediatric intensive care unit with three pediatricians and 60 pediatric critical-care nurses specializes in critical care. The nurse-to-patient ratio for the majority of patients in this unit is one to one. The unit features immediate availability of all pediatric medical and surgical specialties, including cardiovascular surgery, hemodialysis, and neurosurgery.

The UMHC is a national and regional center for bypass operations and surgery for obesity. Dr. Henry Buchwald has performed over 1,400 jejunoileal bypass and gastric bypass operations, the most obesity operations in the world. Other subspecialties in the Department of Surgery include cardiovascular, colorectal, craniofacial, extremity replantation, general, pediatric, thoracic, and transplant.

In the Clinic of Family Practice and Community Health, a Human Sexuality Program offers individual, joint, and group therapy for sex-related problems. Professional education seminars (for example, Sexual Attitude Reassessment) are available for doctors, nurses, ministers, social workers, and others.

The newly formed Minnesota Heart and Lung Institute provides comprehensive care for patients who suffer from medically or surgically treatable heart and lung disease. Through the institute cardiac and thoracic surgery of all kinds are available, along with diagnosis and treatment of coronary artery disease using angioplasty and catheter-measured blood flow.

The Obstetrics and Gynecology Clinic offers artificial insemination, childbirth education, family planning, family sex education, gynecologic oncology and chemotherapy treatment, high-risk obstetric treatment, in vitro fertilization, prenatal detection, sibling preparation, ultrasound, and urodynamics.

The Adolescent and Adult Health Psychology Service provides individual, couple, marital, and family counseling and psychotherapy. Psychotherapy services are available for adults, teenagers, and children. Services are offered to children and teenagers in the areas of behavior disturbances, learning difficulties, and personality. Adults are seen for personality, general ability, aptitude, interest, and educational achievement testing.

The Community University Health Care Center is a community clinic that began as a joint venture with the city of Minneapolis and became a University Hospital project in 1984. More than 20,000 pediatric and adult patient visits were made to the clinic's medical, dental, and mental-health facilities in 1985.

The Spinal Cord Center, the University Kidney Stone Center, the Minnesota Heart and Lung Institute, and the Sports Medicine Institute are four of the latest special facilities added to UMHC.

## Specialties

Anesthesiology, Dentistry, Dermatology, Laboratory Medicine and Pathology, Medicine, Neurology, Neurosurgery, Obstetrics/Gynecology, Ophthalmology, Organ Transplant, Orthopedics, Pediatrics, Psychiatry, Radiology, Surgery, Therapeutic Radiology, and Urology.

Clinics specialize in adult cardiac disorders, allergy, arthritis, cancer, cerebral vascular diseases, chest diseases, colonoscopy, dementia, diabetes, endocrine disorders, gallstones, gastrointestinal diseases, general medicine, genetics, hematology, hypertension, infectious diseases, lipid disorders, liver diseases, chronic obstructive lung disease, male impotence, multiple sclerosis, neuromuscular diseases, renal disorders, sexual dysfunction, and urinary tract disease.

---

**STATISTICAL PROFILE (1985–86)**

Number of Beds: 593
Bed Occupancy Rate: 67%
Average Number of Patients: 399
Average Patient Stay: 8.2 days
Annual Admissions: 17,663
Births: 602
Outpatient Clinic Visits: 224,446
Emergency Room/Trauma Center Visits: 14,551

Hospital Personnel:
  Physicians: 389 full-time; 179 part-time
  Medical Fellows and Medical Fellow Specialists: 1,147
  Registered Nurses: 1,400
  Total Staff: 4,408

Other clinics include Alcohol and Drug Abuse, Family Practice and Community Health (including a Human Sexuality Program), Genetics/Eye, Genetics/Skin, Neurofibromatosis, and Pediatric Oncology.

## Well-known Specialists

Dr. Nancy Ascher, surgery; specialist in liver transplantation.

Dr. Clara Bloomfield, oncology; specialist in leukemia and lymphomas.

Dr. Henry Buchwald, surgery; specialist in operations to treat obesity.

Dr. Frank B. Cerra, surgery; specialist in therapies using nutrient mixes and specialized formulas to reduce multiple system organ failure, which accounts for the majority of deaths in intensive care units.

Dr. Paula Clayton, specialist in manic-depressive illness, chief of psychiatry.

Dr. Donald J. Doughman, specialist in anterior segment eye disease and cornea transplantation.

Dr. Thomas Ferris, specialist in kidney disease.

Dr. Stuart Jamieson, heart transplant surgery; director of the heart-lung transplantation program.

Dr. B. J. Kennedy, oncology; specialist in breast cancer.

Dr. David Knighton, surgery; specialist in treating nonhealing wounds in diabetics, transplant patients, paraplegics, and others, founder of the first clinical wound healing center in the country.

Dr. David Knopman, neurology; pioneer researcher in Alzheimer's disease and other memory disorders.

Dr. Ronald P. Messner, rheumatology; specialist in arthritis, director of the rheumatology and clinical immunology departments.

Dr. Alfred Michael, pediatric nephrology; specialist in chronic renal failure in children.

Dr. John Najarian, specialist in transplantation, chief of surgery.

Dr. Jack Oppenheimer, endocrinology; specialist in thyroid diseases.

Dr. Norma Ramsay, specialist in bone marrow transplantation.

Dr. David Sutherland, surgery; specialist in pancreas transplantation.

Dr. George Tagatz, specialist in female infertility, professor of obstetrics and gynecology.

Dr. Roby Thompson, orthopedic surgery.

Dr. Theodore Thompson, specialist in neonatal intensive care.

Dr. Leo B. Twiggs, specialist in gynecologic cancer and laser treatment of precancerous conditions.

## Research

Almost $40 million in research grants are given to members of the UMHC medical staff; more than $30 million comes from the NIH alone. The hospital is the site of an NIH-funded Clinical Research Center, where special studies of Alzheimer's disease, asthma, diabetes, children's hypertension, and several other ailments are conducted.

In cardiology there are studies of the effects of a variety of drugs in the treatment of heart disease and nonsurgical techniques to correct arrhythmia and blocked arteries. In psychiatry there are special studies of anorexia nervosa, bulimia, and depression as well as a search for genetic links that will make it possible to identify those at risk for Alzheimer's disease.

# Admission Policy

Anyone is eligible to be a patient at UMHC. Although most patients from outside the Minneapolis area are referred by their physicians, anyone can call the Referral Information Center and be directed to the appropriate clinic or department. The general number is 612-626-3000, but there are two toll-free numbers for those calling from outside the metropolitan area. In Minnesota, the number is 800-462-5301; out-of-state patients can call 800-328-5517.

There are financial requirements for some procedures and for most out-of-state residents. For those needing assistance, there are numerous county welfare programs as well as state-funded programs just for the hospital. Although the hospital is a state institution, it is largely self-supporting, with only 6 percent of its operating revenue coming from state taxes.

---

**ROOM CHARGES (per diem)**
Private: $295
Semiprivate: $295
Ward (four to a room): $265
ICU: $765

**ESTIMATED COSTS OF ORGAN TRANSPLANTATION**
Heart: $75,000; preevaluation is $7,500.
Kidney: $46,000; preevaluation is $5,000.
Liver: $140,000; preevaluation is $7,500.

**AVERAGE COST PER PATIENT STAY:**   $9,388

**MAILING ADDRESS**                    **TELEPHONE**
Harvard Street at East River Road    612-626-3000
Minneapolis, MN 55455

---

# Barnes Hospital
## ST. LOUIS, MISSOURI

Most physicians in this part of the country believe Barnes Hospital is the premier teaching and research hospital in the Midwest. Moreover, every national survey we've run across ranks Barnes as one of the top ten major medical centers in the country. So it's no wonder that 40 percent of the 36,000 patients admitted here annually come from outside metropolitan St. Louis. What they come for is the most advanced kind of medical care available anywhere, especially for the treatment of cancer, diabetes, glaucoma and retinal problems, and heart disease, as well as joint replacements and cornea, heart, heart-lung, kidney, and liver transplants. Equipped with virtually every modern medical tool—lasers, PET and CAT scanners, magnetic resonance imaging, a lithotriptor, and so on—Barnes is clearly one of the most technologically advanced hospitals in the nation.

Founded in 1914 through a bequest from a wealthy St. Louis businessman, Barnes is today the primary teaching hospital of the Washington University School of Medicine and the central facility in a 26-building medical complex that includes another first-rate teaching hospital (Jewish Hospital) and the highly regarded St. Louis Children's Hospital. There are three separate buildings for research, one for outpatient care, and another for rehabilitation. But Barnes Hospital, with more than 1,000 beds, 1,100 doctors, and 1,500 registered nurses, is the hub of activity for the entire center.

In fact, there are so many services here and everything is so up to date, we were certain that the exasperating problems patients associate with large teaching hospitals would be immediately apparent. In a sense we were right, since by the hospital's own admission billing problems are often horrendous and by most accounts the food isn't very good. But when it comes to the issues patients care about most, we were a bit astounded to learn just how good the Barnes staff is.

For the last two years the hospital's ongoing patient survey has consistently shown that over 97 percent of the respondents believe they received good care at Barnes; frequently that figure was even higher. One reason almost every patient thinks so positively about Barnes is the quality, courtesy, and concern of the nursing staff. During 1985, for example, 98 percent of those responding to the patient survey approved of the nursing care they received here.

This is not entirely surprising considering that all newly hired nurses at Barnes must go through an intensive six-week orientation; formal classroom work and additional preceptor training are required for intensive care unit duty. Many nurses here have bachelor's degrees, and the hospital encourages further education by providing tuition reimbursement. Turnover is relatively low (20 percent) for a large urban teaching hospital.

The people who run Barnes seem proud of the entire staff, and every issue of the hospital's quarterly magazine includes letters from former patients praising the medical care and attention they received. Here are two typical examples:

"I am a nurse supervisor at another local hospital. I think Barnes is to be commended for their excellent care and professionally manned staff. From the minute I arrived until discharge, I got nothing but attention, concern and wonderful communication. You all really have your act together."

"I have been a patient in nine other hospitals and I can definitely state that the care I received at Barnes far surpassed all others. As a patient, I was given the impression and I believe your employees were concerned about me. I felt everything that was done for me, was done out of caring and trying to make my stay as pleasant as possible—no wonder Barnes is rated as one of the top hospitals in the United States."

This concern for patients' needs carries over into the financial aspects of hospitalization. In recent years Barnes has annually provided over $8 million worth of charity care, not including bad debts or uncollected bills. In addition, Barnes helps transplant patients meet the enormous costs they incur through a Transplant Patient Care Fund. For the relatives of severely ill patients who have traveled a long distance, the hospital offers a few rooms free of charge at the Barnes Lodge; this is, however, a small facility, housing only five families. Although expansion has begun, families shouldn't count on these rooms being available.

Barnes also offers a host of important medical specialties. Patients come from all over the world for cardiology and cardiothoracic surgery, especially surgery for Wolff-Parkinson-White syndrome, heart malformations, difficult coronary artery bypass, and esophageal cancer. Barnes's 15-bed Cardiac Care Unit is the only one anywhere with a PET scanner within the unit.

Ophthalmologists at Barnes have pioneered treatments for diabetic retinopathy, glaucoma, and other conditions. Barnes has received recent national recognition for research into treatment for macular degeneration and ocular histoplasmosis. All kinds of ophthalmologic laser surgery are performed here, and Barnes is the home of the St. Louis Eye Bank.

Specialists in otolaryngology have done important work in dizziness, extracochlear implants, neck and throat cancer, sclera tympanoplasty, sleep apnea, and tongue cancer.

The Burn Center at Barnes was one of the first in the country, developing techniques that have since become standard procedure at other hospitals.

Plastic and reconstructive surgery is a pioneered specialty at Barnes, with national referrals for reimplantation of severed parts, facial reconstruction necessitated by both congenital and accidental causes, sex reassignment, and hand surgery.

In neurology and neurosurgery Barnes specialties include Alzheimer's disease, brain surgery, epilepsy (including mapping the brain to detect and eliminate errant electrical activity centers that cause seizures), immunology and rheumatology (at the Howard Hughes Center), multiple sclerosis, and muscular dystrophy (at the Jerry Lewis Center). In conjunction with otolaryngology, skull base tumors are treated. And in conjunction with ophthalmology, orbital and other eye area tumors receive attention.

In the urology department Barnes is particularly noted for work in bladder and prostate cancers, kidney stones, and testicular impotency.

A full range of specialists and services treat patients with cancer, including bone cancer, breast cancer, Hodgkin's disease, cancer of the larynx, leukemia, liver cancer, lung cancer, skull base tumors, and testicular cancer. An Outpatient Transfusion Center and the Pheresis Center allow cancer patients to receive blood transfusions as outpatients and thus remain in their homes.

Patients from hundreds of miles away are referred to Barnes's high-risk pregnancy program, which helps women who have delayed pregnancy until later in life as well as those with preexisting medical complications, such as diabetes, heart or kidney disease, and hypertension, and those expecting multiple births.

The Health Education and Screening Center and the Community Outreach Program focus on educating the public; their offerings include a television series, printed materials, a speaker's bureau, community forums, and doctors' seminars, all sponsored by Barnes Hospital.

Barnes Home Health helps assure continuity of care after patients leave the hospital and in some cases can even provide an alternative to hospitalization or shorten the stay in the hospital.

In April 1984 Barnes acquired Sutter Clinic in downtown St. Louis, which became Barnes/Sutter and now offers a variety of services, including breast cancer screenings, disability evaluations, and executive physicals, at two locations.

## Specialties

Anesthesiology, Cardiology, Dentistry, Dermatology, Neurology, Neurosurgery, Medicine, Obstetrics/Gynecology, Oncology, Ophthalmology, Otolaryngology, Pathology, Psychiatry, Radiology, and Surgical Pathology.

Surgical specialties include general, cardiothoracic, oral-maxillofacial, orthopedic, plastic and reconstructive, transplants, and urologic surgery.

Other specialties include burn treatment, high-risk pregnancy, retina surgery, and surgery for throat cancer.

STATISTICAL PROFILE

Number of Beds: 1,083
Bed Occupancy Rate: 79%
Average Number of Patients: 857
Average Patient Stay: 8.7 days
Annual Admissions: 35,587
Births: 3,034
Outpatient Clinic Visits: 64,814
Emergency Room/Trauma Center Visits: 41,590

Hospital Personnel:
    Physicians: 1,121
    Residents: 479
    Registered Nurses: 1,500
    Total Staff: 4,087

# Well-known Specialists

As with the other top-rated hospitals in this book, any list of highly regarded physicians is bound to be limited and therefore potentially misleading. Any doctor who becomes a senior staff member at a hospital such as Barnes is necessarily among the best professionals in his or her specialty. With that caveat in mind, here are the names of a handful of physicians at Barnes who have been publicly recognized for their work.

Dr. Charles B. Anderson, vascular surgery; pioneer of pretransplant blood transfusions to desensitize kidney transplant patients, general surgeon in chief.

Dr. R. Morton Bolman, specialist in heart and heart-lung transplants.

Dr. William J. Catalona, specialist in cancer of the bladder and prostate, urologist in chief.

Dr. James Cox, specialist in surgery for heart arrhythmias, including Wolff-Parkinson-White syndrome; cardiothoracic surgeon in chief.

Dr. M. Wayne Flye, director of the liver and kidney transplant program.

Dr. Virgil Loeb, oncology; current chairman of the American Cancer Society.

Dr. William Monafo, director of the Burn Center and head of emergency medicine, which runs a Level I trauma unit.

Dr. Burton Sobel, chief cardiologist; with his associates led the team that developed the drug TPA (tissue plasminogen activator).

Dr. Paul Weeks, specialist in reattaching hands and fingers, plastic and reconstructive surgeon in chief.

## Research

In 1985 the Washington University School of Medicine received research grants totaling $52.5 million, almost 85 percent from the federal government. Researchers here have made many important discoveries related directly to clinical treatment. The PET scanner, for example, which enables cardiologists to find blood-starved or permanently damaged heart tissue without surgery, was developed here. So, too, were both TPA, the well-known but still experimental drug that dissolves clots in blocked coronary arteries, and the surgical procedure for helping victims of heart attack arrhythmias, which employs a computer to pinpoint the origin of the abnormal heartbeat.

The best known and arguably the most important research being done here is the work of Dr. Paul Lacy, a pathologist, and his former student, Dr. David Scharp, a surgeon at Barnes. Their attempts to find a way of implanting the insulin-producing cells (called islets of Langerhans) found in a normal pancreas but missing in those of diabetics represents the best hope for a new kind of diabetes therapy.

Barnes is also the site of an NIH-funded Clinical Research Center, where experimental treatment of patients with diabetes, pituitary tumors, sickle-cell disease, and several other diseases is carried out in a separate and highly controlled environment.

## Admission Policy

Because Barnes is so highly regarded, many of its patients have been referred by physicians not affiliated with the hospital; patients come from all over the country. Patients can also refer themselves by calling the hospital directly. Barnes maintains a toll-free telephone number for doctors and patients wishing referrals: 800-392-0936.

Except for those requiring either emergency care or treatment in the burn center, hospital policy clearly states that prospective patients must provide some guarantee of payment. The hospital's Patient Accounts Department works to help many people find the means to pay, sometimes obtaining money from the hospital's charity budget, sometimes assisting them in getting adequate insurance coverage for special procedures such as transplants.

---

**ROOM CHARGES (per diem)**
Private: $230
Semiprivate: $205
ICU: $470–$700

**AVERAGE COST OF ORGAN TRANSPLANTATION**
Heart Transplant: $49,200; required deposit: $50,000
Liver Transplant: $71,300; required deposit: $125,000
Kidney Transplant: $29,000; required deposit: $25,000
Heart-Lung Transplant: Protocol not yet set but probably will be
similar to liver.

**MAILING ADDRESS**        **TELEPHONE**
Barnes Hospital Plaza      314-362-5000
St. Louis, MO 63110

# Hospital for Joint Diseases
# Orthopaedic Institute
**NEW YORK, NEW YORK**

At the turn of the century, when the Hospital for Joint Diseases opened in northern Manhattan, orthopedic surgery was in its infancy and doctors could offer very little hope for patients with arthritis, bone cancer, curvature of the spine, or many other orthopedic problems. Today the Hospital for Joint Diseases Orthopaedic Institute, an international resource for orthopedic research, patient care, and education, can help many of these patients. The Institute is the largest orthopedic specialty hospital in the country; its Department of Rehabilitation Medicine provides more than 100,000 occupational and physical therapy treatments a year.

The Institute's tradition of specialized care for different kinds of rheumatic diseases is upheld by its innovative clinics and research projects. For example, a new clinic helps people with lupus erythematosus. A Pediatric Rheumatology Clinic was established in 1984. And plans are under way for a new center devoted to the diagnosis, treatment, and study of psoriatic arthritis.

The Center for Orthopaedic and Metabolic Bone Diseases offers comprehensive evaluation and management of patients with both benign and malignant disorders of the musculoskeletal system. This division is currently performing limb salvage surgery—including state-of-the-art bone transplantation and custom modular implants—which can greatly help patients with cancer of the musculoskeletal system.

The Institute's Pediatric Orthopaedic Surgery Service is one of the busiest in the city and the largest in the world, treating between 25 and 50 children at any given time. Children are referred here from as far away as Europe, Latin America, and Asia.

The Comprehensive Arthritis Service utilizes the combined skills of the hospital's medical and surgical services as well as allied health professionals to provide fully coordinated care for both inpatients and outpatients with arthritis.

Other specialized centers help athletes and dancers. The Center for Sports Medicine provides conditioning programs, physical therapy, surgery, and other treatments needed to solve special orthopedic problems. The center has one of the most active services in arthroscopic surgery.

The two-year-old Orthopaedic-Arthritis Pain Center is the only nationally accredited inpatient pain center in the New York metropolitan area. Approximately 50 percent of its patients have resumed a full range of life activities.

The Center for Neuromuscular and Developmental Disorders treats people with cerebral palsy, muscular dystrophy, polio, scoliosis, spina bifida, and a wide variety of other disorders. Most of its patients are children. Other programs for children include the Center for Neuromuscular and Developmental Disorders, the Preschool Program, and the center's Communication Laboratory, which has the country's most sophisticated instrumentation for training children with impairments.

The Institute's Back School is a model program for patients with chronic or acute back pain and related problems who are recovering from back surgery. Attendance expanded from 14 patients in 1983 to 138 patients in 1984, its second year.

The Institute tested several new methods in 1984 to contain the spiraling costs of health care. For example, preadmission testing was improved, enabling physicians to gain quicker access to clinical and diagnostic information. As a result of these methods, the average length of a patient's hospital stay was reduced by approximately one day in 1984, representing substantial savings for patient and hospital alike.

## Specialties

Anesthesiology, Adult Orthopedics, Arthritis, Back Pain, Chronic Pain, Hand and Foot Surgery, the Lupus Clinic, Neuromuscular and Developmental Disorders, Osteoporosis, Pathology, Pediatric Orthopedics, Radiology, Rheumatology, Scoliosis, Sports Medicine/Arthroscopy, and Tumor Surgery.

---

**STATISTICAL PROFILE**

Number of Beds: 230
Bed Occupancy Rate: 80%
Average Number of Patients: 185
Average Patient Stay: 9.8 days
Annual Admissions: 6,715
Outpatient Clinic Visits: 31,400

Hospital Personnel:
  Physicians: 35
  Residents: 50
  Registered Nurses: 211
  Total Staff: 1,050

---

## Well-known Specialists

Dr. Jill Buyon, director of the Systemic Lupus Erythematosus Service.
Dr. Victor Frankel, orthopedic surgery; chief of the medical staff, chairman of the Department of Orthopedics.

Dr. Neil Kahanovitz, chief of the Spine Service.

Dr. William B. Lehman, director of the Pediatric Orthopaedic Surgery Service.

Dr. Peter LoGalbo, director of the Pediatric Rheumatology Clinic.

Dr. Mark Pitman, chief of the Center for Sports Medicine.

Dr. David Present, chief of Orthopaedic Oncology and the Metabolic Bone Disease Center.

Dr. Gary Solomon, medical director of the Comprehensive Arthritis Service.

Dr. Steven Stuchin, surgical director of the Comprehensive Arthritis Service.

Dr. Robert Winchester, chairman of the Rheumatic Diseases Department.

## Research

The growing importance of research at the Hospital for Joint Diseases Orthopaedic Institute was recognized in 1985 by the NIH and other funding agencies, which awarded research grants of close to $2 million, an increase of more than 500 percent in research grants since 1983.

Aided by a grant from Johnson & Johnson Products, Inc., researchers in the Pediatric Orthopaedic Service are investigating the use of biodegradable bone implants, which do not require surgical removal when children outgrow them. Preliminary results are quite promising.

Researchers led by Dr. Mark Pitman are also investigating techniques of transplanting healthy cartilage cells grown in cell culture as a possible way to repair cartilage damage. The team hopes that eventually cartilage transplantation will help repair knee injuries as well as cartilage damage caused by arthritis.

At the Pain Center scientists are analyzing the components of pain by studying the physical, psychological, and behavioral symptoms of pain patients.

## Admission Policy

All Joint Diseases patients must be referred by a physician. However, those who do not have a physician can call the Admission Center (212-598-6530) to receive the names of three physicians who specialize in their problem. Patients can then make an appointment with any one of these physicians, who can refer them to the hospital.

The hospital accepts all forms of insurance, including Medicare, Medicaid, and worker's compensation. Self-paying patients are required to make a deposit, the amount of which varies according to the procedure and expected length of stay in the hospital.

Indigent care at Joint Diseases amounts to approximately $800,000 a year.

**ROOM CHARGES** (per diem)
Private: $565
Semiprivate: $465

**AVERAGE COST PER PATIENT STAY:**    $7,439

**MAILING ADDRESS**        **TELEPHONE**
301 East 17th Street    212-598-6000
New York, NY 10003

# The Hospital for Special Surgery

**NEW YORK, NEW YORK**

Strangely enough, this hospital was first brought to our attention by an orthopedist who lives hundreds of miles from New York. Like many people, we thought The Hospital for Special Surgery (HSS) was simply part of New York Hospital. In fact, HSS is an autonomous hospital that has a strong affiliation with New York Hospital—Cornell Medical Center; it provides orthopedic and rheumatological service for that institution. More than 40 percent of the over 5,000 inpatients who come here each year are from outside New York, and many are from overseas.

Established in 1863, HSS is the oldest orthopedic hospital in the United States. It is a leader in orthopedics and rheumatology and provides ambulatory and inpatient care for adult and pediatric patients with the entire range of musculoskeletal injuries and diseases.

Patients come to HSS for what is indeed "special surgery." For example, over 1,500 total joint replacements are performed here annually. This operation, which HSS has pioneered over the past twenty years, is performed on patients suffering from advanced osteoarthritis, rheumatoid arthritis, and other diseases that have caused such severe deterioration of the joints that no therapy or drug can relieve the pain or restore mobility. In addition, HSS deals with spinal disc problems, scoliosis, sports injuries, orthopedic problems of children, foot problems, and bone cancer (doctors here staff Memorial Sloan-Kettering's Bone Tumor Service [see page 205]).

Improved surgical procedures in certain areas of orthopedics and rehabilitative procedures have reduced the average stay of an HSS patient to less than eleven days. Custom prosthetic joint replacements are designed and manufactured at HSS for patients whose unique problems cannot be addressed by the standard commercially available implants.

Arthroscopic surgery is also provided. Many patients on whom this procedure is performed can return home the same day.

The hospital has been a leader in implementing a program of autologous blood donations. In 1985 approximately 25 percent of the blood used for transfusions during surgery at HSS came from the patients themselves. The hospital also employs a cell saver program, whereby blood removed from the wound during surgery is collected, filtered, and returned to the patient while the operation is in progress.

Recognizing that there is a need to inform the public about the prevention of musculoskeletal, orthopedic, and rheumatic disorders, HSS offers extensive community education programs. The Osteoporosis Center is the hospital's most recent public education effort. The program educates people about the seriousness of the disease, screens high-risk individuals, and provides recommendations for prevention. Classes, lectures, seminars, health fairs, tours, and screening clinics are offered on arthritis, back problems, nutrition, scoliosis, and stress management.

The Sportsmedicine Performance and Research Center provides modern therapeutic techniques and technology, as well as patient education aimed at sports injury avoidance. The center also evaluates dancers' injuries and offers recommendations on how to avoid potential injury; it is one of the few organizations that provides this vital service.

The Back Treatment and Learning Center is a recently established outpatient service that offers a structured, personalized program of physical therapy emphasizing proper body mechanics, exercise, posture, stress management, and weight control to people with chronic back pain.

In addition to New York Hospital, HSS is affiliated with Cornell University Medical Center. It is the site of Cornell Medical College's residency program in orthopedic surgery, a four-year program to which more than 300 medical school graduates apply each year. Only eight are admitted. Medical staff at HSS hold faculty appointments at Cornell Medical College and medical staff appointments at New York Hospital.

## Specialties

All orthopedic and rheumatic conditions.

---

**STATISTICAL PROFILE**

Number of Beds: 192
Bed Occupancy Rate: 82%
Average Patient Stay: 10.7 days
Annual Admissions: 5,200
Outpatient Clinic Visits: 82,000
    Private Physician: 46,000
    Ambulatory Center: 36,000

Hospital Personnel:
    Physicians: 90
    Residents: 31
    Registered Nurses: 115
    Licensed Practical Nurses: 43
    Total Staff: 950

# Well-known Specialists

Dr. Charles Christian, rheumatology; physician in chief and director of rheumatic diseases.

Dr. John Insall, orthopedic surgery; specialist in knee replacement surgery.

Dr. Joseph Lane, orthopedic surgery; chief of Metabolic Bone Disease Unit, medical director of Osteoporosis Center, specialist in osteoporosis.

Dr. David Levine, orthopedic surgery; specialist in scoliosis.

Dr. Leon Root, orthopedic surgery; medical director of Rehabilitation Services, specialist in back pain and children's orthopedics.

Dr. Philip D. Wilson, surgeon in chief, specialist in orthopedic surgery.

# Research

Sixty-two scientists and scientific consultants conduct basic and applied research in musculoskeletal disorders at HSS.

In rheumatology HSS scientists are investigating how the immune system can turn on the body, attacking its own cells. This mechanism is thought to be one of the major causes of diseases such as lupus and rheumatoid arthritis. In orthopedics physicians work on the diseases they treat most often—bone cancer, osteoarthritis, osteogenesis imperfecta, osteomalacia, osteoporosis, and spinal stenosis.

A series of interrelated projects investigate how bone mineral first forms in the body, how it changes with age and disease, and what controls both normal and abnormal bone growth. These studies apply to diseases such as hypertrophic osteoarthritis and osteoporosis. Other projects focus on the effect of certain vitamins, especially D, on the mineralization process, on how joint cartilage receives nutrition, on joint motion and gait analysis, on how ligaments help stabilize joints, and on how bones and joints heal and are repaired.

Currently HSS is researching the use of allograft transplants to replace ligaments in the severely injured knee. Work is also progressing on the development of synthetic ligaments that would restore an injured knee to more normal function, allowing the resumption of activity and curtailing the progression of arthritis.

# Admission Policy

A person can become a patient at HSS by calling to schedule an appointment with an HSS physician or with one of the 25 subspecialty services in the Ambulatory Care Center. A patient is assured access to treatment regardless of the source of payment.

To obtain a referral for a private physician, telephone 212-606-1000. To make an appointment with a subspecialty service, call 212-606-1267.

**ROOM CHARGES (per diem)**
Private: $420
Semiprivate: $260

**AVERAGE COST PER (SURGICAL) PATIENT STAY:**    $9,950

**MAILING ADDRESS**        **TELEPHONE**
535 East 70th Street     212-606-1000
New York, NY 10021

# Memorial Sloan-Kettering Cancer Center

**NEW YORK, NEW YORK**

By all accounts Memorial Sloan-Kettering is one of the most famous cancer treatment and research centers in the world. By any standard, it is also one of the best. Located on Manhattan's Upper East Side and consisting of Memorial Hospital and Sloan-Kettering Institute, it attracts patients from around the world. Almost 60 percent of Memorial's patients come from beyond New York City; more than 1,000 a year are from other countries. Add to this the fact that about 40 percent of all patients here are self-referrals, and one can sense just how widespread Memorial's reputation has become and why its occupancy rate consistently hovers around 90 percent.

Every known form of cancer is treated here; indeed, many were first identified here, just as many of the standard surgical, chemical, and radio therapies were developed here. Founded in 1884 as the New York Cancer Hospital, Memorial was the first institution in this country devoted exclusively to the care of cancer patients. During the first part of this century, physicians here made important contributions in the use of radiation; in 1926 they developed the first implantable radiation source for use in the treatment of cancer. In 1946 physicians here began pioneering work in chemotherapy with the announcement that certain agents developed for chemical warfare were effective against several kinds of cancer. Memorial physicians have also led the way since 1951 in the development of the leading oncological surgical techniques in use today. In basic research too scientists at Sloan-Kettering have played a crucial role in uncovering the nature of cancer, including the first identification of a genetic base for cancer susceptibility in 1965.

With over 138,000 patient visits or admissions annually, Memorial is one of the largest cancer centers in the United States. In addition, more than 11,000 surgical procedures and over 65,000 radiation treatments are performed here each year. Such facts and figures could lead one to believe that this is simply a large, impersonal academic medical center where patient care is subordinated to research. But in fact treatment here is personal, intense, and of the highest quality.

In recent years Memorial has made major strides in developing new procedures for virtually every form of cancer, at every stage and for every age group. Substantial progress has been made in the treatment of lymphomas, adult leukemia, breast cancer, testicular cancer, thyroid cancer, prostate cancer—indeed, in almost all cancers.

Today, as center investigators continue to refine the techniques of surgery, radiation therapy, and chemotherapy, combinations of these three forms of therapy are increasingly improving cure rates. With this improvement in survival rates, Memorial physicians are committed to preserving healthy tissue and normal body function whenever possible.

A prototype of this new combined approach is the treatment of breast cancer. In the past, the standard therapy for breast cancer was radical or modified mastectomy. Today Memorial is able to offer women with early-stage breast cancer a more conservational form of treatment—lumpectomy. Recent studies suggest that this multidisciplinary approach to the treatment of breast cancer is as effective as mastectomy. After five years, 85 percent of all patients are free of their disease.

Refinements of therapy by Memorial physicians have made possible the preservation of body function in the treatment of a number of other cancers, including colon and rectal cancers, testicular cancer, cancer of the larynx, and soft-tissue sarcomas. For the patient, this may mean preventing a colostomy, retaining normal sexual function, saving the voice, or avoiding amputation.

Some of the most dramatic results have been achieved with childhood cancers. Between 70 and 75 percent of all children over the age of two with leukemia, for example, will be cured by chemotherapy alone, with an additional 10 percent cured by such other measures as bone marrow transplants (compared to only 15 to 20 percent in 1960.) These dramatic improvements are largely a result of the recognition of different forms of leukemia affecting children, the development of combination therapies, and the expertise with which doctors at Memorial deliver chemotherapy.

About 1,600 children are in active treatment at Memorial Sloan-Kettering at any given time, with more than 1,100 admissions to the center each year. There are 15,000 outpatient visits each year, which translates into 57 to 60 visits a day in the Pediatric Day Hospital. In 1985, 460 new pediatric patients came to Memorial.

More than a decade ago Memorial established one of the world's first bone marrow transplantation programs. Today that program is among the most comprehensive efforts of its kind in the world, and about 100 transplant procedures are done each year. Because of a technique developed here to prevent graft-versus-host disease, the number of patients who can benefit from bone marrow transplantation has increased significantly. As a result of this technique, bone marrow transplantation is no longer restricted to the 40 percent of patients who have a closely matched sibling for a donor.

Another special feature at Memorial is the Pain Service. When it started in 1982, it was the first of its kind in the country, and it has since become a model for other hospitals that must treat patients with the often acute, chronic, and intractable pain associated with cancer.

As impressive as all these services are, the most extraordinary aspect of

Memorial, and, we think, the key to understanding its preeminent role in cancer care, is the availability of more than 500 "clinical investigative protocols" that go beyond those regarded as standard. In other words, these treatments are experimental and may involve some risk. They are, of course, never recommended unless Memorial physicians have reason to believe they will help, nor are they ever initiated without the patient's full understanding and consent. According to Dr. Samuel Hellman, physician in chief at Memorial, "Patients should understand their disease and the treatment proposed. They should understand what potential advantages it has and what the potential complications are. They should be participants in the medical decisions."

This attitude pervades all the patient-care services here, but there is also a full range of services to help patients deal with other cancer-related problems. The most important of these is the Psychiatric Oncology Service, the first and one of only a few in the country, which offers professionally run support programs for patients and their families. These include patient-to-patient counseling and continued communication between the hospital and patients who have gone home.

Nurses compete for places on Memorial's staff. Once hired, nurses here take part in a one-month intensive orientation program tailored to their area of specialization in cancer nursing. It is a self-directed program combining reading materials, videotapes, workshops, and practice sessions designed to promote an understanding of the concepts and skills needed to care for cancer patients. The multidisciplinary approach to patient care is stressed, with an emphasis on the coordinating role of the nurse.

Memorial also employs several full-time patient representatives to answer questions about hospital policies, explain patients' rights, and act as advocates on a patient's behalf if there are disagreements with any department or service. In addition, each floor at Memorial has a specially trained social worker who can help with problems such as housing for patients' families, transportation, and even bill payment.

## Specialties

Anesthesiology, Bone Marrow Transplantation, Brachytherapy, Cardiology, Chemotherapy, Clinical Chemistry, Clinical Immunology, Critical Care Medicine, Dental Service, Dermatology, Endocrinology, Epidemiology, Gastroenterology, Hematology-Lymphoma, Infectious Diseases, Medical Imaging, Medical Physics, Medicine, Neurology, Nuclear Medicine, Nutrition, Pain Service, Pathology, Pediatrics, Psychiatric Service, Pulmonary Medicine, Radiation Oncology, Solid Tumor Service, and Surgery (which offers specialized services for breast cancer, gastric and mixed tumors, gynecology, head and neck cancer, neurosurgery, orthopedics, pediatrics, plastic and reconstructive surgery, rectal and colon surgery, thoracic surgery, and urology).

---

**STATISTICAL PROFILE**

Number of Beds: 565
Bed Occupancy Rate: 89%
Average Number of Patients: 515
Average Patient Stay: 10.6 days
Annual Admissions: 17,322
Outpatient Clinic Visits: 138,023

Hospital Personnel:
  Physicians: 345
  Residents: 104
  Clinical Fellows: 147
  Registered Nurses: 822
  Total Staff: 5,289

---

## Well-known Specialists

Dr. Joseph R. Bertino, medical oncology, head of the Chemotherapy Research Program.

Dr. Murray F. Brennan, specialist in surgical oncology, chairman of the Department of Surgery.

Dr. Alfred M. Cohen, chief of the Rectal and Colon Service.

Dr. William R. Fair, specialist in prostatic cancer, chief of the Urology Service.

Dr. Kathleen M. Foley, chief of Pain Service.

Dr. Zvi Y. Fuks, specialist in radiation oncology, chairman of Radiation Therapy.

Dr. Samuel Hellman, radiation oncology; physician in chief.

Dr. Jimmie C. B. Holland, pioneer in psychiatric oncology, chief of the Psychiatric Service.

Dr. David W. Kinne, surgery; chief of the Breast Cancer Service.

Dr. John Mendelsohn, specialist in medical oncology, chairman of the Department of Medicine.

Dr. Herbert F. Oettgen, chief of clinical immunology.

Dr. Richard J. O'Reilly, chairman of pediatrics, head of the Bone Marrow Transplant Service.

Dr. Jerome Posner, specialist in tumors of the nervous system, chairman of the Department of Neurology.

Dr. Sidney J. Winawer, chief of the Gastroenterology Service.

## Research

Memorial Sloan-Kettering receives about $70 million a year in research funding, making it one of the most heavily endowed institutions in the world. About 130 scientists work directly in research full time as members of the

Sloan-Kettering Institute; in addition virtually all 345 physicians on staff at Memorial Hospital are also engaged in research. Thus, one of the great assets of this cancer center is the interaction between its laboratories and clinical areas, which provides opportunities for immediate application of research findings. For example, clinical trials are under way with immunotherapy agents such as interferons, interleukins, and tumor necrosis factor, which was first discovered at the center. They are now being studied individually and in combination with other agents to determine their maximum therapeutic potential.

Cytodifferentiation agents—simple chemical entities that induce malignant cells to lose their chemical properties—have been under study at the center since 1971. Monoclonal antibodies, specially engineered products that can recognize with great specificity the surface features that distinguish one cell from another, are now being applied as powerful clinical tools for the diagnosis and treatment of cancer. For example, Memorial Sloan-Kettering clinicians have conducted trials on a monoclonal antibody—identified at the center in 1978—directed against melanoma cells. This work is the first evidence of a monoclonal antibody causing major regression of a solid tumor.

## Admission Policy

Anyone who suspects he or she has cancer or has been diagnosed as having cancer should contact Memorial Sloan-Kettering either through his or her physician or by contacting the hospital's Patient Referral Service (212-794-7177). However, not everyone with cancer is assured admittance. We learned that if the patient has been or is being treated elsewhere and the doctors at Memorial determine that the treatment already being received is the best available, the patient may not be admitted here. The same is true for some terminal cases, for whom Memorial is considered less desirable than a hospice or another alternative.

According to the hospital, there is no financial requirement for American citizens (foreign nationals are generally required to pay a deposit). About $11 million a year is allocated for free care.

---

**ROOM CHARGES (per diem)**
Private: $470
Semiprivate: $425

| **MAILING ADDRESS** | **TELEPHONE** |
|---|---|
| 1275 York Avenue | 212-794-7722 or |
| New York, NY 10021 | 212-794-7177 |

# The Mount Sinai Medical Center
**NEW YORK CITY, NEW YORK**

The commonplace observation that everything in New York is done on a slightly larger scale than anywhere else clearly applies to its vast network of hospitals. According to the Greater New York Hospital Association, an average of 60,000 patients are treated daily in New York City. Within the city limits alone there are 31 major teaching hospitals; 18 more are within an hour's drive. Some of these hospitals—St. Luke's/Roosevelt, and Albert Einstein, for example—have nationally famous programs in numerous medical areas, while others—including Bellevue, Kings County, and Harlem Hospital—attempt to offer first-class medicine in the face of socioeconomic problems associated more with certain cities in India than in the center of the world's wealthiest nation.

Of course, in New York the close juxtaposition of wealth and want can be seen everywhere. For the people at The Mount Sinai Medical Center, which exists exactly on the border of upper Fifth Avenue opulence and lower East Harlem poverty, it is a daily fact of life. Perhaps more so these days, since the entire Sinai complex is being rebuilt and modernized at a cost of some $488 million; this is the largest hospital reconstruction project in U.S. history. Slated to be completed in 1991, the new Mount Sinai will be dominated by a ten-story patient-care pavilion designed by I. M. Pei and destined to be both aesthetically and medically extraordinary. Some believe it will be the most up-to-date facility on the East Coast.

Still, that's all in the future, and today some of Mount Sinai's older buildings leave a lot to be desired in terms of patient amenities. We suggest that those contemplating admission here try to determine beforehand what their accommodations will be like. On every other level of patient concern, however, Mount Sinai does extremely well, including patient satisfaction with medical care (87 percent of respondents rated it "excellent" in the latest survey by the hospital). One obvious reason for this is the exceptional nursing staff, 70 percent of whom hold bachelor's degrees; moreover, the screening process for nurses is so rigorous that only one in three applicants is judged qualified. This selectivity reflects the standard of excellence sought in every area of the medical complex, from the highly regarded medical school and the much-sought-after residency program to medical research, in which Mount Sinai holds a preeminent place nationally and internationally.

At first glance Mount Sinai's commitment to research is its most impressive aspect; over 500 physicians and scientists are working in more than 700 programs funded at over $52 million. But for tens of thousands of New Yorkers, Mount Sinai is first and foremost a hospital that offers some of the best medical care available anywhere, a hospital with a long tradition of excellence in medicine and in service to the city.

First opened in 1855 as Jews' Hospital, it was founded by wealthy philanthropists in response to the needs of the ever-increasing number of recently arrived Jewish immigrants. By 1866 the hospital was treating patients of all races and creeds, including many veterans of the Civil War, so the name was changed to Mount Sinai. Over the next half century, the hospital developed a reputation for leadership in medicine. In the 1880s and 1890s, pediatrics was made a separate discipline here, teaching was brought to the hospital bedside, and Tay-Sachs disease (a genetic disease that often affects Jews) was identified.

During this century doctors at Mount Sinai participated in a series of medical breakthroughs, including the pioneering of radiotherapy in 1911, the perfection of blood transfusion techniques in 1915, and the discovery of serum against typhoid fever in 1934 and an influenza vaccine in 1977. Especially strong departments in gastroenterology (Crohn's disease was first identified here), gynecology, and psychiatry have developed over the last fifty years and remain vital elements in the hospital's vast array of medical specialties.

With the exception of heart and liver transplantation, which will be available soon, Mount Sinai offers just about every patient service from neonatology to geriatrics, from expertise in pediatric cardiology to one of the best-known programs in Alzheimer's disease. Some highlights follow.

The care and treatment of cancer patients is one of Mount Sinai's most highly valued services. Over 2,500 new cases are seen here each year, and almost 20 percent of the hospital's discharges are cancer patients. As an NIH-designated Clinical Cancer Center, Mount Sinai provides the most up-to-date forms of treatment. In addition to drugs and radiation, the hospital recently became one of the first to utilize hyperthermia. Not surprisingly, Mount Sinai is the home of one of the most highly regarded oncology research programs in the country.

Mount Sinai is also a leading regional provider of obstetric services, offering diagnostic testing to ensure safe pregnancies, the most advanced fetal-testing techniques, and a complete program for high-risk pregnancies that includes one of the city's best neonatal intensive care units (820 premature babies were born here in 1985, and 30 others were transferred from other hospitals). There is also an active in vitro fertilization program.

In pediatric medicine Mount Sinai has a large number of special programs, including allergy, asthma, cancer, dermatology, gastroenterology, and neurology. The Juvenile Diabetics Unit is well known in the area for its team approach in teaching youngsters how to live with their illness and how to control and understand their blood sugar levels. In recent years the hospital's department of pediatric cardiology has gained recognition for treating infants with heart defects. Mount Sinai is one of only a few hospitals in the country to use a special color-coded echocardiography technique, and cardiologists here have introduced noninvasive procedures for diagnosing infant heart defects.

The Adolescent Health Center has six component programs: an outpatient unit, a family education program, a counseling program for drug-abusing youth, an alternative school, a mental-health counseling program, and a 15-bed inpatient unit. The staff of 34 full-time and 12 part-time workers handles about 500 patient visits a week. Because few teenagers can afford medical treatment at market rates, the center has a sliding fee scale based on the family's income. Counseling for teenagers and their families is free under the Community Youth Program.

The Department of Geriatrics and Adult Development's system of health care for older people includes a clinic, an inpatient unit, a rehabilitation unit, a long-term home health-care program, and a multidisciplinary consultation team. There are special programs for falls and immobility, osteoporosis, psychiatry, and urinary incontinence. This department was ranked first in a list of the best hospital programs for the elderly published in *Good Housekeeping* in 1985.

Through its more than 100 ambulatory care clinics and special programs, Mount Sinai records over 250,000 outpatient visits every year. In addition to the most popular ones—dentistry, obstetrics, otolaryngology, pediatrics, and psychiatry—the hospital has outstanding clinics for patients with ALS, cleft palate, cystic fibrosis, diabetes, myasthenia gravis (with 2,000 patients this is the largest program in the world), osteoporosis, Parkinson's disease, and sickle-cell disease. There is an internationally known Center for Jewish Genetic Diseases that provides diagnosis and treatment to victims of Gaucher's disease and Tay-Sachs disease; genetic counseling is also offered to families seeking to avoid passing these diseases on to the next generation.

The Mount Sinai School of Medicine is one of the country's few medical schools to have been established by a hospital rather than a university. Chartered in 1963 and formally affiliated with the City University of New York in 1967, the school admitted its first students in 1968. Mount Sinai now graduates about 130 students a year.

In addition to its standard program, the medical school, in conjunction with the Graduate Center of the university, offers a Ph.D. program in the biomedical sciences and a combined M.D./Ph.D. program. The medical school has five New York area affiliates: the Beth Israel Medical Center, the Veterans Administration Medical Center in the Bronx, City Hospital Center in Elmhurst, the Jewish Home and Hospital for Aged, and the Joint Diseases North General Hospital.

## Specialties

Allergy, Anesthesiology, Cardiology (Adult and Pediatric), Dentistry, Dermatology, Endocrinology, Gastroenterology, Genetics, Geriatrics, Hematology/Oncology, Internal Medicine, Kidney Transplantation, Neonatology,

Neurology, Neurosurgery, Nuclear Medicine, Obstetrics/Gynecology, Occupational Medicine, Ophthalmology, Orthopedics, Otolaryngology, Pathology, Pediatrics, Physical Medicine and Rehabilitation, Plastic Surgery, Preventive Medicine, Psychiatry, Radiology, Rheumatology, Sports Medicine, Surgery, Thoracic Surgery, and Urology.

---

**STATISTICAL PROFILE**

Number of Beds: 1,112
Bed Occupancy Rate: 84.5%
Average Number of Patients: 940
Average Patient Stay: 10.1 days
Annual Admissions: 33,537
Births: 3,625
Outpatient Clinic Visits: 257,129
Emergency Room/Trauma Center Visits: 48,735

Hospital Personnel:
  Physicians: 1,400
  Residents: 671
  Registered Nurses: 1,535
  Total Staff: 7,000

---

## Well-known Specialists

Dr. Arthur H. Aufses, Jr., chairman of general surgery department.
Dr. Richard L. Berkowitz, specialist in perinatology, chairman of obstetrics/gynecology.
Dr. Edwin Brown, neonatology; director of the neonatal intensive care unit.
Dr. Lewis Burrows, surgery; specialist in kidney transplantation.
Dr. Robert N. Butler, psychiatry; chairman and founder of the geriatrics department.
Dr. Carmel Cohen, gynecology; specialist in cervical cancer.
Dr. Kenneth Davis, psychiatry; director of the Alzheimer's Disease Research Center.
Dr. Fredda Ginsberg-Fellner, specialist in juvenile diabetes.
Dr. Richard Golinko, pediatric cardiology.
Dr. Randall Griepp, chief of cardiothoracic surgery.
Dr. Valentin Fuster, chief of cardiology.
Dr. Kurt Hirschhorn, well-known researcher and clinician in medical genetics, chairman of pediatrics.
Dr. James F. Holland, internationally acclaimed chairman of oncology.

Dr. Roy Jones, oncology.

Dr. Jerome Waye, gastroenterology; specialist in inflammatory bowel disease.

## Research

Since Mount Sinai has one of the most extensive lists of research programs in the country, we cannot hope to describe even a fraction of it. Suffice it to note that virtually all the clinical services here are backed up by some kind of intensive research. Major programs exist in cardiology, dentistry, dermatology, endocrinology, geriatrics, neurology, neurosurgery, obstetrics/gynecology, oncology, orthopedics, otolaryngology, pediatrics, psychiatry, radiotherapy, rehabilitation medicine, surgery, and urology. Special clinical studies in diabetes, hypertension, obesity, and Parkinson's disease, among others, are conducted in the hospital's NIH-funded Clinical Research Center.

In recent years the NIH has also given extensive support to several long-range studies at Mount Sinai Medical School. In 1985 a $5.5-million grant was awarded to the National Alcohol Research Center here, which has been funded by the NIH for the last ten years. Only nine such centers exist in the nation. Mount Sinai's doctors and scientists have demonstrated alcohol's toxic effects on the liver, as well as confirmed the fact that alcoholism is biologically based and not the result of weakness or psychological aberration.

Also in 1985 the National Institute on Aging awarded $3.1 million for Mount Sinai to establish its regional Alzheimer's Disease Research Center. Only a few other institutions were chosen to create such centers.

In oncology the hospital's clinical research is underwritten in large part by the National Cancer Institute and covers the whole spectrum of cancers. The best known (and to some the most controversial) research is conducted by Dr. James Holland, an internationally famous cancer researcher and clinician, who is also chief of oncology. Dr. Holland and his staff have undertaken extensive clinical trials using experimental drugs (including interleukin-2) on specially selected patients. Over 1,300 patients (many of them diagnosed as terminal) have participated in the program. Dr. Holland's work with leukemia patients, begun in 1966, has led to a dramatic increase in survival rates for those with this disease.

## Admission Policy

Patients can be admitted to Mount Sinai in various ways. The majority of admissions are elective, referred either by one of the 150 clinics or by a private physician. Patients can also be admitted directly through the Adult or Pediatric Emergency Room. In addition, there is an active Ambulatory Surgery Program.

Prospective patients wishing office visits with Mount Sinai physicians can either call their offices directly or call a computerized referral service that helps select specialists with offices throughout the New York metropolitan area: 800-MD-SINAI. The service is staffed daily by a registered nurse. (In September of 1987 Mount Sinai opened a separate facility with private offices for 350 physicians, who are available to prospective patients.)

Mount Sinai expects patients to have insurance but will make alternative financial arrangements whenever possible. Despite the hospital's stature as one of New York's premier hospitals, only 85 percent of its patients had some form of medical insurance in 1985. In that year the hospital performed $7.5 million worth of charity care and incurred $9.5 million in bad debts.

---

**ROOM CHARGES (per diem)**
Private: $475–$670
Semiprivate: $410–$415
ICU: $720
Neonatal ICU: $530
Private Maternity: $610–$640
0041Semiprivate Maternity: $375
Nursery: $150

**AVERAGE COST PER PATIENT STAY:**   $651 a day

**MAILING ADDRESS**         **TELEPHONE**
One Gustave Levy Place    212-650-6500
New York, NY 10029

# The Presbyterian Hospital
# Columbia-Presbyterian
# Medical Center

**NEW YORK, NEW YORK**

Many doctors around the country consider Presbyterian New York's foremost hospital. Given the kinds of medical services offered here, this should not be surprising. Presbyterian is, for example, the leading organ transplant center in the Northeast, a federally designated Comprehensive Cancer Center, and the site of the largest stroke patient caseload in the world. Over 35 percent of the people hospitalized here come from outside New York City. As the principal teaching hospital of one of the country's oldest and most prestigious medical schools, Presbyterian offers highly specialized care based on the most up-to-date research in almost every area of medical science. Presbyterian receives more outside funding for research than all but three other medical schools.

To the people of New York and its environs, however, Presbyterian is much more than a highly prestigious academic center—it is an indispensable community resource. Over the last decade the medical center has reached out to the surrounding community with a wide range of primary and specialty care programs, including family planning, education about and treatment of lead poisoning among children, and treatment for a wide range of psychiatric disorders. It is also constructing a 300-bed community hospital and a network of doctors' offices to help alleviate a desperate shortage of inpatient and primary-care treatment facilities caused by the closing of five local hospitals in the last fifteen years.

Community service and tertiary-care medicine aren't often seen in such stark juxtaposition, but Presbyterian's success demonstrates that they can be combined. A staggering 780,000 patient visits have been recorded here each year, most in doctors' private offices and in the vast array of clinics and centers available to anyone needing care.

The Presbyterian Hospital is actually a corporate title that includes not only Presbyterian Hospital itself but also The New York Orthopaedic Hospital, Babies Hospital, Sloane Hospital for Women, The Edward Harkness Eye Institute, The Squier Urological Clinic, and the world-famous Neurological Institute.

Neurology has been one of the most important specialties of Presbyterian for almost eighty years. Renowned for its work in child neurology, epilepsy, neuromuscular disease, and strokes, the medical center is today the world headquarters for the Parkinson's Disease Foundation and one of four major sites participating in the Stroke Data Bank Study funded by the NIH. Surgery

**215**

for stroke victims, a vital part of the comprehensive program here, is performed by the department of neurological surgery, which is also highly regarded in all areas of neurosurgery, including brain tumors and arteriovenous malformations.

Cardiology is another department with a long and distinguished history, which includes a Nobel Prize for medicine and credit for developing many of the techniques used in the treatment of heart disease. Today, for example, the Arrhythmia Control Center is regarded as one of the most sophisticated programs of its kind. Other services include open-heart surgery (739 were performed in 1985) and pacemaker evaluation and insertion, as well as cardiac imaging and mapping.

Given this history, it was a natural step for Presbyterian to become one of the nation's most highly respected centers for heart transplantation. Over 120 transplants have taken place here since the late 1970s, with an ever-increasing success rate and the lowest infection rate of any hospital doing cardiac transplants. Presbyterian is also a recognized leader in heart transplantation for children.

The success of the heart transplant program tends to overshadow the medical center's impressive kidney transplant program, which has been in place for over twenty years. More than 50 kidney transplants are performed here annually, and well over 90 percent of the transplanted kidneys are still functioning after five years. Heart-lung and liver transplant programs are in the final stages of preparation.

The diagnosis and treatment of cancer is another area in which Presbyterian has achieved special status. As a federally designated Comprehensive Cancer Center, the medical center is equipped to provide the latest treatments for almost every kind of cancer, including Hodgkin's disease and melanoma. The newly formed Radiation Oncology Department offers access to the most up-to-date forms of radiation therapy, in conjunction with a full range of medical and surgical options. Federal funds also support research in cancer. In recent years, for example, new tests to detect and/or treat breast cancer and lymphoma were developed here. Each year over 2,000 new cancer patients come to Presbyterian, making this one of the largest cancer centers in the region.

Obstetrics/gynecology and pediatrics also have long and distinguished histories here. Both Sloane Hospital for Women and Babies Hospital were founded in the late 1880s and became part of Presbyterian sixty years ago. Today the High Risk Pregnancy Program and the Perinatal Center serve as important referral centers for the tristate area of New York, New Jersey, and Connecticut. The neonatal intensive care unit has an outstanding national reputation; in a study of 12 such units in academic medical centers, Presbyterian was ranked first. Approximately 95 percent of two- to three-pound babies treated here survive and, consequently, hundreds of women with difficult pregnancies come to the medical center every year.

Other programs for women range from in vitro fertilization to a newly formed menopause clinic, while in pediatrics the entire gamut of major childhood diseases—asthma, cystic fibrosis, and juvenile diabetes, to name a few—are treated here. There are also special programs for children with arthritis, cancer, heart disease, liver disease, and sickle-cell anemia, among many others.

Other major specialties at Presbyterian include ophthalmology, orthopedics, psychiatry, and surgery.

Having said all these remarkable things about this clearly outstanding institution, we must point out that the hospital spokesperson had no meaningful response to our questions about satisfaction among former patients. The hospital has not, as of this writing, commissioned a formal survey of patient satisfaction.

On the other hand, from what we could find out about the nursing staff, the quality of care appears to be quite good. Most of the nurses are educated at the bachelor's level or beyond, and, in the ambulatory care, critical care, and emergency services departments, prior experience is a requirement. Critical-care nurses receive extensive training here, including special supervised work in areas such as cardiology, general surgery, neonatology, neurology, and neurosurgery.

One final note. By 1988 construction of a 745-bed replacement facility as well as thorough renovation and upgrading of the existing buildings on the medical center campus should be completed.

## Specialties

Allergy, Anesthesiology, Cardiology (Adult and Pediatric), Dentistry, Dermatology, Endocrinology, Gastroenterology, Geriatrics, Hematology, Immunology, Infectious Diseases, Medical Genetics, Nephrology, Neurological Surgery, Neurology, Obstetrics/Gynecology, Oncology, Organ Transplantation, Ophthalmology, Orthopedic Surgery, Otolaryngology, Pathology, Pediatrics, Plastic and Reconstructive Surgery, Psychiatry, Radiation Oncology, Radiology, Rehabilitation Medicine, Rheumatology, Surgery, Urology, and Vascular Surgery.

There are special clinics for adult psychiatry, ambulatory chemotherapy, anorexia nervosa, anxiety, arrhythmia control, brain tumors, cocaine abuse, colorectal cancer laser treatment, Cooley's anemia, corneal disorders, corneal transplants, depression evaluation, dystonia clinical research, eating disorders, eye day surgery, family planning, genetic counseling, geriatric care, glaucoma treatment, gynecologic cancer, headaches, infertility, kidney stones, lead poisoning, lithium, lupus, multiple sclerosis, oral surgery, the Pacemaker Program, pain management, pediatric rheumatology, prosthetics, psoriasis, retinoblastoma, sickle-cell anemia, sleep disorders, and stroke rehabilitation.

---

**STATISTICAL PROFILE**

Number of Beds: 1,291
Bed Occupancy Rate: 88%
Average Number of Patients: 1,136
Average Patient Stay: 9.2 days
Annual Admissions: 44,319
Births: 4,363
Outpatient Clinic Visits: 338,800, with an additional 278,000 in
    doctors' offices
Emergency Room/Trauma Center Visits: 120,000

Hospital Personnel:
    Physicians: 1,171
    Residents: 398
    Registered Nurses: 1,200
    Total Staff: 6,600

---

# Well-known Specialists

Dr. Maxwell Abramson, director of otolaryngology.
Dr. R. Peter Altman, director of pediatric surgery.
Dr. Arthur D. Bloom, pediatrics; director of clinical genetics.
Dr. Frederick O. Bowman, Jr., director of cardiac surgery.
Dr. Charles J. Campbell, ophthalmology.
Dr. James D. Cox, director of radiation oncology.
Dr. Darryl DeVivo, pediatric neurology.
Dr. Harold Dick, director of orthopedic surgery.
Dr. Nas Eftekhar, specialist in hip and joint replacement.
Dr. Robert Glickman, gastroenterology.
Dr. Leonard Harber, specialist in photosensitive disorders, director of dermatology.
Dr. Mark Hardy, surgery; director of organ transplantation.
Dr. Donald A. Holub, medicine and endocrinology.
Dr. L. Stanley James, pediatrics.
Dr. John K. Latimer, urology.
Dr. Francis A. L'Esperance, ophthalmology.
Dr. James R. Malm, cardiac surgery; specialist in pediatric as well as adult heart surgery.
Dr. Jay Mohr, neurology; director of stroke center.
Dr. Charles S. Neer II, specialist in shoulder and elbow repair.
Dr. Harold Neu, specialist in infectious diseases.

Dr. Carl Olsson, urology; specialist in prostate and bladder cancer.

Dr. Herbert Pardes, director of psychiatry, former director of the NIH.

Dr. Keith Reemtsma, specialist in cardiac surgery, especially heart transplantation, director of surgery.

Dr. Eric Rose, director of cardiac transplantation.

Dr. Mortimer G. Rosen, director of obstetrics/gynecology.

Dr. Lewis P. Rowland, director of neurology.

Dr. Bennett M. Stein, director of the department of neurosurgery.

Dr. Frank E. Stinchfield, orthopedic surgery.

Dr. I. Bernard Weinstein, director of the Comprehensive Cancer Center.

# Research

Since the turn of the century, Presbyterian's physicians and scientists have made many contributions to the development of modern medicine. Beginning with the invention of the oxygen tent in 1910 and the founding of one of the first cancer research institutes in 1911 and continuing through the discovery of the first serum therapy for bacterial meningitis in 1938 and the development of standard medical practices such as the Apgar test for newborns, the amniocentesis procedure for detecting genetic defects in a fetus (first done here in 1959), and L-dopa treatment for victims of Parkinson's disease, the tradition of clinical research here has solid roots. In 1956 the Nobel Prize in medicine was awarded to two Presbyterian physicians for their studies of the heart's interior and for their demonstration of a practical method for using a catheter to diagnose heart conditions. Today, of course, cardiac catheterization is used worldwide.

The depth of commitment to medical research can be seen in several simple facts: in 1985 alone physicians and scientists here published almost 2,500 articles; they received over $90 million in research grants. Just a bare outline of the research programs would take several pages, so we've confined ourselves to some of the best known.

In pediatrics the medical center has heavily funded studies of cystic fibrosis and sickle-cell and Cooley's anemia. In pediatric cardiology a joint effort with General Electric Company is developing noninvasive techniques for the diagnosis of congenital heart disease.

In adult cardiology there are two nationally famous research programs, one for arrhythmia, the other for atherosclerosis; the latter is one of only eight special research centers in the country funded by the NIH. Because of its expertise in heart disease, the medical center was also selected as a site for a national study of TPA (tissue plasminogen activator), a new clot-dissolving drug.

Important programs exist in every major department. In neurology continuing studies of ALS, Alzheimer's disease, muscular dystrophy, and myasthenia gravis keep Presbyterian in the forefront of research in these areas. In ophthalmology clinical research programs study everything from optic nerve disease to the risks and complications of extended-wear contact lenses. In neurosurgery physicians have established a new program for the biopsy of deep cerebral tumors, and they participated in a national study of cerebral bypass surgery. In urology the National Institute of Child Health and Human Development is currently funding a study of the causes of male infertility, while the National Cancer Institute is supporting research into prostate cancer.

Since the medical center is a Comprehensive Cancer Center, oncology research is extensive and includes almost every medical department. The center recently received a $1-million grant from the American Cancer Society to continue its investigations into the causes and prevention of cancer. The new Department of Radiation Oncology continues the far-reaching work of radiological researchers, who receive over $3 million annually for basic and clinical research. New kinds of radiation treatment, new radiosensitized drugs, and combinations of radiation and chemotherapy are being investigated, with particular emphasis on cancers of the brain, lung, prostate, and upper aerodigestive tract.

There are two NIH-funded Clinical Research Centers here as well, one adult and one pediatric. Their studies include investigations of ways to improve the diagnosis and treatment of cardiac arrhythmia, new therapies for parkinsonism, and the relation of so-called Type A behavior and coronary heart disease. Sleep disorders, male infertility, and psoriasis are some of the other adult subjects being studied here; infant nutrition and sudden infant death syndrome are under investigation in the pediatric unit.

## Admission Policy

Admission to all the facilities that make up Presbyterian Hospital can be arranged through the patient's own physician. (The referral number for doctors to call is 212-305-5222 or 800-247-CPMC for those in New York, 800-227-CPMC for out-of-state doctors.) Patients can also call the hospital directly at the general number and make an appointment to be seen by one of the doctors.

Although officially there is a financial requirement for admission for elective procedures, the hospital rarely turns away anyone needing care; in 1985 it provided $12 million worth of indigent care.

**ROOM CHARGES** (per diem)
Private: $440–$740
Semiprivate: $415
ICU: $1,000–$1,200

**AVERAGE COST PER PATIENT STAY:**    $4,887

**MAILING ADDRESS**              **TELEPHONE**
New York, NY 10032-3784    212-305-5156

# The Rockefeller University Hospital

**NEW YORK, NEW YORK**

The Rockefeller University Hospital is a clinical research center offering the most modern and complete medical care available, at no charge, to patients with conditions under study at the hospital.

The hospital is staffed by full-time, salaried research physicians working in their own laboratories and at the bedside but also in collaboration with the university's other basic scientists. Opened in 1910, the hospital of what was then called The Rockefeller Institute for Medical Research (founded in 1901) was the first clinical research center in the country where human disease was studied in a setting of rigorous, scientific inquiry. In the 1950s the hospital served as a model for the Magnuson Clinical Center of the NIH (see page 127). Similar facilities established with federal funding at more than 80 medical schools were also modeled on the university's hospital. While supported in part as an NIH General Clinical Research Center, The Rockefeller University Hospital is the only facility in the United States exclusively devoted to clinical research that is sustained in large part by private resources.

According to Dr. Attallah Kappas, vice-president and physician in chief, "We follow our patients as long as our studies require and, beyond that, as long as is necessary to assure a continuity of good clinical care. But clinical care per se is not the primary function of this hospital. The raison d'être for this hospital is to make discoveries in medical science that permit other clinicians to carry on more effective programs of prevention and treatment of disease."

Scientists at institutions all over the world are well aware of the research achievements of Rockefeller University faculty members. One prominent biologist, Robert Morison, recently a visiting professor at MIT, has said, "Although it is difficult to measure such things . . . the output of really significant high-quality research per person, per dollar, or per square foot at Rockefeller has been higher than that of any other medical research institute in the country."

Besides its clinical and research responsibilities, the hospital plays a major role in preparing M.D.'s to become accomplished laboratory scientists; the physicians here are supported during their postdoctoral training through the hospital's privately funded clinical scholars program.

The faculty at the university includes 600 members, of which approximately 100 have Rockefeller Hospital appointments. A survey published recently by the National Academy of Sciences rated the Rockefeller faculty among the nation's five most distinguished in biochemistry, cellular/molecular biology, microbiology, and physiology.

The Rockefeller University educational program for medical research is unusual in several aspects. Faculty generally outnumber students by a ratio of at least two to one. The laboratory—not the classroom—is the principal site of learning. And the program has no formal departments and virtually no prescribed curriculum.

Encouraged to plan their own courses of study, students must fulfill only two major program requirements. They must demonstrate competence in three broad scientific areas of their own choosing, and they must complete a doctoral thesis based on significant investigation conducted under the supervision of a faculty member. Students present their doctoral theses at lectures open to the scientific community and the public.

The university's highly selective graduate program rarely admits more than 20 students a year. Enrollment is limited to approximately 125 students, including a small group in the Rockefeller University—Cornell University Medical College joint M.D./Ph.D program integrating scientific and medical interests that was launched in 1972. By 1984 the university had graduated nearly 450 men and women. Approximately 95 percent of these graduates are engaged in full-time research and teaching at academic, corporate, and governmental organizations. Two have won Nobel Prizes. Nearly 100 are full professors, six hold endowed chairs, and 30 head departments or research programs at leading institutions in the United States and abroad.

Rockefeller patients are drawn not only from the New York metropolitan area but from all over the world.

---

**STATISTICAL PROFILE**

Number of Beds: 40
Bed Occupancy Rate: 100%
Average Number of Patients: 40
Average Patient Stay: varies with study
Annual Admissions: 500
Outpatient Clinic Visits: 5,000

Hospital Personnel:
   Physicians: 100
   Registered Nurses: 15
   Total Staff: 181

---

## Specialties

The hospital has inherited the flexibility of organization unique to Rockefeller University. There are no conventional hospital departments, and laboratory programs tend to be defined in terms of scientific disciplines. They span fields such as biochemistry, dermatology, endocrinology, immunology, metabolism, microbiology, and pharmacology.

Conditions currently under investigation, among more than 40 discrete clinical entities, include coronary and peripheral vascular insufficiency, endocrine-related cancers, gastrointestinal disorders, chronic active hepatitis, immune deficiency, lupus, lymphatic leukemia, multiple sclerosis, poisonings from metals and environmental chemicals, the genetic acquired porphyrias, reproductive disorders, acute rheumatic fever, rheumatoid arthritis, and skin cancers and other cutaneous diseases, as well as problems of alcoholism, diabetes mellitus, jaundice, obesity, and sickle-cell disease.

## Well-known Specialists

Dr. Jan Breslow, pediatrics and biochemistry; currently a researcher on cholesterol.

Dr. D. Martin Carter, dermatology.

Dr. Christian de Duve, biochemical cytology; Nobel laureate who discovered lysosomes, the subcellular particles that function as the digestive system of the cell.

Dr. Vincent P. Dole, researcher on methadone treatment and the causes of alcoholism in conjunction with his wife, Dr. Marie Nyswander, psychiatrist.

Dr. Gerald Edelman, Nobel laureate who deciphered the structure of the key molecule of immunity.

Dr. Emil C. Gotschlich, bacteriology and immunology; researcher who helped develop meningitis vaccines.

Dr. Hidesaburo Hanafusa, viral oncology.

Dr. Attallah Kappas, authority on liver and metabolic disease, biochemical and clinical pharmacology, and environmental medicine, vice-president and physician in chief.

Dr. Joshua Lederberg, president of the university, Nobel laureate who elucidated the organization of genetic material in bacteria.

Dr. Torsten N. Wiesel, head of the Laboratory of Neurobiology, Nobel laureate who advanced understanding of how the brain processes visual information.

## Research

The nature of basic research and the unusual structure of Rockefeller University make it difficult to categorize campus research groups. Many if not most scientific and medical problems span a number of scientific disciplines. Scientists in a single laboratory often have expertise in varied fields, and investigators in different laboratories often collaborate.

Broadly speaking, ten Rockefeller laboratories are currently devoted primarily to clinical research within the hospital, while some 45 others conduct basic research spanning a wide range of fields, including biochemistry, cell biology, molecular biology, the neurosciences, molecular parasitology, physics, plant biology, and virology.

More than 15 laboratories are conducting investigations relevant to determining the causes and nature of cancer. Other research is being done on aging, atherosclerosis, chemical metabolism, dermatology, diabetes mellitus, genetic and metabolic diseases such as porphyrias, heart disease, immunology, microbiology, reproduction, and tyrosinemia.

## Admission Policy

Patients are virtually always referred to The Rockefeller University Hospital by a physician. The hospital mails to 30,000 physicians a list of conditions under study by its clinical staff. Patients who have the listed conditions may be referred by their physicians for possible admission.

For general information regarding patient referral, physicians can call the program director at 212-570-8521.

---

**ROOM CHARGES** (per diem)
Care is provided throughout the study period without charge to the patient. When a patient is discharged, a report of all findings is sent to the referring physician.

**MAILING ADDRESS**            **TELEPHONE**
1230 York Avenue              212-570-8000
New York, NY 10021-6399

---

# Strong Memorial Hospital University of Rochester

**ROCHESTER, NEW YORK**

Strong Memorial Hospital is the primary teaching hospital for the University of Rochester Schools of Medicine and Dentistry and of Nursing and serves as a regional referral center for the ten-county area of western New York between Rochester and the Pennsylvania border. One of the most respected hospitals in the Northeast, Strong is particularly well regarded by its former patients—as demonstrated in a 1985 patients' survey conducted by the hospital. Over 96 percent of all respondents would return to Strong if they required hospitalization in the future.

Strong provides special care to severely burned patients in a nine-bed unit equipped with a hydrotherapy tub room and an operating room. The Burn Unit coordinates the services of medical, nursing, surgical, physical and occupational therapy, and psychiatric staff.

The Pediatric Intensive Care Unit is the only one of its kind in central western New York State. A six-bed unit, it provides around-the-clock care for critically ill infants, young children, and teenagers. The Special Care Nursery, which provides neonatal intensive care, is divided into three sections: a 12-bassinet neonatal intensive-care section, an 8-bassinet "suspect" section for babies suspected of having a contagious disease or infection, and a 20-bassinet section for premature babies.

Strong's specialized Pediatrics Services also include the region's Birth Defects Center, pediatric cardiology, a cystic fibrosis program, pediatric gastrointestinal nutrition, genetics, infectious diseases, pediatric neurology, sudden infant death syndrome, and the Rochester Adolescent Maternity Program. The Adolescent Medicine Unit offers a variety of services geared to teenagers and has a special interest in treating eating disorders, such as anorexia nervosa and bulimia. Each pediatric unit contains a playroom, and a special classroom on the pediatric floor allows patients away from school for extended lengths of time to keep up with their education.

Strong's department of psychiatry is well known. The newly renovated facility here houses the department's outpatient clinics, treatment areas, research laboratories, faculty and staff offices, and inpatient care units. Services are designed to respond to every kind of mental-health-care need and to function in close association with the other medical center departments nearby. Outpatient services include the Alzheimer's Disease and Memory Disorders Clinic, the Child and Adolescent Psychiatry Clinic, the Family and Marriage Clinic, the Methadone Maintenance Treatment Program, the Stress Clinic, and the Tourette Syndrome Clinic. The department also houses the offices and facilities of the Pain Treatment Center, the area's only comprehensive pain facility, which treats chronic pain from a multidisciplinary approach. The Alcoholism and Alcohol Abuse Program is certified as an outpatient clinic by the New York State Division of Alcoholism.

Two adult intensive care units, each divided into four sections, provide facilities for coronary and respiratory patients and others requiring complex and closely monitored care.

Occupational and physical therapy facilities in the 20-bed rehabilitation unit represent a major expansion for Strong. Patient rooms here are larger, three are equipped with hoists to move paralyzed patients, and corridors and rooms alike are designed to allow for wheelchairs and other large equipment used in rehabilitation. Strong and the University of Rochester Medical Center have been designated by the U.S. Department of Education as one of fewer than 20 Spinal Cord Injury Centers in the country.

Strong's Ambulatory Surgical Center has accommodations for 24 patients. A wide variety of medical and surgical procedures are performed here, including blood transfusions, chemotherapy, pacemaker battery replacements, and X-ray studies.

The Magnetic Resonance Center is sponsored jointly by Strong, Genesee Hospital, and Rochester General Hospital, under the aegis of the New York State Department of Health; it makes magnetic resonance imaging available to the population of Rochester and the surrounding ten counties.

The Strong Heart Program at the University of Rochester Medical Center is a unique preventive service that utilizes the skills of a heart specialist, behavioral psychologist, nurse practitioner, and nutritionist to identify people at risk for cardiovascular disease. This program seeks to help high-risk individuals cope with stress, quit smoking, and develop exercise and nutrition programs. After a physical examination and laboratory test, the patient's heart attack risk profile is assessed. The Cardiac Rehabilitation Program works with people who have undergone heart surgery or have heart disease in an effort to improve their heart function and fitness level. It utilizes state-of-the-art monitoring techniques and the latest knowledge in exercise and patient education and encourages participation by the patient's family.

Strong was the first hospital in upstate New York to begin using a lithotriptor to treat patients suffering from kidney stones. Operated under the auspices of the Department of Urology, the lithotriptor is part of Strong's Kidney Stone Treatment Center. Also under the auspices of the Department of Urology is Strong's Sperm Bank and Andrology Program, which provides a variety of services, including artificial insemination and sperm testing and analysis.

The Department of Obstetrics and Gynecology supervises the region's only in vitro fertilization program, which is open to married couples from throughout New York State.

Established in 1920, the University of Rochester School of Medicine and Dentistry offers programs leading to the M.D. degree and to the M.S. and Ph.D. degrees in basic biomedical science. The School of Nursing became an independent school of the university in 1972, after almost fifty years as a department within the medical school. The school offers programs of study leading to the B.S., M.S., and Ph.D. degrees in nursing as well as a post-doctoral clinical scholars program.

The Office of Continuing Professional Education is a clearinghouse of information for more than 4,000 physicians in upstate New York; it provides a catalog of regularly scheduled education programs available at the medical center and its affiliated hospitals.

## Specialties

Medical services at Strong cover a wide spectrum of specialties, the best known being Emergency Care, Oncology, Orthopedics, Pediatrics, and Psychiatry.

The University of Rochester Cancer Center includes special departments in gynecologic oncology, medical oncology, nursing oncology, pediatric hematology/oncology, psychosocial oncology, and radiation oncology.

Other special programs include kidney transplantation, diabetes self-management, the Strong Heart and Cardiac Rehabilitation programs, the dialysis unit, medical and surgical intensive care units, a pediatric intensive care unit, neonatal intensive care, long-term care, a burn unit, and in vitro fertilization. Specialties within the Department of Orthopedics include the Regional Spinal Cord Injury Center, sports medicine, joint replacement and hand surgery, and a comprehensive musculoskeletal program.

The psychiatry specialties include an affective disorders program, an alcoholism and substance abuse program, a behavioral and psychosocial med-

---

**STATISTICAL PROFILE**

Number of Beds: 741
Bed Occupancy Rate: 86%
Average Number of Patients: 650
Average Patient Stay: 9 days
Annual Admissions: 26,987
Births: 3,218
Outpatient Clinic Visits: 132,555
Emergency Room/Trauma Center Visits: 36,967

Hospital Personnel:
  Physicians: 1,028
  Residents: 273
  Registered Nurses: 1,500
  Total Staff: 4,802

icine program, a child and adolescent program, a community and preventive unit, emergency services, general adult ambulatory care (groups, family, geriatric, and adult), general inpatient care, neuropsychiatry, and a partial hospitalization program.

## Well-known Specialists

Dr. John Baum, rheumatology.
Dr. Abraham T. K. Cockett, urology.
Dr. John J. Condemi, allergy.
Dr. Richard B. Freeman, nephrology.
Dr. Robert C. Griggs, neurology.
Dr. Robert M. Herndon, neurology; specialist in brain research.
Dr. Robert J. Joynt, neurology.
Dr. Philip Rubin, radiation oncology.
Dr. Seymour I. Schwartz, gastrointestinal surgery.
Dr. Paul N. Yu, cardiology.

## Research

Doctors and scientists at Strong Memorial Hospital and the University of Rochester's School of Medicine work closely in all areas of medical research. Together, these institutions receive almost $45 million a year in research funding, 90 percent of it from federal sources. The Cancer Center alone receives over $2 million annually, and the Clinical Research Center over $1 million from NIH. The research staff also participates in several other national programs funded by NIH, including the well-publicized projects for AIDS and Alzheimer's disease. Other major research programs that reflect some of the hospital's most important clinical services are studies of eating disorders, multiple sclerosis, schizophrenia, spinal cord injuries, and the transplantation drug cyclosporine.

In recent years the research programs at Rochester have achieved some very promising results in several areas. A long-term study of cystic fibrosis, for example, led to the recognition of a genetic marker in adults that can be identified and which might discourage couples from having children who are bound to develop this disease. Several potentially important drugs are being developed and tested here, including surfactant, which relieves respiratory distress syndrome in premature infants, and rimantadine, which is used to prevent the flu and as a very effective treatment for those already infected.

Several very interesting experimental research projects here are still in the animal model stage. The most promising appears to be the brain cell transplantation program, in which Parkinson's disease has actually been reversed in monkeys.

# Admission Policy

Patients may be admitted to Strong through a clinic, the emergency room, or physician referral.

There is no financial requirement for admission.

---

**ROOM CHARGES (per diem)**
Private: $241
Semiprivate: $200
ICU: $500

**MAILING ADDRESS**       **TELEPHONE**
601 Elmwood Avenue       716-275-2644
Rochester, NY 14642

---

# University Hospital
# New York University Medical Center
**NEW YORK, NEW YORK**

In a city well known for self-promotion and self-congratulations, it's strange to discover that the hospitals in New York, even those with world-class reputations, keep low profiles. Unlike hospitals in other parts of the country, New York hospitals do little advertising to the general public. Consequently, the availability of specialized, hard-to-find medical services is made known through an informal network of physicians and hospital professionals. This may help explain why University Hospital at New York University (NYU) Medical Center, virtually unknown outside New York City except among doctors, is consistently filled almost to capacity. In fact, the hospital's occupancy rate has been over 90 percent for several years running, a nearly unheard of statistic for the average private hospital.

But University Hospital is not an average facility—it is the flagship hospital of a medical enterprise that includes one of the nation's best municipal hospitals (Bellevue) and one of the leading medical schools in the world. Since the faculty of the NYU School of Medicine serves as the medical staff of University Hospital, it's not surprising that people come here from all over the metropolitan area and, for some of the more specialized services, from around the nation and overseas.

What they find here, in addition to a group of highly regarded physicians, is a modern facility equipped with every technological device available, and a nursing staff that is among the most stringently screened in the country. Over 70 percent of the nurses here have bachelor's degrees. Not one negative comment has been made about the nursing staff either in the state inspection process or by the Joint Commission on the Accreditation of Hospitals.

Patients can come to University Hospital for treatment of almost every kind of illness (organ transplantation is not yet offered, although application for approval has been filed with the state). The hospital has achieved national recognition in specialties including dermatology, geriatrics, pediatric neurosurgery (which has its own division), otolaryngology (this is one of the few hospitals performing multichannel cochlear implants), and rheumatology. University Hospital is also a regional center for the study and treatment of heart disease, and over 1,000 open-heart procedures are performed here each year. In addition, over 2,000 births take place here annually, many of them the result of high-risk pregnancies.

Some of the best known services at University Hospital are available on an outpatient basis. The Day Surgery Unit, for example, the first ambulatory surgical unit on the East Coast, offers elective surgery for more than 200 procedures without requiring an overnight hospital stay. Approximately 4,066 patients were seen here in 1985. (The phone number is 212-340-7213.)

The Institute for Reconstructive Plastic Surgery treats problems ranging from aesthetic (cosmetic) surgery to severe deformities resulting from the cancer-related removal of large areas of tissue and bone (breast reconstruction, for example) and posttraumatic problems of injuries and burns. The Variety Center for Craniofacial Rehabilitation, located in this institute, treats severe congenital facial deformities (for instance, cleft palate) and other disorders. Specialists at the institute also do microsurgery and reconstructive surgery of the hand. Patients are seen by appointment only. (The phone number is 212-340-5834.)

The Harris Skin and Cancer Pavilion offers outpatient clinics for the diagnosis and treatment of skin conditions ranging from acne, hair loss, and psoriasis to more serious disorders, such as skin cancer. The medical center's department of dermatology, which staffs this clinic, is the oldest such department in the nation and is internationally renowned for advances in research in and treatment of skin cancer. (The phone number is 212-340-5245.)

The care and treatment of cancer victims is a major service at University Hospital, and almost 2,000 new cancer patients are admitted every year. Funded by the National Cancer Institute, the Kaplan Cancer Center offers the most up-to-date clinical services, including chemotherapy, hormonal therapy, radiation therapy, and surgery. According to the hospital, NYU physicians are best known for treating breast cancer, cancers in children, lung cancer, ovarian cancer, and skin cancer. Melanoma is the subject of an internationally recognized program that has treated the largest number of patients in the world while developing new surgical and medical procedures for this disease.

Cancer patients have access to two of NYU's most important services, the innovative Cooperative Care Unit and the world-famous Rusk Institute of Rehabilitation Medicine. Although these facilities handle patients with all kinds of illnesses, their services are particularly beneficial to cancer patients.

The Cooperative Care Unit (called Co-op) was created in 1979 to provide cost-effective health care in a more humane hospital environment in which families can play an active role in the patient's care. This "wellness environment" is best described as a cross between a traditional acute-care hospital and an ambulatory facility. Criteria for admission and continued stay in Co-op are identical to those of a traditional acute-care hospital except that a patient must not require constant nursing observation and must be able to move independently or with the aid of crutches, a walker, or a wheelchair. Patients either enter the unit directly (for example, for chemotherapy or for an invasive diagnostic procedure such as cardiac catheterization) or they are transferred from other wings of the hospital.

Central to the co-op care approach is the care partner, usually a relative or close friend, who lives with the patient between four and twenty-four hours a day as needed but pays nothing for room and board. The care partner is trained by the hospital staff to provide many of the services traditionally handled by nurses.

The environment of Co-op Care differs from that of a traditional hospital. Patient rooms contain pairs of twin beds (rather than steel-framed hospital beds), bathrooms are unencumbered by regulation hospital paraphernalia, and meals are served in a communal dining room, located on a separate floor near a lounge and recreational area. Nursing stations are also on a separate floor, along with an educational center and treatment rooms.

As closely as possible, the Co-op environment simulates the situation the patient will encounter upon leaving the hospital; visiting is unrestricted, patients wear street clothes, and patients themselves are responsible for maintaining the medication prescribed by their physician. Visits with physicians are by appointment, not interruption. The education center provides patients, care partners, and families with tapes and materials explaining the illness, treatment, and follow-up; and trained staff are available to meet with family members.

Co-op Care has been remarkably cost effective; the average patient bill in this unit is 40 to 45 percent less than that for a similar stay in the traditional hospital environment. In addition, the co-op care approach has been shown to foster better patient compliance with the prescribed medical regimen. The program has become a model for an increasing number of health-care institutions.

The Rusk Institute is the world's largest university-affiliated center for treating and training disabled adults and children. As an outpatient facility it records over 5,000 patient visits a year. Established in 1948 as the first facility of its kind by Howard H. Rusk (considered the father of rehabilitation medicine), the institute treats patients referred from all over the world. The Jerry Lewis Center for Neuromuscular Diseases, which treats patients suffering from 40 different neuromuscular diseases, is part of the institute.

Treatment at Rusk is based on the team approach, involving specialists in physiatry, physical therapy, psychology, occupational therapy, social services, speech pathology, and vocational rehabilitation, all working in conjunction with medical specialists in other divisions of the medical center. The total-care approach takes into consideration the psychological aspects of rehabilitation and the patient's vocational requirements. Rusk has pioneered the development of support services, including a breast cancer support group that has become the model for such groups and the Cancer Rehabilitation Service, which provides continuity of care and support for cancer patients and their families during all phases of treatment. This service is available both to cancer patients of the medical center and by referral.

## Specialties

Allergy/Immunology, Anesthesiology, Cardiology, Dermatology, Diagnostic Radiology, Emergency Medicine, Endocrinology, Family Practice, Gastroenterology, Hematology, Infectious Diseases, Internal Medicine, Nephrology, Neurological Surgery and Pediatric Neurosurgery, Oncology, Orthopedic Surgery, Otolaryngology (includes Otology and Plastic and Reconstructive Surgery), Pathology, Pediatrics, Physical Medicine and Rehabilitation, Plastic Surgery (includes Craniofacial Surgery, Hand Surgery, and Microsurgery), Preventive Medicine, Psychiatry, Pulmonary Diseases, Rheumatology, Sports Medicine, Surgery, Therapeutic Radiology, Thoracic Surgery, Urology, and Vascular Surgery.

Dental specialties and subspecialties include Dental Anesthesiology, General Practice Dentistry, and Oral Surgery.

---

**STATISTICAL PROFILE**

|  | University Hospital | Rusk |
|---|---|---|
| Number of Beds: | 726 | 152 |
| Bed Occupancy Rate: | 92% | 95% |
| Average Number of Patients: | 668 | 144 |
| Average Patient Stay: | 9 days | 50 days |

Annual Admissions:   approximately 25,000 for both hospitals
Births:   19,722
Outpatient Clinic Visits:   2,300 for both hospitals
Emergency Room/Trauma
   Center Visits:   21,441 for both hospitals

Hospital Personnel:
   Physicians: 1,235
   Residents: 687
   Registered Nurses: 1,150
   Total Staff: 7,528 plus 3,264 volunteers

---

## Well-known Specialists

Dr. Alejandro Berenstein, specialist in embolization, developer of a nonsurgical procedure to treat certain vascular disorders, professor of radiology.

Dr. Jean-Claude Bystryn, director of the Melanoma Research Program, professor of dermatology.

Dr. Noel Cohen, specialist in multichannel cochlear implants, professor and chairman of the department of otolaryngology.

Dr. Eugenia Doyle, pediatric cardiology; professor of pediatrics.

Dr. Fred J. Epstein, pioneer in developing a procedure for removing tumors from the spinal cords of children and infants, director of the division of pediatric neurosurgery.

Dr. Eugene Flamm, professor of neurosurgery, director of the spinal cord injury project.

Dr. Alvin Friedman-Kien, conductor of clinical studies using interferon to treat genital warts and herpes, specialist in the treatment of AIDS, professor of dermatology and microbiology.

Dr. Martin Kahn, cardiology; professor of clinical medicine.

Dr. Alfred Kopf, specialist in skin cancers, clinical professor of dermatology.

Dr. Abraham Lieberman, professor of neurology, chairman of the medical advisory board of the American Parkinson's Disease Association, director of the Leon Lowenstein Parkinson's Disease Foundation and Treatment Program.

Dr. Joseph McCarthy, professor of plastic surgery, director of the Institute for Reconstructive Surgery.

Dr. Barry Reisberg, specialist in Alzheimer's disease, associate professor of psychiatry.

Dr. William W. Shaw, associate professor of surgery, head of the microsurgery team at NYU-Bellevue, one of the foremost limb reimplantation units in the country.

Dr. Frank Spencer, cardiac surgery; chairman of the department of surgery.

Dr. Arthur Upton, professor and chairman of the department of environmental medicine, former director of the National Cancer Foundation.

Dr. Fred Valentine, immunology; associate professor of medicine, director of the AIDS Treatment Evaluation Unit, conductor of clinical trials to treat melanoma with immunotherapy.

## Research

In recent years more than 1,000 NYU biomedical projects—studying everything from the basic chemistry of life to problems of air pollution in cities—have received more than $50 million in annual funding from governmental and nongovernmental sources.

Some of the most important research done here reflects the hospital's best-known clinical services, in cardiology, cardiovascular surgery, neurosurgery, reconstructive plastic surgery (especially microsurgery), rehabilitation medicine, and rheumatology. As a federally funded cancer center, NYU conducts both basic and clinical research in almost every area of oncology. In addition to its melanoma program, NYU has physicians and scientists doing specialized research in the treatment of breast and ovarian cancers. They also participate in several nationwide clinical trial programs exploring new drug and radiation therapies for all kinds of cancers, and several do special trials for brain tumors and gastrointestinal tumors. Cancer research at NYU accounts for over 40 percent of the total research budget.

Other major research programs include studies of depression in the elderly and Alzheimer's disease (the largest study of Alzheimer's was conducted here), hypertension, Parkinson's disease, sexually transmitted diseases, and stroke.

The AIDS Treatment Evaluation Unit was established in 1986 with a $10-million contract from the NIH. It is one of the largest programs of clinical trials evaluating drugs used to treat the AIDS virus and the infections and cancers contracted by people with AIDS. The medical center has been in the forefront of research on AIDS since the first patients were identified in 1980; in fact, scientists here were the first to describe the clinical syndrome later identified as AIDS. Currently basic and clinical research in AIDS at NYU is conducted by almost 40 physicians and scientists.

Environmental medicine at NYU involves a diverse series of studies carried out through the Institute of Environmental Medicine. One of the largest (funded by a $406,000 grant from the Charles A. Dana Foundation) examines the prevention, early diagnosis, and treatment of environmentally related diseases. Other studies focus on chemical and radiation carcinogens, radon exposure, and toxicology; and there is a series of epidemiology-biostatistical investigations in AIDS and Karposi's sarcoma, breast cancer, colon cancer, melanoma, radiation exposure, and radon exposure, among other topics.

Vaccine development is another important part of the research at NYU. A vaccine to combat malaria began clinical trials in 1986; it was developed at the medical center's Department of Medical and Molecular Parasitology, the only department of its kind in the country. Clinical work continues on development of a vaccine to prevent secondary recurrences of melanoma.

## Admission Policy

Patients must be admitted to University Hospital by an NYU physician. However, anyone can call the general number (212-340-7400), ask for the appropriate department, and set up an appointment with an NYU doctor.

The hospital accepts self-paying patients as well as those covered by Medicare, Medicaid, and other third-party payers. Emergency patients are treated immediately in the emergency room.

Rusk patients must be referred by a physician.

**ROOM CHARGES (per diem)**
Private: $437 (regular); $470 (deluxe)
Co-op Care: $254 (twin); $387 (suite)
Semiprivate: $341
Ward (four-bedded): $330
ICU: $639

**AVERAGE COST PER PATIENT STAY:**    $6,762 (University Hospital)
$23,750 (Rusk)

**MAILING ADDRESS**        **TELEPHONE**
560 First Avenue        212-340-5505
New York, NY 10016

# Duke University Medical Center

**DURHAM, NORTH CAROLINA**

Education is an integral aspect of most of the hospitals we have included in this book, because the increasing specialization in medicine has brought a corresponding need for postgraduate training for physicians. In the past few decades Duke University has become a formidable training ground for specialists.

Each year about 800 M.D.'s and Ph.D's receive advanced training here in the clinical and basic sciences. Another 150 trainees are in paramedical programs. In addition, about 50 nurses are in a new specialized master's in nursing curriculum that prepares them for advanced clinical practice and administration.

Medical training is similarly impressive; the Duke University School of Medicine is one of the finest in the country. Admission is highly selective; in 1984, for example, there were 3,100 applicants for 112 openings.

In addition to being on the staff of the hospital, Duke's physicians hold appointments at the medical school and usually do research in their field. Consequently, patients benefit from Duke's educational facilities and from its extensive corresponding research.

Duke University Hospital is the major private tertiary-care center in the Southeast. In some clinical subspecialties, such as bone marrow transplantation and open-heart surgery, patients are referred from all over the world. The range of services available at Duke covers just about every medical specialty and subspecialty.

One of the major areas of concern here is children's health and related pediatric problems. The Children's Medical and Surgical Center was designed as a compact, child-oriented unit within Duke University Hospital with quick access to the specialists and facilities of the entire medical center. Duke is a major center for the treatment of children with severe combined immunodeficiency disease (SCIDS) and a major referral center for children with cardiac disease. It has one of the most modern facilities available anywhere for pediatric cardiac catheterization, as well as a first-rate neonatal intensive care unit for treating premature infants. The pediatric metabolism lab is the only one in the country devoted entirely to the analysis of clinical samples, and its high-tech equipment can diagnose rare metabolic diseases and Reye's syndrome. The Child Guidance Clinic is the home of the Durham Community Guidance Clinic for Children and Youth, a service of the Department of Psychiatry.

In other areas of psychiatry Duke is a major referral center for patients with eating disorders, in particular anorexia nervosa. Duke also offers an interdisciplinary approach to the treatment of chronic pain.

The Duke Diet and Fitness Center is part of the Department of Community and Family Medicine and is one of the best-known facilities in North Carolina. The program concentrates on self-education so participants can develop a weight control and exercise program that can be maintained after they leave. The program focuses on four areas: medical, behavioral, dietary and nutritional, and fitness. Participants are asked to spend at least four weeks in Durham, although six to eight weeks are recommended.

Duke has had a kidney transplant program for nearly twenty years, and heart and liver transplant programs were initiated in 1984. Duke is a regional referral center for microsurgery and replantation of severed limbs. Plastic surgeons specialize in breast reconstruction, treatment of cleft palate, and the specialized treatment of patients in the Burn Unit.

The Duke Comprehensive Cancer Center houses inpatient and outpatient programs in oncology and treats more than 6,000 patients a year. The center is the only federally designated facility of its magnitude between Washington, DC, and Birmingham, Alabama; it is one of about 20 such facilities in the country. Autologous bone marrow transplants are used to treat recalcitrant cases of breast cancer, leukemia, lymphoma, and melanoma. Other innovative techniques include hyperthermia to enhance the effectiveness of chemotherapy. Extensive radiation therapies are also available.

Duke specialists use a number of procedures, including in vitro fertilization, to treat couples with infertility problems. The obstetrics/gynecology department offers clinics for patients with pelvic pain, premenstrual syndrome, sexual dysfunction, and sexually transmitted diseases. A lab for prenatal diagnosis of disease includes facilities for chorionic villi sampling. Duke is a major regional referral center for high-risk obstetric patients.

The Duke University Eye Center is a clinical and research unit, the only one of its scope between Baltimore and Miami. The chairman of ophthalmology originated the technique of vitrectomy, in which the clouded vitreous humor of the eye is removed and replaced with clear fluid. Other specialists here use innovative procedures to treat a variety of unusual eye diseases. For instance, the retinal tack, a Duke invention, has been used in several patients to smooth out badly folded and torn retinas. Duke is one of the few places in the country to perform epikeratophakia, which involves suturing a lens onto an eye.

The large Neurosciences Division includes an extensive study of Alzheimer's disease and certain inherited neurological disorders, such as Huntington's disease and muscular dystrophy. A special program offers a comprehensive approach to people who have or are at risk of heart disease. Several physicians specialize in the treatment of rheumatoid diseases, especially the myriad types of arthritis. The Hypertension Center treats and educates patients with this "silent killer."

The Center for the Study of Aging and Human Development, the first and longest continuously funded such center in the country, studies what happens—biologically, psychologically, economically, and socially—as people grow older. The center has conducted many long-term studies, including the first longitudinal study in normal aging. The Geriatric Evaluation and Treatment Clinic provides initial assessment and continuing care, refers patients to specialty clinics when necessary, and works with family members.

As would be expected in an institution of this size and breadth, Duke has extensive facilities for diagnostic and therapeutic radiology. The Emergency Room has a Level I trauma rating and two helicopter ambulances (Life Flight) to transport trauma victims and acutely ill patients within a radius of 150 miles.

Eight compression chambers provide hyperbaric oxygen therapy for a number of conditions, such as acute cyanide and carbon monoxide poisonings, gas gangrene, and certain soft-tissue infections. Duke is part of the national Divers Alert Network, providing immediate care, transportation, and compression chamber treatment for diving accident victims in the southeastern United States.

Other major specialty clinics are devoted to diabetes, epilepsy, prosthetics and orthotics, pulmonary rehabilitation, sickle-cell anemia, stroke, and swallowing disorders.

Medical personnel from Duke serve the 484-bed Veterans Administration Medical Center; Lenox Baker Children's Hospital, a 40-bed rehabilitation center for children; and Sea Level Hospital, a 75-bed community hospital in eastern North Carolina. Duke personnel staff outreach programs that cover the state.

The range and diversity of services at Duke is even more impressive when one considers that at the time of its founding North Carolina ranked forty-fourth in the nation in personal income, and medicine in the state was practically a cottage industry. The original 400-bed hospital opened in 1930, funded by James Buchanan Duke, a Durham native who had become a major U.S. industrialist. In his will he designated $4 million to be used to erect a medical school, hospital, and nurses' residence at Duke University.

Today almost 80 percent of Duke's patients come from North Carolina; the rest come from the other states and from around the world.

## Specialties

Clinical services include Allergy, Anesthesiology, Audiology, the Burn Unit, Cardiology, Dermatology, Endocrinology, Family Planning, Gastroenterology and Hepatology, Genetics, Geriatric Psychiatry, Gynecology, Hematology, Hyperbaric Medicine, Infectious Diseases, Infertility, Internal Medicine, Maternal Fetal Medicine, Medical Speech Pathology, Metabolism, Nephrology, Neurosurgery, Nuclear Medicine, Obstetrics, Occupational Medicine, Occupational Therapy, Oncology, Ophthalmology, Oral Surgery, Orthodontics, Orthopedics, Otolaryngology, the Pain Clinic, Pathology, Pediatrics, Pediatric Surgery, Physical Therapy, Plastic and Maxillofacial Surgery, Proctology, Psychiatry, Psychoanalysis, Psychology,

Pulmonary Disease, Radiology, Rehabilitation Medicine, Rheumatic and Genetic Disease, Speech and Hearing, Surgery, Thoracic Surgery, Trauma Surgery, and Urology.

There are major programs in aging, cancer, cardiovascular disease, childhood diseases, eye diseases, genetics, immunology, mental illness, and organ transplantation—as well as the specialists and facilities to care for most other illnesses.

---

**STATISTICAL PROFILE (1985–86)**

Number of Beds: 1,008
Bed Occupancy Rate: 88%
Average Number of Inpatients: 843
Average Patient Stay: 9 days
Annual Admissions: 33,600
Births: 1,960
Outpatient Clinic Visits: 305,000
Emergency Room/Trauma Center Visits: 36,000

Hospital Personnel:
  Physicians: 550 staff
  Residents and Fellows: 780
  Registered Nurses: 1,780 plus 200 in the operating rooms
  Total Staff: 7,000

---

## Well-known Specialists

Dr. Brenda Armstrong, pediatric cardiology.
Dr. Robert Bast, oncology.
Dr. Randy Bollinger, liver and kidney transplantation.
Dr. Rebecca Buckley, pediatric immunology; specialist in severe combined immunodeficiency syndrome.
Dr. Barney Carroll, psychiatry.
Dr. R. Edward Coleman, diagnostic radiology.
Dr. John Falletta, pediatric oncology.
Dr. Henry Friedman, pediatric oncology; specialist in pediatric brain tumors.
Dr. Joseph C. Greenfield, Jr., cardiology.
Dr. Charles Hammond, infertility.
Dr. Arthur Haney, infertility.
Dr. Samuel Katz, pediatric infectious diseases and immunizations.
Dr. Robert Machemer, ophthalmology; specialist in vitrectomy.
Dr. Blaine Nashold, neurosurgery; specialist in pain.

Dr. Jerry Oakes, pediatric neurosurgery.

Dr. William Peters, oncology; specialist in autologous bone marrow transplantation.

Dr. Sheldon Pinnell, dermatology.

Dr. Edward Pritchett, cardiology.

Dr. Leonard Prosnitz, radiation oncology.

Dr. Charles Roe, pediatric genetics and metabolism.

Dr. Allen Roses, neurology; head of the Alzheimer's disease program.

Dr. David C. Sabiston, Jr., cardiothoracic surgery.

Dr. Donald Serafin, plastic surgery and microsurgery.

Dr. James Urbaniak, orthopedic surgery and microsurgery.

Dr. Andrew Wechsler, heart transplantation.

Dr. Redford Williams, behavioral medicine.

## Research

In 1985–86 Duke received about $51 million for sponsored research and research training. The two major thrusts in research here are molecular genetics and the neurosciences.

Cancer research is the major priority, calling on the cooperative efforts of scientists from endocrinology, genetics, hematology, immunology, molecular biology, pharmacology, radiology, surgery, and virology.

More specifically, work proceeds at Duke in the molecular genetics of normal and cancerous cells; the mechanisms of carcinogenesis by viruses, chemicals, and radiation; immunology, with emphasis on understanding the body's defenses against cancer induction, growth, and spread; new techniques for employing monoclonal antibodies for the more precise diagnosis of cancer and, it is hoped, for treatment; and studies of biological response modifiers, substances produced by the body, like interferon, that boost immunity to cancer.

Important areas of clinical research are the use of PET and magnetic resonance imaging scanners in diagnosing cancer and studying the metabolism of tumors; hyperthermia to enhance response to chemotherapy and radiation; bone marrow transplantation (Duke is one of the few places in the country where autologous bone marrow transplants are performed); evaluation of new chemotherapeutic agents to treat cancer; use of lasers for palliative removal of tumors; and intraarterial chemotherapy using an implantable pump.

## Admission Policy

There are three ways to enter Duke University Hospital: preadmission (patients referred to Duke by their personal physicians are scheduled for hospitalization by their Duke physicians), through the emergency/trauma center, or after examination in one of Duke's clinics.

There is no financial requirement for patients entering through the emergency room. Nonemergency patients must have some kind of insurance. If insurance does not cover the estimated bill, a deposit is required. If a deposit is not possible, the patient may receive a waiver from a physician or hospital administrator. A waiver may also be granted if the service would be a significant teaching case. Duke provides more than $20 million annually in charity discounts and uncollectible debts.

---

**ROOM CHARGES (per diem)**
Private: $248
Semiprivate: $248
Ward:
  $310 for psychiatric departments; one to six in a room
    (depending on treatment plan)
  $248 for delivery room suites with six per room
ICU: $550–$1,120
The Diet and Fitness Center Program costs approximately $2,000
  for the first four weeks, not including fees for laboratory studies or
  room accommodations. (Most participants stay in local hotels.) The
  cost of each additional four weeks is approximately $1,420.

**AVERAGE COST PER PATIENT STAY:**   $7,717

**MAILING ADDRESS        TELEPHONE**
Durham, NC 27710    919-684-8111

---

# The North Carolina Memorial Hospital

## CHAPEL HILL, NORTH CAROLINA

In the early 1950s Dr. Nathan Womack, the chairman of surgery at the University of North Carolina, created the world's first intensive care unit at The North Carolina (NC) Memorial Hospital. Because of this, intensive care has always been of major interest here. In December 1985 the concept rose to a new level of sophistication with the opening of the Esley O. Anderson, Jr., Pavilion, a six-story, $18.6-million critical-care center that includes 41 intensive care beds.

North Carolina Memorial is the teaching hospital for the University of North Carolina (UNC) at Chapel Hill School of Medicine. While the hospital is not part of the medical school, its medical staff is composed of faculty from the medical and dental schools.

The hospital is a 600-bed teaching and referral center providing general, comprehensive medical care as well as highly specialized treatment for all types of rare and complex problems. It offers diagnostic and treatment services for people referred from throughout North Carolina and from surrounding states. It also serves the primary-care needs of residents of Orange County and several neighboring counties.

Nursing care at NC Memorial is provided by an 80 percent licensed staff. Approximately 70 percent of the registered nurses have a bachelor's, graduate, or doctoral degree.

Special facilities continue to expand to meet the needs of this complex medical center. The emergency room, already designated a Level I Trauma Center, has recently been renovated and expanded. The Magnetic Resonance Imaging Facility began operating in early 1986. The Radiation Oncology Center, currently being organized, will serve inpatients and outpatients. The center will also house research facilities and a motel unit. The hospital began a heart transplant program in October 1986.

The NC Jaycee Burn Center is one of the most comprehensive burn facilities in the country. Patients receive acute and intermediate care, physical therapy and rehabilitation, and reconstructive surgery. The staff also provides emotional support and psychiatric counseling for patients and their families.

The hospital offers a full range of gynecologic and obstetric services, including in vitro fertilization. The staff uses many medical and surgical techniques to treat infertility.

The elderly and disabled are helped through Lifeline, a service providing quick access to medical assistance when needed. Subscribers wear a small button on a chain around their necks. If they need help, they can press the button and transmit a signal to the emergency room at NC Memorial, where staff will make sure appropriate medical care is provided.

To lower costs and improve services, NC Memorial offers Day-Op, an ambulatory surgical program. Under an innovative new Outpatient Admissions Program, patients are allowed to stay in the hospital for up to twenty-three hours as outpatients. This program is designed for those who may not be well enough to go home after a minor surgical or diagnostic procedure but are not sick enough to be admitted as inpatients.

North Carolina Memorial is the patient-care heart of one of the most comprehensive health science complexes in the country. This complex includes five professional schools—dentistry, medicine, nursing, pharmacy, and public health—with a combined enrollment of 3,000 students; a number of prestigious centers and institutes, and one of the largest health sciences libraries in the South. The hospital's history goes back to October 1949, when construction was begun on a 400-bed hospital that would serve as both a community hospital and a teaching facility for the UNC at Chapel Hill School of Medicine.

Current plans at NC Memorial include the installation of a lithotriptor in early 1987 and the opening of a Ronald McDonald House to host families of critically ill children. Carolina Air Care, the hospital's air ambulance service, began operation in July 1986.

---

**STATISTICAL PROFILE**

Number of Beds: 593
Bed Occupancy Rate: 79%
Average Number of Patients: 468
Average Patient Stay: 7.4 days
Annual Number of Admissions: 21,555
Births: 1,669
Outpatient Clinic Visits: 282,840
Emergency Room/Trauma Center Visits: 32,123

Hospital Personnel:
  Physicians: 560
  Residents: 425
  Total Staff: 3,739

---

## Specialties

Anesthesiology, Dermatology, Family Medicine, Hospital Dental Service, Medicine, Neurology, Obstetrics/Gynecology, Ophthalmology, Pathology, Pediatrics, Psychiatry, Radiology, Rehabilitation, and Surgery.

There are over 160 outpatient clinics offering services ranging from general medical care to treatment for highly specialized problems.

North Carolina Memorial is recognized nationally for expertise and innovation in caring for a variety of medical problems, including arthritis, autism, burns, cancer, coagulation disorders, cystic fibrosis, genetic disorders, growth disorders, infertility, and neuromuscular diseases. The hospital is also a major center for the care of high-risk mothers and infants.

## Well-known Specialists

Dr. Watson A. Bowes, specialist in high-risk pregnancies.
Dr. Philip A. Bromberg, chief of pulmonary medicine, director of Cystic Fibrosis Research Center.
Dr. Ernest Craige, well-known cardiologist.
Dr. Stanley Mandel, surgery; head of kidney transplant program.
Dr. Joseph Pagano, director of Lineberger Cancer Research Center.
Dr. Don W. Powell, chief of digestive disease and nutrition.
Dr. John T. Sessions, well-known gastroenterologist.
Dr. Luther Talbert, obstetrics/gynecology, specialist in infertility problems.
Dr. John Winfield, chief of rheumatology/immunology, director of the Arthritis Research Center.
Dr. Robert Utiger, endocrinology; director of Clinical Research Unit.
Dr. Clayton Wheeler, chairman of dermatology.

## Research

Medical researchers at UNC have the advantage of access to a federally funded Clinical Research Unit, and, according to Dr. Robert D. Utiger, director of the unit, there are usually about 60 active projects here at any one time. In 1985 there were 100 publications by faculty members based on work done in whole or part on the unit.

At the Lineberger Cancer Research Center, scientists investigate chemical carcinogenesis, cancer cell biology, drug development, immunology, recombinant DNA, and viruses.

The Arthritis Research Center coordinates research into the causes and treatment of this disease. The center also sponsors research seminars to educate physicians on the latest advances in arthritis care. In late 1985 the center, one of two federally funded arthritis centers in the Southeast and of only a few across the United States, was awarded a $1.6-million grant from the National Institute of Arthritis.

The Center for Thrombosis and Hemostasis studies blood and clotting disorders. The Comprehensive Hemophilia Diagnosis and Treatment Center, a part of the research center, follows the treatment and progress of 400 hemophiliacs throughout the Southeast.

The Cystic Fibrosis Research Center studies the causes of this disease and is one of the first three such centers in the United States.

Research is conducted in all departments and in other centers such as the Alcohol Studies Center, the Biological Sciences Research Center, and the Center for Environmental Health and Medical Sciences. The study of aging has become an important research effort at the UNC School of Medicine, in conjunction with the UNC Schools of Nursing, Pharmacy, and Public Health.

## Admission Policy

Patients without regular doctors can come to the clinics at NC Memorial for diagnosis and treatment of almost any problem. No appointment is needed to be seen in the following Walk-In Clinics: General Medicine Screening Clinic, Medicine Evening and Weekend Clinic, Pediatric Screening Clinic, Psychiatric Emergency Clinic, and Surgery Screening Clinic. Appointments are required in the hospital's other clinics. In many cases patients do not have to be referred by physicians; they may make their own appointments by calling Central Appointments at 919-966-2231.

In addition to traditional emergency services, NC Memorial operates a twenty-four-hour care and counseling service for rape victims and a computer-based poison identification system that may be reached at 919-966-4721.

---

**ROOM CHARGES** (per diem)
Private: $205
Semiprivate: $197

**MAILING ADDRESS**       **TELEPHONE**
Manning Drive          919-966-3366
Chapel Hill, NC 27514

---

# The Cleveland Clinic Foundation
## CLEVELAND, OHIO

In medical circles around the country, the Cleveland Clinic is regarded as one of the finest institutions in the world. Hyperbole comes easily because almost everything about the Cleveland Clinic is out of the ordinary. To state, for example, that it is on the cutting edge of medical practice doesn't quite say enough considering that in 1985 alone the physicians here performed over 3,100 heart operations, including 2,500 bypass procedures. The Department of Cardiology, treating and evaluating about 6,000 patients a year, is the largest such department in the world. One fourth of the hospital, including a 351-bed cardiovascular wing, is set aside for heart patients. In addition, the Department of Thoracic and Cardiovascular Surgery performed these 2,500 bypass operations with a mortality rate of less than 1 percent, even though the foundation's case complexity rate is in the top 1 percent of the country.

In recent years the clinic has also done over 1,000 kidney transplants, 24 heart transplants, nine liver transplants, two pancreas transplants, approximately 700 cornea transplants, and 700 artificial joint replacements. It has pioneered less-than-radical surgery for breast and thyroid cancer and a surgical stapling technique that helps preserve normal bowel function in nine out of ten rectal cancer patients.

The foundation has created one of the foremost epilepsy diagnostic, treatment, and research programs in the country. A testing site for new drugs, the foundation is working to increase the percentage of patients who respond to medical treatment. Some difficult cases require surgery, for which the foundation has helped develop sophisticated testing techniques that allow surgeons to pinpoint—and remove—the source of seizures in the brain. Although difficult cases make up only 2 percent of the epileptic population, 20 percent of these surgeries are performed here.

The clinic is one of four U.S. medical centers that cooperated on the design and testing of cementless replacement joints. These prostheses are expected to last longer than earlier cemented models; they feature a porous metal coating that allows bones to grow into them, locking the implants in place.

It is an understatement to report that many of the clinic's doctors are considered among the top people in their fields. The only thorough survey of the "best doctors" in America (a study conducted by John Pekkanen) named 31 physicians from the Cleveland Clinic. Many well-known, university-affiliated hospitals had a maximum of 10 or 12 doctors on the list.

As in other high-powered institutions, the quality-assurance program at the clinic employs up-to-date computer-based techniques. Here, however, the head of the program is a practicing physician, not a nurse or trained administrator. In addition, all department heads and program directors are responsible for quality-assurance matters.

However, according to the clinic, the best assurance of quality care rests with the highly selective process employing extensive peer review that is used to determine which doctors practice here. Annual professional review of all staff members ensures that physicians continue to maintain the highest standard of care.

The Cleveland Clinic Foundation is the second largest medical group practice in the world. In a manner similar to that at the Mayo Clinic, doctors here pool services. Each staff physician is a specialist in one or more areas of medicine. None has an outside practice, and none sees patients at any other hospital. (The doctors jointly benefit by earning salaries that range from $60,000 to $250,000.)

The clinic was founded just after World War I by four Cleveland physicians—Drs. Frank Bunts, George W. Crile, William Lower, and John Phillips. The group practice concept was considered revolutionary at the time, but three of the founders had already discovered its advantages near the battlefields of France. In 1921 a new four-story clinic building was officially opened.

Since then the clinic has evolved as a multifaceted organization consisting of four major divisions: the clinic, the hospital, the educational division, and the research division. All four divisions are included in the private, not-for-profit practice of medicine. As a consequence, in 1979 Congress recognized The Cleveland Clinic Foundation—its official name—as a center of medical excellence, a National Health Resource.

The foundation's Division of Education was incorporated as a postgraduate medical school in 1935 and was one of the first institutions to promote continuing medical education. Today it is recognized as the largest postgraduate medical facility in the United States that is not connected with a medical school or university.

Located on a one-hundred-acre campus on Cleveland's East Side, The Cleveland Clinic Foundation consists of 22 buildings, including the recently expanded hospital, a new 12-story outpatient clinic, and a 400-room hotel for patients and their families. There is even a specially designed building for the nuclear imaging scanner.

As a testimony to the level of patient satisfaction, almost 95 percent of the patients surveyed by the foundation said that the clinic was better than other facilities in terms of the skill of the doctors, the medical technology available, and the handling of complex problems. Also, 95 percent said they would recommend Cleveland Clinic, and over 96 percent expressed satisfaction with their experience here.

## Specialties

The foundation provides care in 38 specialties and 67 subspecialties. The divisions of anesthesiology, laboratory medicine, medicine, radiology, research, and surgery have formed "centers of excellence," assembling the diverse talents of many specialists. It is clear from the foundation's success in focusing on cardiovascular disease that this approach stimulates a more rapid exchange of ideas between physicians and scientists. Thus far six centers of excellence have been established: Cancer, Cardiovascular Diseases, Digestive Diseases, Musculoskeletal Disorders, Neurosensory Disorders, and Urogenital and Reproductive Disorders.

The foundation has earned international acclaim for pioneering work in the artificial heart, bone marrow transplantation, coronary angiography, coronary bypass surgery, hemodialysis, hypertension, kidney dialysis and transplantation, pediatric intensive care, and retinal vascular disease.

---

**STATISTICAL PROFILE**

Number of Beds: 1,008
Bed Occupancy Rate: 80%
Average Number of Patients: 740
Average Patient Stay: 8.3 days
Annual Admissions: 31,336
Outpatient Clinic Visits: 460,648
Emergency Room/Trauma Center Visits: 10,565

Hospital Personnel:
  Physicians: 401
  Residents: 585
  Registered Nurses: 1,158
  Total Staff: 8,132

---

## Well-known Specialists

Dr. Lester S. Borden, orthopedic surgery.
Dr. John P. Conomy, neurology.
Dr. Richard G. Farmer, gastroenterology.
Dr. Victor W. Fazio, colorectal surgery.
Dr. Ray W. Gifford, Jr., hypertension and nephrology.
Dr. Froncie A. Gutman, ophthalmology.

Dr. Robert E. Hermann, general surgery.
Dr. John R. Little, neurosurgery.
Dr. Floyd D. Loop, thoracic and cardiovascular surgery.
Dr. Andrew C. Novick, urology.
Dr. Robert W. Stewart, thoracic and cardiovascular surgery.
Dr. Harvey M. Tucker, otolaryngology and communicative disorders.

## Research

There are over 347 funded research projects at the Cleveland Clinic. A research staff of 42 scientists, supported by 150 technical personnel, conducts studies in artificial organs, cardiovascular diseases, and cellular and molecular biology.

The foundation has been a pioneer in the development of the artificial heart and kidney dialysis and in the identification of the hormones that affect blood pressure and hypertension and their links to hardening of the arteries. Among the innovations at the foundation are the first artificial kidney, built in the late 1940s and housed in an old Maytag washing machine, and the first heart bypass operation, performed in 1967.

Current projects include research into the causes of cancer and into the control and prevention of ALS and other neurosensory disorders. Research related to the clinic's best-known specialties includes the development of blood purification techniques to help liver transplant patients, work on laser catheterization to unclog narrowed arteries, and testing of TPA (tissue plasminogen activator), a genetically engineered drug to dissolve blood clots.

## Admission Policy

Physicians from around the country refer thousands of patients to the Cleveland Clinic, but anyone can call and make an appointment with one of its doctors. In fact, the clinic makes it easy to get an appointment: Central Appointment Services at 216-444-5641 will refer prospective patients to the appropriate department. One can also call a toll-free number: 800-321-5398 (out of state) or 800-362-2306 (in Ohio). There is even a separate department to deal with the special needs of international patients; they should write or call Patient Facilitated Services at 216-444-5902.

Unlike many university-affiliated medical institutions described in this book, the Cleveland Clinic does make clear that they like patients to have a full-coverage health insurance policy or Medicare. From patients without coverage, they want a deposit and a discussion of how the bill will be paid. Prospective patients with limited insurance or some form of disability or welfare insurance are asked to call the admitting financial coordinator (216-444-6579) to make the necessary arrangements.

**ROOM CHARGES** (per diem)
Private: $373–$398
Semiprivate: $348
Ward: $324
ICU: $872–$983; $598 for coronary step-down
Room Charges at the Clinic Inn:
  Single: $56–$77
  Double: $66–$88
  American Plan: $80–$110 (includes three meals)
  Luxury Suites: $550–$1,000 (includes all meals, a butler, stocked
    bar, and airport limo)
  *Note*: Patients staying at the inn before admission receive a 15
percent discount if they stay in ordinary rooms.

**MAILING ADDRESS**          **TELEPHONE**
9500 Euclid Avenue      216-444-2200
Cleveland, OH 44106

# University Hospitals of Cleveland

**CLEVELAND, OHIO**

In a poll reported in the April 17, 1982, issue of *Family Circle Magazine*, University Hospitals of Cleveland (UHC) was named among the top 20 hospitals in the United States. The magazine polled private practitioners, medical school faculty members, health educators, foundation officials, and medical writers. Part of UHC's reputation must have derived from the fact that many new technological advances are to be found here.

This was the first hospital in the United States to house the superconducting whole-body magnetic resonance imaging scanner. More recently UHC acquired a Siemens 1.0 Tesla Magnetom, one of the first of its kind in the United States. Research with these machines will establish their clinical capabilities as well as explore proton imaging, spectroscopy, image display techniques, and hardware and software applications.

The UHC lithotriptor enables over 1,000 patients a year to avoid kidney surgery. Ophthalmologists use a new Barraquer cryolathe, a computer-assisted microscopic cutting machine, to reshape the eye's cornea. The hospitals' Ireland Cancer Center has access to two magnetic resonance imaging units and a CAT and a PET scanner, making it one of the best-equipped facilities in the nation for cancer detection.

Located in the University Circle Section of Cleveland, UHC is an academic medical center composed of five hospitals that operate under one management. The hospitals are Lakeside and Hanna Hospitals, general medical and surgical facilities; Rainbow Babies and Children's Hospital; MacDonald Hospital for Women, a maternity and gynecology hospital; and Hanna Pavilion, a psychiatric hospital. Many UHC physicians also have offices in the University Suburban Health Center in the suburb of Euclid and the University Hospitals Center in Willoughby. The whole medical center is affiliated with, but separate from, the adjacent Case Western Reserve University School of Medicine. The hospitals' attending physicians are all faculty members at the medical school.

The highest quality care for women with normal and problem pregnancies is provided at the MacDonald Hospital. Programs include alternative methods of delivery, a high-risk pregnancy unit, and a midlife health center dealing with the problems of menopause. There is direct linkage on several floors with Rainbow Hospital.

Rainbow Babies and Children's Hospital is a special facility for infants, children, and adolescents, the only treatment center in northern Ohio providing acute and continuous care for children with serious diseases and handicapping conditions. Rainbow maintains 30 divisions and 39 specialty centers, providing medical and surgical treatment for more than 85,000

**253**

children annually. The 220-bed hospital has a staff of approximately 1,000, including 70 physicians, 151 clinical faculty, 90 doctors in training, and 300 registered nurses. Through numerous programs families are encouraged to participate in the care of their children to provide as near to normal an environment as possible during their hospital stay. In addition to its role as a principal pediatric referral center for Ohio, Indiana, and Pennsylvania, Rainbow is a leading world center for the care of children with cystic fibrosis. It has the only diagnostic cardiology unit for children in northern Ohio, and its Pediatric Cardiology and Cardiothoracic Surgery divisions provide a nationally renowned program for training pedatric cardiologists.

Complicated major surgery, as well as ambulatory surgery, is performed in Lakeside Hospital, which consists of 28 operating rooms and 280 medical and surgical beds, including the cardiac monitoring unit, surgical intensive care unit, and medical intensive care unit. The medical center was a world pioneer in heart surgery through the work of the late Dr. Claude Beck from the 1920s onward and today remains a respected center for heart surgery.

University Hospitals of Cleveland was one of five Ohio health-care facilities to join a statewide organ transplant consortium, the first of its kind in the nation. As a member of the consortium, UHC will perform heart, heart-lung, liver, and pancreas transplants. The hospitals and physicians have agreed to contribute 25 percent of related institutional gifts and professional fees to a fund to help defray the patients' costs. Other major departments at Lakeside Hospital include dialysis, neurology, oncology, orthopedics, pulmonary medicine, and urology.

Cancer is a major specialty at UHC. Under the direction of Dr. Nathan Berger, chief of the Division of Hematology/Oncology, the Ireland Cancer Center serves as an umbrella organization for all facets of oncological activity at UHC. This comprehensive multidisciplinary approach benefits not only the patient but also the physician, the researcher, and support staff, as well as concentrating resources. In patient care various disciplines are brought together. Specialized oncology nurses, dieticians, social workers, and therapists join physicians to form teams devoted to breast cancer, colon cancer, digestive tract tumors, female reproductive tract tumors, head and neck tumors, leukemia and lymphoma, lung cancer, melanoma, muscle and bone tumors, and radiation therapy.

For patients suffering from cancer pain, UHC Pain Center provides a multidisciplinary support staff of specialists in pain control. The center also treats patients with all other varieties of pain, including those with headaches, low back pain, and pain from medical conditions such as diabetes.

The emotionally disturbed and the mentally ill are treated at the Hanna Pavilion, an 80-bed psychiatric hospital that includes a children's unit, adolescent area, outpatient clinics, and private offices for psychiatrists and psychologists.

The elderly are helped at the Geriatrics Center for Clinical Assessment, Research, and Education. A joint effort of UHC and the Veterans Administration Medical Center, the center was developed in 1984 to address multiple needs of the elderly, taking into account psychiatric, social, and environmental factors.

Providing community services is another function of UHC. At the Health Enhancement Center a group of professionals committed to the development of communty wellness offers programs such as Smoke Stoppers, Be Trim, and Aerobics.

The origin of today's UHC complex was the establishment, in 1863, of the "Home for the Friendless." Lakeside Hospital, dedicated in 1931, was the original hospital of University Hospitals. In 1967 the original Lakeside Hospital was expanded. Rainbow Babies and Children's Hospital dates back to the founding of Rainbow Cottage in 1887 and Children's Hospital in 1902. In 1972 Rainbow Hospital joined Babies and Children's Hospital.

University Hospitals was also a leader in the formation of a health-maintenance organization with four other hospitals and the School of Medicine at Case Western Reserve. Planning for this organization was made possible by a $1.2-million grant from the Robert Wood Johnson Foundation. The grant, the largest of 12 given nationally, was awarded to set up a health-maintenance organization for the area's Medicaid population.

## Specialties

Anesthesiology, Cardiology, Clinical Pharmacology, Critical Care, Dermatology, Emergency Services, Endocrinology, Family Medicine, Gastroenterology, Geographic Medicine, Geriatrics, Hematology and Oncology, Human

---

**STATISTICAL PROFILE**

Number of Beds: 874
Bed Occupancy Rate: 83%
Average Number of Patients: 704
Average Patient Stay: 7.5 days
Annual Admissions: 27,696
Births: 3,106
Outpatient Clinic Visits: 171,443
Emergency Room/Trauma Center Visits: 58,461

Hospital Personnel:
  Physicians: 1,020
  Residents: 566
  Registered Nurses: 1,246
  Total Staff: 3,902

Genetics, Infectious Diseases, Medicine, Nephrology, Neurology, Obstetrics/Gynecology, Ophthalmology, Orthopaedics, Otolaryngology, Pathology, Pediatrics, Psychiatry, Pulmonary Medicine, Rheumatic Diseases, Radiology, and Surgery.

## Well-known Specialists

Dr. Ralph J. Alfidi, director of the Department of Radiology.

Dr. Nathan A. Berger, director of the Ireland Cancer Center.

Dr. David Bickers, director of the Department of Dermatology.

Dr. Robert B. Daroff, director of the Department of Neurology.

Dr. Alexander S. Geha, chief of the Division of Cardio-Thoracic Surgery.

Dr. Kingsbury C. Heiple, director of the Department of Orthopaedics.

Dr. John H. Kennell, chief of the Division of Child Development.

Dr. Herbert Y. Meltzer, director of the Mental Health Clinic Research Center.

Dr. Robert A. Ratcheson, chief of the Division of Neurosurgery.

Dr. Oscar D. Ratnoff, medicine.

Dr. Leon Speroff, medical director of the Department of Obstetrics and Gynecology.

## Research

There are 100 research laboratories located throughout the UHC complex, with headquarters in the Wearn Building. Combined with Case Western Reserve University (CWRU), UHC forms the state's largest biomedical research center. Hospital physicians work with CWRU School of Medicine scientists to identify incidence, causes, progressions, treatments, and effects of various types of cancer. For example, leuprolide, a new drug tested at UHC, has been found effective in the treatment of prostate cancer and has been submitted to the Food and Drug Administration.

Ophthalmology is another important area under investigation here. Opticrom, a new eye drug that prevents conjunctivitis, was recently licensed for use in the United States after having been studied for seven years at UHC.

The hospital is also the site of an NIH-funded Clinical Research Center, where specialized studies are conducted in numerous areas including breast cancer, sleep disorders, childhood hypoglycemia, and, most significantly, in cystic fibrosis (in 1986 CWRU received over $800,000 for studies of this disease).

## Admission Policy

Arrangements for most admissions to UHC, other than obstetric and gynecologic, are made in advance between the physician and the Humphrey Building Admitting Reservations Office, although patients can be admitted through the emergency room or by a physician. Obstetric and gynecologic patients are admitted to MacDonald Hospital, and arrangements are made through the Admitting Office there.

---

**ROOM CHARGES (per diem)**
Private: $600
Semiprivate: $575
ICU: $1,200

**AVERAGE COST PER PATIENT STAY:**    $6,225

**MAILING ADDRESS**          **TELEPHONE**
2074 Abington Road          216-844-1000
Cleveland, OH 44106

---

# Hospital of the
# University of Pennsylvania
**PHILADELPHIA, PENNSYLVANIA**

As do most of the hospitals cited in this book, the Hospital of the University of Pennsylvania (HUP) conducts a survey to evaluate its services from the point of view of the patients. The results of HUP's survey are just about the highest of any we've reviewed. Of the 1,050 HUP patients surveyed in fiscal year 1985, 90 percent responded that they were very satisfied with their overall experience and another 9 percent were satisfied.

Strict quality-assurance programs and excellent nursing services account for part of these ratings, but it is perhaps the humanistic attitude of the professional staff at HUP that is the major factor in patient satisfaction. An example of this attitude is apparent in the waiting rooms. Responding to extensive research indicating that the most anxiety-producing time for the family of a patient is the period during which their relative is in the operating room, nurses here have organized a direct phone line from the operating room to the waiting area to convey information to family members every two hours during the surgical procedure. If there is a delay in the holding area or the procedure is canceled, calls are made immediately. In addition, a direct phone line is set up for family members to call in from anywhere in the hospital.

Coupled with this humanistic approach, HUP offers a full range of acute, general care services, filling the health-care needs of West Philadelphia and serving as a referral center for the Delaware Valley and beyond for complex medical problems.

Medicine is the largest clinical department in the hospital, administering the Rodebaugh Diabetes Center, the clinical component of the University of Pennsylvania Diabetes Center, and the Stone Evaluation Center, a referral center for the northeastern United States for patients with a history of kidney and other types of stones. The Cardiovascular Section has developed the electrocardiographic procedure known as signal averaging, providing physicians with a dependable way of predicting who could be at risk of sudden death from heart attack, and the Pennsylvania peel, a surgical procedure that uses cardiac mapping to locate the source of tachycardia so that the inner lining of the heart may be peeled away in that area, leaving healthy tissue intact.

In the Department of Surgery, HUP physicians perform 100 kidney transplants a year, and the Division of Plastic Surgery is among the world's foremost in cleft-palate and cleft-lip surgery and in craniofacial reconstruction. Work in pancreas as well as islet transplantation is offering hope to diabetics. The Division of Cardiothoracic Surgery has made pioneering advances in the surgical treatment of irregular heart rhythms.

The University of Pennsylvania Cancer Center is one of only twenty or so Comprehensive Cancer Centers designated by the NIH. The center specializes in surgical oncology and offers a hospice program to improve the quality of life for cancer patients and their families.

Its Breast Cancer Program has earned an international reputation for the treatment of early breast cancer with lumpectomy and radiotherapy as an alternative to mastectomy. In conjunction with the Breast Cancer Program, the Radiation Therapy Department of HUP, one of the most active in the country in both treatment of patients and training of radiation therapists, has a national reputation in research in and treatment of breast cancer following lumpectomy.

The world-renowned Pigmented Lesion Clinic and Melanoma Program is one of the foremost patient-care and research efforts in the evaluation and treatment of moles. The clinic, in the Department of Dermatology, is the largest facility in the United States for the diagnosis and treatment of melanoma. The hospital is the only major medical center between New York and Washington, DC, using Mohs surgery for the removal of cutaneous malignant tumor tissue. It is also one of the few centers in the United States using phototherapy to treat psoriasis and other light-related diseases.

The In Vitro Fertilization Program in the Department of Obstetrics and Gynecology treats couples afflicted with a wide variety of reproductive disorders that may result in infertility. As of March 1986, 33 babies have been born in this program. Known for its work in infertility, the Division of Human Reproduction was among the first to attempt to treat tubal disease with microsurgery. High-risk obstetrics involving patients threatened by diabetes mellitus, Rh factor, and premature or preterm birth is another major area of concentration.

One of the best facilities for hip replacement and revision, HUP is also renowned for ambitious multidisciplinary efforts in its metabolic bone disease unit. Capacitive coupling, using electrical impulses to stimulate bone growth in nonunion fractures, was developed in the Department of Orthopaedic Surgery. Joint transplantation, available in only three other centers in North America, is being developed at the Joint Reconstruction Center.

The Department of Psychiatry provides comprehensive consultation, evaluation, and management of all psychiatric disorders, including acute psychoses. A number of specialty programs, including Affective Disorders, Brain and Behavior Research, Geropsychiatry, and Pain Management, provide advanced diagnostic evaluation and acute care, both inpatient and outpatient. Cognitive therapy, a technique for relieving negative emotions, was developed here.

New programs in Dental Medicine include an interdisciplinary group of dentists and physicians specializing in the diagnosis and treatment of facial pain and temporomandibular joint disease; a section on cosmetic and functional deformities of the teeth, mouth, and jaws; and the use of maxillofacial prosthetics to replace facial structures lost to disease, surgery, or accident.

The Otorhinolaryngology Department has pioneered developments for successful cochlear implants. The Smell and Taste Center's 12-stage air-dilution human olfactometer—the only one in the world—provides computer-based measurement of nasal airflow and taste functions, allowing researchers to study the smell and taste functions.

The Institute for Environmental Medicine serves as a regional focus for hyperbaric therapy. Besides research, these facilities are used for the emergency treatment of patients requiring exposure to increased oxygen pressures, as in the treatment of air embolism, the bends, carbon monoxide poisoning, or gas gangrene. They are also used for elective treatment of specific chronic defects of healing, such as in osteoradionecrosis and osteomyelitis.

The hospital's Emergency Department is one of the busiest in the city. Adjacent to the emergency room is a walk-in clinic where patients with nonurgent medical problems are treated on a first-come, first-served basis.

Every member of HUP's medical staff has an academic appointment in the University of Pennsylvania School of Medicine or the School of Dental Medicine, and most are involved in research.

Established in 1874, HUP was the first university-owned hospital in the United States built to serve specifically as a clinical teaching facility. One hundred years later a major expansion program was initiated. Projected for completion in 1987, the project involves a 15-level clinical services tower, which will include a state-of-the-art surgical suite with expanded critical-care units; a new psychiatric unit; improvements in pathology and laboratory medicine; expanded facilities for radiation therapy, respiratory care therapy, and student health; along with a new kitchen and cafeteria facilities serving patients and staff.

## Specialties

There are 18 clinical departments at HUP: Anesthesia, Dental Medicine, Dermatology, Emergency Medicine, Environmental Medicine and Hyperbaric Therapy, Medicine, Neurology, Obstetrics/Gynecology, Ophthalmology, Orthopaedic Surgery, Otorhinolaryngology and Human Communication, Pathology and Laboratory Medicine, Pediatrics, Physical Medicine and Rehabilitation, Psychiatry, Radiation Therapy, Radiology, and Surgery.

In addition, outpatient services include Allergy, Cardiology, Diabetes, Endocrinology, Gastroenterology, General Medicine, Geriatric Internal Medicine, the Health Evaluation Center, Hematology/Oncology, the Immunization Program, Occupational Health Programs, Pulmonary, Renal-Electrolyte, Rheumatology, the Travelers Program, Urology, and the Walk-In Clinic.

The Health Evaluation Center provides periodic physical examinations to individuals in the professional and business community in the Delaware Valley, ensuring ongoing medical care for those who wish to have a primary physician at HUP.

---

**STATISTICAL PROFILE (1985–86)**

Number of Beds: 686
Bed Occupancy Rate: 80.7%
Average Number of Patients: 553
Average Patient Stay: 7.7 days
Annual Admissions: 26,110
Births: 3,224
Outpatient Clinic Visits: 300,000
Emergency Room/Trauma Center Visits: 50,000

Hospital Personnel:
  Physicians: 700
  Residents: 650
  Registered Nurses: 740
  Total Staff: 4,400

---

# Well-known Specialists

Dr. Clyde F. Barker, vascular, transplant, and general surgery.
Dr. Stanley Baum, radiology; specialist in cardiovascular radiology.
Dr. Carl T. Brighton, M.D., Ph.D., orthopedic surgery; specialist in non-union of fractures.
Dr. Laurence E. Earley, nephrology.
Dr. William J. Erdman II, physical medicine and rehabilitation.
Dr. Robert L Goodman, radiation therapy; specialist in radiation oncology.
Dr. Martin S. Greenberg, dental and oral medicine.
Dr. Sheldon Jacobson, emergency and internal medicine.
Dr. Leonard Jarett, pathology and laboratory medicine; specialist in diabetes.
Dr. Thomas W. Langfitt, neurosurgery.
Dr. Gerald Lazarus, dermatology; specialist in psoriasis.
Dr. Luigi Mastroianni, Jr., obstetrics and gynecology; specialist in reproductive endocrinology and infertility.

Dr. Frederick Murtagh, neurosurgery.

Dr. Charles Nichols, ophthalmology.

Dr. George Peckham, pediatrics; specialist in neonatology.

Dr. Donald H. Silberberg, neurology; specialist in multiple sclerosis.

Dr. James B. Snow, Jr., otorhinolaryngology; specialist in head and neck surgery.

Dr. Alan J. Wein, urology; specialist in neurourology, incontinence, urologic oncology, and reconstructive surgery.

Dr. Peter C. Whybrow, psychiatry; specialist in thyroid disorders related to mood disorders.

Dr. Harry Wollman, anesthesiology.

# Research

Research at the University of Pennsylvania School of Medicine is conducted in many areas. Diabetes research is a combined effort of the Rodebaugh Diabetes Center and the George Cox Medical Research Institute. Transplants of the pancreas and the islets of Langerhans are being studied as a means to combat diabetic complications. In fact, HUP is the first hospital in the Philadelphia area to perform pancreatic transplants.

Members of the Department of Human Genetics, part of a joint U.S.-Canadian team of scientists, are working on isolating the gene that causes the most common form of muscular dystrophy, analyzing it, and determining why genetic defects cause this disease.

The hospital has been awarded an NIH grant to become a national computer resource center for three-dimensional imaging. Magnetic resonance imaging, CAT scans, and ultrasound are being combined with state-of-the-art computer programs to create three-dimensional images of the insides of the body.

A recent study of the Obesity Research Group links fatness and obesity to biologic parents and indicates that early childhood experience has little influence on whether a person will grow up obese.

The hospital's Premenstrual Syndrome Treatment Program was the first in Philadelphia designed to help women with this condition. An interdisciplinary team of specialists provides medical treatment, psychological counseling, and nutritional education while conducting research into causes of and treatments for the disorder.

The Department of Surgery is studying heart augmentation, a technique whereby a spare muscle is removed from the body, treated with electric shocks to strengthen it, attached to a major artery, and connected to a pacemaker so that it will contract like a healthy heart and pump additional blood. This technique could help people with severe congestive heart failure.

Other special areas of research include Alzheimer's disease, multiple sclerosis, and psoriasis.

# Admission Policy

All patients at HUP must be admitted by a staff physician. Self-referring patients and physicians should call 215-662-4000.

Although HUP does not have a specific number of beds or a specific dollar amount of indigent care, the hospital has an open-door policy, so that no one in need of medical attention is turned away because of money.

---

**ROOM CHARGES** (per diem)
Private: $611
Semiprivate: $543
ICU: $965 per day

**MAILING ADDRESS**          **TELEPHONE**
3400 Spruce Street          215-662-4000
Philadelphia, PA 19104

# The Milton S. Hershey Medical Center Pennsylvania State University

HERSHEY, PENNSYLVANIA

The concept of replacing the function of the human heart with a mechanical substitute is far from new but few hospitals in the country have been as involved with artificial organs as the University Hospital at The Milton S. Hershey Medical Center of the Pennsylvania State University. In medical circles one of the best known artificial organs is the Penn State heart, developed seven years ago by Dr. William S. Pierce and members of a research team of The Pennsylvania State University Colleges of Medicine and Engineering. A prototype of the heart was first used in December 1976; since then Dr. Pierce has performed about 40 operations using the heart. The air-powered artificial heart made its debut in October 1985; it was designed specifically as a "bridging device" until a human donor heart becomes available.

In addition to the Penn State heart, the University Hospital is involved with three other major artificial organ projects: a ventricular-assist pump, an electric long-term ventricular-assist device designed for complete implantation, and an electric total artificial heart. These devices are expected to be ready for clinical use in the next decade.

Yet research is only one part of the work performed at The Hershey Medical Center. Its more immediate purpose is to serve as a full-service tertiary-care institution, the only one between Pittsburgh and Philadelphia. Hershey is a referral center for patients throughout Pennsylvania; it also provides primary care for residents of the surrounding area. In patient care Hershey has many established centers of excellence and comprehensive programs.

For example, the Neonatal Intensive Care Unit serves as the regional center for central Pennsylvania, treating critically ill newborns whose problems range from premature and respiratory distress to congenital heart defects requiring open-heart surgery. The hospital is one of four to participate in the Neonatal Surgery Program of the Pennsylvania Department of Health, established to treat infants with congenital malformations of the intestinal, respiratory, and urinary tracts. The neonatal unit has 26 bassinets, and more than 700 infants are referred here annually from more than 50 hospitals in 20 counties. The hospital also owns and operates its own mobile neonatal intensive care unit to transport sick infants.

The Pediatric and Adult Heart Surgery Program has been designated as one of four official centers in the commonwealth for state-sponsored programs in child cardiac care. Patients with either congenital or acquired diseases are managed in the program, and more than 500 operations are performed annually.

The Child Psychiatry Unit provides comprehensive diagnostic assessment and intensive treatment for children aged three to thirteen who suffer from a variety of behavior and conduct disorders, including anorexia nervosa, autism, child abuse, depression and suicide, hyperactivity, learning disorders, and childhood psychosis. This unit, in addition to promoting a homelike atmosphere, includes several innovative design features, such as a closed nursing observation area for viewing children with special medical problems and audiovisual therapy—taping children and their parents together—for assessing and monitoring treatment.

Adult cancer is treated by faculty from many departments. Scientific programs have been established in the divisions of endocrinology, gynecologic oncology, hematology, oncology, otorhinolaryngology, and plastic and reconstructive surgery. Established protocols and investigative methods are used to treat more than 1,000 new patients each year with the primary diagnosis of cancer.

The hospital also serves as the center for the Central Pennsylvania Oncology Group, an outreach program that includes 91 physicians and nurses affiliated with 32 community hospitals.

The Department of Obstetrics and Gynecology offers a wide range of outpatient and inpatient diagnostic and treatment regimens, including evaluations for problems relating to endocrinology-infertility, menopause, and premenstrual syndrome. For women who have gynecologic cancer, the department provides complete services, including evaluation and all forms of treatment. In addition, the staff's clinical expertise includes family-centered care for normal and high-risk pregnancies, family planning, general gynecology, and gynecologic urology.

The University Hospital is the designated site of the Capital Area Poison Center, which serves residents throughout southcentral Pennsylvania. As a service of the hospital, the poison center maintains comprehensive information on product formulation and treatment of poisons. An affiliate of the American Association of Poison Control Centers, the center functions as an information and referral network for seven area hospitals. In 1984 it responded to more than 6,400 calls.

The Short Stay Unit offers treatment on an outpatient basis, which is usually more convenient and less costly for the patient. The Pain Management Clinic, a program of the Department of Anesthesiology, is part of this unit. The clinic combines various specialties in the diagnosis and treatment of persistent pain. The two main techniques used are transcutaneous electrical nerve stimulus (TENS) and biofeedback. The use of TENS produces relief from pain and also prompts the release of endorphins, a natural bodily substance that inhibits the transmission of pain by the nerves. Biofeedback teaches patients to control parts of the body not normally under conscious control. This technique helps in the management of pain and can even alter the perception of pain.

Within the psychiatric department, the Sleep Disorders Clinic and Laboratory is one of the most advanced of its kind in the world. It has achieved breakthroughs in the diagnosis and treatment of insomnia, narcolepsy, and night terrors, as well as sleep apnea.

Senior citizens receive complete psychiatric and medical examinations, as well as neuropsychological testing, in the comprehensive psychogeriatric outpatient program that is part of the psychiatric department. The University Hospital is designing an inpatient geriatric psychiatry unit as well as developing a partial hospitalization program for geriatric patients.

In 1982 the Pennsylvania State University assumed control of The Elizabethtown Hospital and Rehabilitation Center, a 55-bed facility providing rehabilitation services for severe and complicated disabilities. Elizabethtown offers comprehensive programs in brain injury, neurodevelopmental disability, pediatric orthopedics, spina bifida, and spinal cord injury. The orthopedic service provides a variety of family-oriented services to correct or prevent deformities in children. The neurodevelopmental service treats learning and developmental problems such as cerebral palsy and traumatic head injury. Adolescent and adult patients with spinal cord injuries and deterioration receive rehabilitation services. There are plans to relocate the hospital to the Hershey campus.

Milton S. Hershey, founder of the Hershey Chocolate Company, established a foundation named for him, which in 1963 awarded Penn State a $50-million trust to establish a medical school, hospital, and related research and graduate programs. Today components of the medical center include the University Hospital, the medical sciences building, the animal research facility, the magnetic resonance imaging facility, the recreation facility, and University Manor apartments for students and resident physicians. In addition, 20 other institutions aid in teaching through major affiliations with the medical center.

## Specialties

Anesthesiology, Family and Community Medicine, Internal Medicine, Medicine, Neonatal Intensive Care, Obstetrics/Gynecology, Pediatrics, Physiology, Psychiatry, and Surgery.

The pediatrics department has particular expertise in treating childhood cancer, cardiac malfunctions, leukemia, and premature birth.

The University Hospital has established state and regional centers in cancer, cardiology, core endocrine testing, duplex scanning technology, hematology, neonatology, spinal cord injury, and sports medicine.

Special services and comprehensive programs are offered in allergy, arthritis, cardiothoracic surgery, child cardiac care, child psychiatry, genetic disorders, hemophilia, high-risk obstetrics, hypertension, infertility, multiple sclerosis, muscular dystrophy, newborn surgical care, pain management, premenstrual syndrome, sleep disorders, tinnitus, and many others.

Specialized services include cardiac rehabilitation, nutritional care, physical therapy, recreational therapy, respiratory therapy, and speech pathology.

---

**STATISTICAL PROFILE**

Number of Beds: 362
Bed Occupancy Rate: 81.9%
Average Number of Patients: 272
Average Patient Stay: 7.9 days
Annual Admissions: 13,899
Births: 774
Outpatient Clinic Visits: 138,415
Emergency Room/Trauma Center Visits: 15,608

Hospital Personnel:
  Physicians: 299
  Residents: 216
  Registered Nurses: 341
  Total Staff: 1,224

---

# Well-known Specialists

Dr. John W. Burnside, author of the fifteenth and sixteenth editions of the classic *Adams' Physical Diagnosis*, chief of internal medicine.

Dr. Roger J. Cadieux, psychiatry; screener of heart transplant and artificial heart recipients to ensure that they will be mentally able to undergo heart surgery, specialist in sleep disorders.

Dr. Dwight Davis, cardiologist for Hershey's heart transplant team.

Dr. M. Elaine Eyster, specialist in AIDS research, professor of medicine.

Dr. Anthony Kales, director of the sleep research and treatment center.

Dr. John L. Penncock, surgery; specialist in heart transplants.

Dr. William S. Pierce, pioneer in developing the Penn State heart and, in March 1985, became the second person in the United States authorized by the FDA to implant an artificial heart, chief of the division of artificial organs.

Dr. John A. Waldhausen, specialist in cardiothoracic surgery and heart research, chairman of the department of surgery.

# Research

As part of Penn State, Hershey conducts basic and clinical research in many fields of medicine. Cancer research here is internationally acclaimed, and awards in this area alone exceed $5 million. In all, federal support for research at the medical center totaled almost $16 million in 1984–85.

A 1979 study by the State University of New York Medical Center of the research productivity of academic departments of pediatrics found that the department at Hershey is, per capita, the most productive in the country.

Research interests within obstetrics and gynecology include exercise and menstrual dysfunction, exercise in pregnancy, earlier detection and better treatment of ovarian cancer, and the cause and treatment of uterine cancer.

A research team headed by Dr. M. Elaine Eyster, professor of medicine and part of Hershey's hemophilia research laboratory, has been involved in AIDS research for the past several years.

Tracheostomies below the voice boxes of 100 people suffering from sleep apnea have had an almost 100 percent cure rate.

# Admission Policy

Most of the patients admitted to Hershey come via doctor referral. However, patients are also admitted through the clinics. Some clinics allow patients to walk in; others require an appointment.

---

**ROOM CHARGES (per diem)**
Private: $265 (All rooms at Hershey are private.)
ICU: $850

**AVERAGE COST PER PATIENT STAY:**  $7,000
The cost of heart and heart-lung transplants averages approximately $75,000 (for inpatient services only), although the figure does vary. If insurance does not sufficiently cover the procedure, a deposit of 20 percent, or $15,000, is required.

| **MAILING ADDRESS** | **TELEPHONE** |
| --- | --- |
| PO Box 850 | 717-531-8521 |
| Hershey, PA 17033 | |

---

# Presbyterian-University Hospital

**PITTSBURGH, PENNSYLVANIA**

To the people who live and work in Pittsburgh, ready access to a number of first-rate hospitals (Mercy, Montefiore, St. Francis, and Shadyside, for example) is an important reason that their city has come to be regarded as one of the most desirable places to live in the nation. Unlike Boston, Houston, or New York, Pittsburgh is not a city most people think of as a leading medical enclave, but doctors and those in hospital administration know that in recent years Presbyterian-University Hospital (known as Presby), the principal teaching institution of the University of Pittsburgh School of Medicine, has emerged as one of America's outstanding medical facilities.

Although Jonas Salk developed his polio vaccine here in the 1950s, until recently Presby was basically a highly regarded teaching hospital and a well-known regional tertiary-care center. However, in 1981 Dr. Thomas Starzl arrived and helped transform the hospital into one of the world's foremost organ transplantation centers. Dr. Starzl was the key figure in designing the techniques used in liver transplantation. He was also instrumental in testing cyclosporine, the drug that suppresses the body's natural tendency to reject a new organ. The significance of his work is enormous, as a dean of the UCLA medical school, where Starzl had originally planned to bring his program, acknowledged: "The loss of Tom Starzl was the greatest recruiting loss at UCLA in thirty years."

What was lost, of course, was the professional prestige a successful transplantation program brings, not to mention the research money from foundations and the media attention that engulfs the whole institution and brings recognition to both the hospital and the medical school. And it has been virtually impossible for the news media to ignore Presby's program. Between 1980 and 1986 there have been over 2,100 transplants at Presby, including 275 heart transplants and an extraordinary 800 liver transplants (253 in 1985 alone, more than half those done in the entire country). Since 1983 there have been 42 heart-lung and 13 pancreas transplants, both very complex and difficult procedures. Even the kidney transplant program, which was begun in 1964, was dramatically affected; it went from 47 operations in 1980 to 204 in 1984. In addition, the hospital uses the Jarvik-7 artificial heart as a bridge device until a human heart for transplant can be found. In the twelve months following the first implant in October 1985, surgeons at Presby implanted eight more temporary Jarvik devices. The hospital is now the country's leader in Jarvik implantation.

Geography has also played an important role in Presby's success as a transplant center. Because Pittsburgh is within an hour's flying time of 70 percent of the country's population, Presby's medical teams have quick access to organs when they become available. The city also boasts one of the best procurement teams in the country; every year it flies over 250,000 miles to transport lifesaving organs.

Having said all this, we have to add a cautionary and somewhat negative note. The fame of this hospital has sent hundreds of very sick people to Pittsburgh in search of organ transplants. Many must be rejected for medical reasons, some for financial ones. The cost of transplantation is so high that the hospital—like other transplant centers—has had to develop a rigid method of guaranteeing payment (see page 274). Unfortunately, a Pittsburgh newspaper discovered that surgeons at the hospital gave certain foreign nationals precedence over Americans for scarce organs. Although the furor has waned and the hospital assures us it was all a regrettable error, now well in the past, we feel obligated to tell prospective patients about the real effects of financial matters in the world of transplant surgery.

Presby does, however, try to assist transplant patients and their families through several hospital-sponsored fund-raising groups. The Cyclosporine Fund, for example, helps needy patients pay for the drug that prevents the body's rejection of the new organ (its annual cost is about $8,000); the Spirit of Life Fund provides aid to patients' families who might not be able to travel to the hospital to provide essential emotional support. The hospital also works closely with several independent groups that offer a variety of postoperative services—including financial, medical, and psychological assistance—to both families and organ recipients.

Although transplantation was the key to putting Presby on the national medical map, it is hardly the hospital's only important specialty. Orthopedic surgery, for example, has a history of pioneering work in developing artificial implants dating back over twenty-five years. Neurosurgery, under the direction of Dr. Peter Jannetta, has achieved international fame in the last few years for discovering microsurgical procedures for relieving dizziness, hypertension, and constant vertigo. Dr. Jannetta is a leading authority on the cranial nerves and has performed over 2,000 operations to relieve facial tics and spasms as well as severe facial pain.

The Pittsburgh Cancer Institute, a comprehensive center for research in and treatment of cancer, is a joint effort of Presby and the other hospitals of the University Health Center of Pittsburgh, the University of Pittsburgh, and Carnegie-Mellon University. The center is the only one in the country focusing research on treatment with biological response modifiers—agents that stimulate the body's natural defenses against cancer.

In addition to medical evaluation and care, the Geriatric Center provides psychiatric assessment and treatment, health education, and individual and family counseling. The Pittsburgh Diabetes Center offers individualized education and training in the self-management of diabetes. Other specialized clinics include the Hypertension Clinic, the Pain Control Center, and the

Sudden Cardiac Death Prevention Center. Presby is also noted for its programs in cardiology, internal medicine, and plastic and reconstructive surgery. Falk Clinic is the ambulatory care facility of the University Health Center.

As you would expect in a place that delivers so many advanced medical services, Presby has easy access to almost every kind of technical device used in a major referral center. The Specialized Neurosurgical Center, the first to use CAT scanning for surgical purposes, has recently purchased what will be the only gamma knife in clinical use in the United States. Developed at the Karolinska Institute in Sweden, it uses radiation to treat deep-seated brain tumors that were once considered inoperable.

Because it is also a regional trauma center, Presby is exceptionally well equipped to deal with emergency situations. Critical-care service includes medical and surgical intensive care units, a neurosurgical continuous care unit, and a coronary care unit. During the past few years the hospital has experienced a 50 percent increase in the number of patients requiring intensive care; growth in the transplantation and trauma services has made this need especially acute. Because both emergency medicine and critical-care medicine are so important here, the hospital sponsers highly regarded training programs in those areas for physicians and nurses from the region. Presby is the site of the largest critical-care training program for physicians in the country.

Obviously, this is a hospital poised for the great leap into the twenty-first century, ready to accept the dramatic changes medical technology is sure to bring about. In such a high-powered setting, it should come as no surprise that the nursing staff is more than a cut above average. For example, over 65 percent of the registered nurses here have a bachelor's degree, and about half of the head nurses have a master's; these figures are almost twice the national norm. In addition, because the hospital does so much critical care, the ratio of registered nurses to beds is almost one to one. While no one would claim that these factors alone guarantee excellent patient care, you can be certain that nursing is not given a backseat here and that the people who choose to be nurses at Presby have a commitment to their profession.

Commitment in fact seems to be the word that best sums up the impression this hospital left on us. A commitment to excellence, of course, but also a willingness to explore the possibilities of medicine without fear of the criticism that's sure to follow. To do this while maintaining the best possible patient care is something very few hospitals can claim. But you don't have to take our word for it; here's the public statement made by the physicians who conducted the Joint Commission on Accreditation of Hospitals survey of Presby: "We cherish the opportunity to see what you are doing here. The Hospital is to be commended for providing really quality care. It has been a pleasure to survey Presby."

## Specialties

Anesthesiology, Cardiology, Dermatology, Emergency Medicine and Trauma, Endocrinology, Gastroenterology, Hematology/Oncology, Hypertension and Clinical Pharmacology, Immunopathology, Infectious Diseases, Medicine, Neurology, Neurosurgery, Nuclear Medicine, Oral and Maxillofacial Surgery, Orthopaedic Surgery, Pathology, Plastic Surgery, Pulmonary Medicine, Radiology, Rehabilitation Medicine, Renal-Electrolyte Medicine, Rheumatology, Surgery, Urological Surgery, and Urology.

---

**STATISTICAL PROFILE**

Number of Beds: 568
Bed Occupancy Rate: 79%
Average Number of Patients: 444
Average Patient Stay: 9 days
Annual Admissions: 17,949
Outpatient Clinic Visits: 30,607
Emergency Room/Trauma Center Visits: 21,560

Hospital Personnel:
  Physicians: 514
  Residents: 502
  Registered Nurses: 562
  Total Staff: 2,500

---

## Well-known Specialists

Dr. Henry Bahnson, heart transplantation.
Dr. Paul Chervenick, hematology.
Dr. Bartley Griffith, heart transplantation.
Dr. Thomas Hakala, urology.
Dr. Robert Hardesty, heart transplantation.
Dr. Peter Jannetta, neurosurgery; specialist in the cranial nerves.
Dr. Dana Mears, orthopedic surgery.
Dr. Thomas Medsger, Jr., rheumatology.
Dr. Oscar Reinmuth, neurology.
Dr. Alan Robinson, endocrinology.
Dr. Robert M. Rogers, pulmonary medicine.
Dr. Thomas Starzl, liver transplantation and immunosuppression in transplant recipients.

# Research

Presby is noted for its research programs in cardiology, hematology/oncology, internal medicine, neurosurgery, orthopedics, and plastic and reconstructive surgery. As expected, extensive research is conducted in transplantation, including improving surgical strategies for liver transplants; designing a carrier for transporting the beating heart and lungs from a donor to a waiting patient; developing a new system for determining the need for transplantation; investigating a promising new antirejection drug; undertaking preliminary study of an artificial lung; and continuing to refine protocols and techniques for improving survival statistics.

The hospital is also active in clinical and surgical research. The Rapid Infusion System replaces lost blood at 15 times the rate of traditional intravenous methods. The pump, developed by a Presby anesthesiologist, has become an essential part of surgeries involving severe blood loss, such as transplantation and traumas. The Food and Drug Administration also recently approved a new treatment for patients with arrhythmic hearts—the implantable cardiac defibrillator, which was developed here.

The Orthopaedic Research Lab focuses on implant materials, new implant surfaces, and substitute bone material as partners in reconstructive surgery. As a leader in orthopedic research for more than twenty-five years, Presby has helped establish the viability of total joint replacement.

The hospital is also the site of an NIH-funded Clinical Research Center, which conducts specialized studies in diabetes, hypertension, and nephrology. The Division of Infectious Diseases conducts research trials with patients who have herpes simplex virus. They are also studying interferon's role in the treatment of herpes zoster, commonly known as shingles. Pain relief, improved treatment of cardiac arrests, and other medical procedures are conducted on the city of Pittsburgh's mobile intensive care units, nicknamed "super ambulances."

# Admission Policy

With the exception of those in the transplant program, prospective Presby patients are admitted either through the Emergency Department or through Falk Clinic, the outpatient facility associated with the hospital. Patients without a physician will have one from the hospital staff assigned to them.

While there is no formally stated policy requiring a prospective patient to show an ability to pay, the hospital administration makes it clear that everyone who can afford to do so is expected to pay. In 1985 Presby underwrote over $3.5 million in charity care and uncollectible accounts, and the people there sound determined to keep that figure stable, at the very least.

*Organ Transplantation Costs*: Organ transplants are enormously expensive. At Presby the cost of just an evaluation to determine whether a patient needs a transplant or is a good candidate to receive one range from $6,000 for heart patients to $12,000 for those with liver conditions. Almost all insurance plans cover these evaluation charges, but patients need to inquire very carefully about their particular plan's coverage for an actual transplant. Presby requires a preoperation letter of credit, proof of insurance coverage for these charges, or a deposit of $78,000 for heart, $125,000 for heart-lung, and $115,000 for liver transplants.

---

**ROOM CHARGES (per diem)**
Private: $351–$419
Semiprivate: $335
ICU:
   Cardiovascular: $789
   Coronary Care: $1,255
   Medical/Surgical: $1,640

**AVERAGE COST PER PATIENT STAY**
$6,730 (not including transplant patients)

**MAILING ADDRESS**    **TELEPHONE**
DeSoto at O'Hara Street   412-647-2345
Pittsburgh, PA 15213

# Wills Eye Hospital

## PHILADELPHIA, PENNSYLVANIA

Although the procedure of extracting cataracts is not new, the operation and the recovery period have changed radically in the past eighty years. In 1910 cataract extractions at Wills Eye Hospital meant three weeks of immobility, with the patient's head surrounded by sandbags. Today the operation is performed on an outpatient basis. In fact, the rise of outpatient, or day surgery, operations represents an enormous revolution in eye treatment. In 1986, 5,746 day surgery procedures were performed at Wills, of which 3,700 were on adults needing cataract extractions and 1,400 were on children requiring correction of eye muscle problems.

Day surgery procedures are performed in Wills's nine operating rooms, where ceiling-mounted microscopes enable physicians to use the most refined techniques and instrumentation available. Recently, part of a floor at Wills was converted into semiprivate recovery rooms to allow day surgery patients to rest for three to six hours after surgery in the company of a relative or a close friend.

Wills is the nation's largest facility devoted solely to eye care and a worldwide referral center for the treatment of both the most common eye problems and the rarest sight-threatening diseases.

Because Wills specializes, it is able to offer state-of-the-art ophthalmologic diagnostic and treatment resources. For example, in 1985 the radiology department installed a high-resolution GE9800 CAT scanner, which provides clear cross-sectional images of microscopic sections of the eye and brain for the diagnosis of eye and orbital trauma and for detecting foreign bodies or tumors in the eye.

An equally important acquisition in 1985 was the PAR Image Analyzer, then only the second of its type in the United States, which provides a computerized analysis of the image of the eye. The analyzer is used in conjunction with the Octopus Computerized Perimetry, which precisely gauges the range of a patient's vision, to diagnose glaucoma.

A phacoemulsification machine, developed by a former Wills resident, removes cataracts with ultrasonic waves.

Also developed by a Wills doctor is an instrument used for a procedure called vitrectomy, frequently used to treat retinal complications.

Wills employs every major laser capability: argon, krypton, and YAG lasers are used to treat a wide range of ocular disorders, such as cancer, diabetic retinopathy, glaucoma, macular degeneration, postcataract complications, and retinal tears.

In 1985 Wills established the Ocular Trauma Center as part of its emergency services. The center provides patients with severe eye injuries access to highly specialized ophthalmologic surgeons on a twenty-four-hour on-call basis. It was also one of twenty-eight regional eye traumas centers named to the National Eye Trauma System, which evaluates the treatment of ocular injuries nationwide.

Wills's Cornea Service is one of nine centers in the United States participating in the Prospective Evaluation of Radial Keratotomy (PERK), an ongoing National Eye Institute study assessing the effects of radial keratotomy on myopia. Results indicate that the procedure effectively reduces nearsightedness with no serious short-term complications, although prediction of long-term success is unreliable.

Much of Wills's success must be credited to its nursing staff, which includes 90 ophthalmologic nurses, who have received extensive training in all aspects of eye care, such as anatomy, diseases, emergency treatment, and surgical procedures. Continuing education programs and participation in clinical studies are all part of the nursing program at Wills. Several staff nurses are also on the faculty at Thomas Jefferson University.

Wills is a major affiliate of Thomas Jefferson and a preeminent center for ophthalmologic education. Thirteen new physicians joined the Wills residency program in 1986, bringing the total enrollment to 38 and making it the largest ophthalmology residency program in the country. In addition, 21 ophthalmologists pursued one- or two-year fellowships in various sub-

---

**STATISTICAL PROFILE**

Number of Beds: 120
Bed Occupancy Rate: 37%
Average Number of Patients: 45
Average Patient Stay: 3.2 days
Annual Admissions: 5,370
Outpatient Clinic Visits: 228,000
Day Surgery: 5,746

*Note*: The bed occupancy rate and average number of patients reflect the major shift toward day surgical procedures in ophthalmology and outpatient laser treatment for major eye diseases.

Hospital Personnel:
Physicians: 259
Residents: 38
Registered Nurses: approximately 90
Total Staff: 460

specialties, including cornea, glaucoma, neuroophthalmology, oculoplastics, oncology, pediatrics, and retina.

Wills also provides continuing education programs for medical students and practicing physicians. During the past year members of the staff published six textbooks and more than 400 scientific articles and delivered over 500 lectures both in the United States and abroad.

Wills also serves the community in more immediate ways. Each spring the hospital sponsors a two-day public eye screening. In 1986 more than 1,000 people were examined, 37 percent of whom needed some kind of follow-up care, including treatment for sight-threatening conditions such as glaucoma and retinal detachment.

## Specialties

General Ophthalmology Service and nine subspecialties: Contact Lens, Cornea, Glaucoma, Neuro-Ophthalmology, Oculoplastics, Oncology, Pathology, Pediatric Ophthalmology, and Retina.

Wills also provides the Low Vision Service, and is a recognized facility for the treatment of ocular emergencies.

## Well-known Specialists

Dr. Raymond Adams, chief of the General Ophthalmology Service.
Dr. William H. Annesley, Jr., director of the Retina Service.
Dr. Joseph H. Calhoun, director of the Pediatric Ophthalmology Service.
Dr. Thomas D. Duane, author of the five-volume standard *Clinical Ophthalmology*, former ophthalmologist in chief.
Dr. Ralph C. Eagle, director of the Pathology Service.
Dr. Jay L. Federman, director of research.
Dr. Zoraida M. Fiol-Silva, director of the Contact Lens Service.
Dr. Joseph C. Flanagan, director of the Oculoplastic Service.
Dr. John B. Jeffers, director of the Low Vision Service.
Dr. Peter R. Laibson, director of the Cornea Service.
Dr. Peter J. Savino, director of the Neuro-Ophthalmology Service.
Dr. Jerry A. Shields, director of the Oncology Service.
Dr. George L. Spaeth, director of the Glaucoma Service.
Dr. William Tasman, specialist in the retina, ophthalmologist in chief at Wills and chairman of the Department of Ophthalmology at Jefferson Medical College of Thomas Jefferson University.

## Research

A major three-year research project by the Wills Neuro-Ophthalmology Service, in conjunction with the Neurology Department of the University of Pennsylvania, was funded by a 1985 grant from the National Multiple

Sclerosis Foundation. The grant is being used to continue research into the disease mechanisms involved in multiple sclerosis, the effects of which frequently become apparent to patients through their vision.

Other ongoing research projects include investigations into the treatment and cause of diabetic retinopathy, the use of lasers in treating glaucoma and in hemangiomas, the use of botulinum toxin in treating blepharospasm and strabismus, the cause of ocular melanoma, photoradiation therapy for ocular cancer, treatment for uveitis, and uveal melanoma. In 1986 research funding at Wills totaled a little over $884,000.

## Admission Policy

Patients can be admitted to Wills through the clinic, through the emergency room, or by physician referral. Anyone can call the General Ophthalmology Service Clinic (215-928-3041) to make an appointment. Or one's ophthalmologist can call Wills and make a referral.

In 1986 the hospital provided $3 million in indigent care and bad debts.

---

**ROOM CHARGES (per diem)**
Private: $515
Semiprivate: $450
Day Surgery: $450

**AVERAGE COST PER PATIENT STAY:**   $4,138

**MAILING ADDRESS**          **TELEPHONE**
Ninth and Walnut Streets   215-928-3000
Philadephia, PA 19107

---

# St. Jude Children's Research Hospital

**MEMPHIS, TENNESSEE**

When St. Jude opened in 1962, less than 4 percent of children with acute lymphocytic leukemia (ALL), the most common form of childhood cancer, survived. By 1965, with protocols developed at St. Jude, the survival figure had risen to a dramatic 17 percent, and today over 50 percent of the children diagnosed with ALL are living cancer-free for five years or more. Some St. Jude patients have been living normal, disease-free existences for as many as twenty years.

St. Jude operates the world's largest childhood cancer research center, treating children from 39 states and 29 foreign countries. It conducts basic and clinical research into catastrophic childhood disease, mainly cancer, and provides patient care. The children who come to St. Jude are afflicted with the most devastating kinds of disease; acute lymphocytic leukemia, Hodgkin's disease, numerous other forms of cancer, and severe infectious diseases.

St. Jude is the first and only institution established for the sole purpose of conducting basic and clinical research into catastrophic childhood diseases. Extensive research is done in the basic biological sciences—biochemistry, immunology, microbiology, pharmacology, tumor cell biology, and virology. Along with this basic research goes intensive clinical study in hematology and oncology.

St. Jude physicians pioneered the concept of treating patients outside the hospital as often as possible. Even in the initial effort to destroy all cancer cells, most children are treated through clinical visits. At this stage, the child visits the hospital daily for treatment, usually for four to eight weeks. When remission is achieved, the child goes on continuation therapy. A child at this stage commutes to St. Jude, sometimes for hundreds of miles, on a weekly basis but also receives treatment from the family doctor. After two and a half to three years, children who remain cancer-free are taken off medication and return to the hospital only for periodic evaluation and follow-up studies.

Unlike general health-care facilities, St. Jude provides continuous and increasingly long-term care to all children in its research studies. An active patient is one who is admitted to a research protocol, a scientific plan of study of illness. The treatment received depends on the state of the patient and the response to therapy.

Of St. Jude's more than 2,400 active patients, about 45 percent are enrolled in a protocol for one of the forms of leukemia, while about 47 percent are being followed by the solid tumor service. Eight percent are enrolled in hematology studies.

Some of these patients have also been the subjects of studies in the departments of psychology and social services. While these departments provide clinical services for families of patients, they also recently completed studies to determine whether long-term survivors of leukemia have permanent neuropsychological dysfunctions. These studies—conducted with the first sizable group of long-term cancer-free patients available—have provided the first description of psychological problems prevailing among children treated for ALL. They offer the initial step toward development of remedial education techniques for long-term survivors. Psychiatry/psychology studies in familial adjustment to the catastrophic diseases of childhood, children's learning difficulties after cancer treatment, and special problems of adolescents with malignant diseases requiring amputation are also under way.

Other areas of research provide more immediate results. For example, new techniques in surgery are helping patients with osteogenic sarcoma, a malignant primary tumor of the bone that was previously treated by amputation. The surgery, involving removal of the diseased section of the bone and replacement with a steel rod while leaving all blood vessels and nerves intact, is followed by chemotherapy and is proving successful.

One of the newest divisions at St. Jude is Tumor Cell Biology. Its goal is to intensify basic research in cancer biology. Members are investigating issues such as the regulation of normal cell proliferation and its pathological counterparts. Studies also examine cell transformation, regulation of oncogenes and transforming proteins, hormonal control of cell division, differentiation of hematopoietic cells, and cell surface receptors.

One of the most important and successful areas of research being conducted is the influenza study of Dr. Robert Webster. His pioneering work

---

**STATISTICAL PROFILE**

Number of Beds: 48
Bed Occupancy Rate: 60%
Average Number of Inpatients: 29
Average Patient Stay: 7 days
Annual Admissions: 1,800
Outpatient Clinic Visits: 21,500

Hospital Personnel:
  Full-time Faculty: 113
  Postdoctoral Fellows: 54
  Registered Nurses: 125
  Total Staff: 900

over the last several years has brought about a totally new understanding of influenza.

St. Jude enjoys a worldwide reputation as a teaching facility. Postdoctoral fellows with an M.D. or Ph.D. degree may enter programs for one to three years in one of the basic biomedical sciences or a clinical subspecialty.

St. Jude is supported primarily by volunteer contributions raised by ALSAC, the national fund-raising organization established by Danny Thomas expressly to support this institution.

## Specialties

Biochemistry, Hematology, Immunology, Infectious Disease, Nutrition, Oncology, Pathology, Pharmacology, Radiology, Radiotherapy, Surgery, Tumor Cell Biology, and Virology/Molecular Biology.

## Well-known Specialists

Dr. William Crist, chairman of hematology/oncology.
Dr. Allan Granoff, deputy director of St. Jude, chairman of virology/molecular biology.
Dr. Walter Hughes, chairman of child health sciences.
Dr. Joseph V. Simone, director of St. Jude.

## Admission Policy

Patients are admitted to St. Jude when referred by their attending physician.

There is no financial needs test. In cases of financial need, St. Jude will pay for transportation and lodging for the patient and one parent. Although the hospital will accept insurance benefits when available, insurance availability is never a criterion for admission.

---

**ROOM CHARGES** (per diem)
Inpatient: $262
Intensive Care: $587
Outpatient: $44

**AVERAGE COST PER PATIENT STAY:**    $850 per day for treatment

**MAILING ADDRESS**          **TELEPHONE**
332 North Lauderdale Street   901-522-0300
Box 318
Memphis, TN 38101

# Vanderbilt University Hospital
# Vanderbilt University Medical Center

**NASHVILLE, TENNESSEE**

Many hospitals tout themselves as being "in the forefront" of modern medicine. But we must emphasize that Vanderbilt is indeed on the "cutting edge"—way ahead of other hospitals in its innovative programs and obvious determination to be responsive to today's health-care needs.

Vanderbilt's Cooperative Care Center, for example, clearly shows the hospital's determination to meet patient needs without unnecessarily escalating costs and reflects, we think, one of the most sensible contemporary trends in health care. One of only two such centers in the country (see also University Hospital, pages 232–33), the Cooperative Care Center here brings family members actively into the care of the patient during hospitalization. A typical patient in this unit is one with a chronic disease, such as diabetes, who is having an acute episode, such as insulin shock. In the center the patient is brought through the episode and then, along with family members, is educated to avoid a recurrence. Long-range preventive steps are planned and implemented. This approach often reduces the cost of a patient's care by at least one-third.

Many other services offered at Vanderbilt are unique to the state and, in some instances, to the United States. Vanderbilt Children's Hospital, for example, is a prototype for about a dozen university hospitals around the country. Although it occupies two floors within Vanderbilt Hospital, Children's Hospital maintains a separate identity. This organization has enabled Children's to have the best of both worlds: the support of a comprehensive teaching and research medical center and the skills and expertise of a dedicated pediatric faculty. During 1984 Children's Hospital became the first member of its type to be admitted to the National Association of Children's Hospitals, which previously admitted only freestanding facilities.

Children's provides a complete range of medical services and treatment for patients from newborns to adolescents. Two of its newest specialty centers are the Division of Medical Genetics and the Children's Kidney Center. Research into many areas of pediatrics is also conducted at Children's Hospital.

One of the newest additions to Vanderbilt's campus is the Vanderbilt Child and Adolescent Psychiatric Hospital, opened in December 1985, which includes specialized treatment programs for a wide range of emotional and medical problems. In addition, the hospital serves as a center for medical education and training and for research into the causes and treatment of psychiatric disorders of children and adolescents.

Such innovative programs are reinforced by traditional medical services and nationally visible biomedical research. The medical center is made up of Vanderbilt University Hospital, the School of Medicine, and the School of Nursing. Patient-care statistics for 1985 indicate that Vanderbilt's principal business is secondary and tertiary referrals from local and regional physicians. Many clinics and centers at Vanderbilt afford patients a variety of medical specialties; we can only describe a select few.

The Parkinson's Disease Center is the only one within a seven-state area and provides diagnostic evaluation, drug treatment—including experimental therapies—and educational facilities for victims and their families. Only about six such treatment and research centers exist nationwide.

The Pain Center operates in conjunction with the departments of anesthesiology, neurology, neurosurgery, psychiatry, and psychology and helps with the management of chronic pain, such as that caused by arthritis or lower-back pain.

Vanderbilt's Institute for the Treatment of Alcoholism (VITA) provides comprehensive treatment that stresses individualized care. Designed for individuals eighteen years and over, the three-week inpatient regimen consists of a variety of therapies, including individual and group counseling, family counseling, and physical, recreational, and social activities.

In addition to cardiac transplants, Vanderbilt performs kidney and cornea transplants, and a pancreatic transplant team is ready to operate whenever a proper donor-recipient pair is identified. Since the inception of the kidney program in 1962, over 1,000 kidney transplants have been performed at Vanderbilt.

A state-of-the-art laser surgery program has recently been developed. A modern ambulatory care facility is currently under construction. Lifeflight, an air ambulance emergency service, provides services for hospital transfers as well as emergency flights to accident locations.

Even the traditional services at Vanderbilt are augmented by the most modern innovations and equipment. For example, Vanderbilt maintains a neonatal intensive care unit called Angel III. An ambulance designed to transport newborn babies with medical problems, Angel III has helped more than 3,000 infants since 1974. The Neonatal Intensive Care Unit in the hospital was the first such unit in the United States when it was founded in 1961. Today this nationally recognized unit treats more than 700 infants each year.

A 20-bed Burn Treatment Center, opened in November 1983, is the first one in middle Tennessee. It is also the largest and the most advanced burn center in the state. The center serves referral patients from the mid-South and emphasizes research and education in addition to patient care.

Medical equipment at Vanderbilt includes a magnetic resonance imager and a high-field magnet, acquired in 1984 from researchers in Switzerland. Researchers hope the magnet will prove effective in the diagnosis of muscular dystrophy and in testing the viability of kidneys about to be transplanted.

Vanderbilt constantly double-checks the services being offered to patients. During the most recent reviews by the Joint Commission on Accreditation of Hospitals and the College of American Pathologists, Vanderbilt was recognized for its outstanding quality-assurance program. This comprehensive program embraces both medical staff and support service department review. All areas, including the clinical service, have individually developed quality-assurance plans and specific monitoring programs.

While patients may not be aware of the significance of these efforts, they are certainly aware of the results. In a January 1986 survey of 400 former patients conducted by Vanderbilt, approximately 90 percent of respondents rated Vanderbilt as either the best or better than any other hospital in the area.

Vanderbilt University was founded in 1873 with a grant from Cornelius Vanderbilt; the medical school issued its first diplomas to 61 doctors in 1875. In the 1920s the school was restructured, and a new hospital was constructed on the Vanderbilt campus. A replacement facility, Vanderbilt University Hospital was opened in September of 1980.

## Specialties

Burn Treatment, Cardiology, Clinical Pharmacology, the Clinical Research Center, the Emergency/Trauma Center, Endocrinology/Metabolism, the Center for Fertility and Reproductive Research, Genetic Counseling, Hypertension, Intensive Care, Kidney Transplants, Neonatal Intensive Care, Neurosurgery, Oncology, Orthopedic Surgery and Rehabilitation, Pediatrics, Psychiatry, Rheumatology, and Surgery.

---

**STATISTICAL PROFILE**

Number of Beds: 661
Bed Occupancy Rate: 80.6%
Average Number of Patients: 494
Average Patient Stay: 8.3 days
Annual Admissions: 20,892
Births: 928
Outpatient Clinic Visits: 165,148
Emergency Room/Trauma Center Visits: 27,476

Hospital Personnel:
  Physicians: 962
  Residents: 433
  Registered Nurses: 997
  Total Staff: 5,227

# Well-known Specialists

Dr. George S. Allen, neurosurgery.
Dr. Harvey W. Bender, thoracic and cardiac surgery.
Dr. Lonnie S. Burnett, obstetrics and gynecology.
Dr. Gottleib C. Friesinger II, cardiology.
Dr. A. Everette James, Jr., radiology.
Dr. W. Scott McDougal, urology.
Dr. John Oates, clinical pharmacology.
Dr. Robert H. Ossoff, otolaryngology.
Dr. C. Leon Partain, radiology; specialist in nuclear medicine and magnetic resonance imaging.
Dr. John L. Sawyers, surgery.
Dr. Dan Spengler, orthopedics and rehabilitation.
Dr. Mildred T. Stahlman, pediatrics and pathology; director of the specialized center for research in newborn lung disease.
Dr. Anne Colston Wentz, obstetrics and gynecology; director of the Center for Fertility and Reproductive Research.

# Research

In 1985 over $47 million in research funding was awarded to Vanderbilt University School of Medicine; 65 percent of this funding was provided by the federal government.

Vanderbilt has 14 research centers, including basic sciences and clinical research, cancer, diabetes, environmental health sciences, general clinical, newborn lung, nutrition, pharmacology and drug toxicology, individual responsiveness to drugs, pulmonary edema–lung vascular injury–lung function, renal function, reproductive biology, and institutional animal resources. There are strong research programs in arthritis, cancer, diabetes, heart disease, lung disease, mental and neurological problems, and reproductive and infertility problems.

Among other cancer studies, research is under way to develop markers for human colon cancer and for classifying leukemia. Clinical investigators are making progress in determining the value of high-dose therapy for improving survival rates in patients with acute myelogenous leukemia, improving the use of bone marrow transplantation, and developing new and improved techniques in radiation diagnosis and therapy. Atherosclerosis, cardiac arrhythmia, and hypertension are major areas of study. For example, in the Vanderbilt Arrhythmia Center a multifaceted approach to research and treatment includes drug therapy, programmed electrical stimulation, pediatric service, surgery, and research utilizing single cells, animals, and human subjects. Also, Vanderbilt research on the use of defibrillators is at the forefront in managing arrhythmias. Clinical research has contributed greatly to improved management of hypertension through drugs.

The Center for Newborn Lung Disease and the Center for Pulmonary Edema have focused on understanding and treatment of lung disease. The Diabetes Research Center, in existence since 1973, was the first one established by the NIH. Its activities include professional training, information dissemination, and research in the diagnosis and treatment of diabetes mellitus and related endocrine and metabolic disorders.

Kidney research is extensive and supports, among other activities, a transplant and dialysis program. Investigations are under way in mental and neurological diseases, especially in the use of drugs to treat disorders such as depression and mania; psychosis and the way antipsychotic drugs work; drug abuse, and various aspects of behavioral pharmacology. At the Child and Adolescent Psychiatric Hospital, mental disorders in adolescents are the focus of research.

In other specific disease-oriented research, scientists study Parkinson's disease and Huntington's disease.

As a result of their individual and group research, Vanderbilt investigators have received many national and international awards and honors. For example, Dr. Earl Sutherland won the 1971 Nobel Prize for medicine for the discovery of cyclic AMP, a chemical regulator that affects growth and behavior. In 1986 Dr. Stanley Cohen of Vanderbilt won the Nobel Prize for his contributions to understanding the substances that influence cell growth and the orderly development of tissues, including the nervous system.

In November 1986 Vanderbilt received a $6.65-million grant from the Office of Naval Research to develop a Free-Electron Laser Center for Biomedical and Materials Research.

## Admission Policy

Patients must be admitted to Vanderbilt by a physician with admitting privileges. They can be admitted through the clinics and Emergency Department but must have or be assigned to a private physician.

All patients treated at Vanderbilt are expected to make adequate advance arrangements for payment of their hospital bills. Payment is defined as verified insurance benefits or receipt of a deposit representing either the patient's portion above coverage limits or payment in full. Exceptions are made when the admission and/or treatment is an emergency as determined by the attending physician. After the emergency condition has ended, the patient comes under the standing financial policies. Exceptions to the financial requirement are also made when the needed services can be obtained only at Vanderbilt.

The only requirement for admission to the burn center is that a patient in Vanderbilt's service area be in need of the care provided. There are no financial restrictions on burn center patients.

The hospital-based helicopter service is available, without restriction, to all residents in the service area in a medical emergency.

**ROOM CHARGES** (per diem)
Private: $220
Semiprivate: $219
ICU: $430–$700, depending on department

**AVERAGE COST PER PATIENT STAY:**    $8,742

**MAILING ADDRESS**        **TELEPHONE**
1161 21st Avenue South    615-322-5000
Nashville, TN 37232

# Baylor University Medical Center
## DALLAS, TEXAS

Baylor has an impressive history of commitment to quality assurance, with significant benefits to its patients. In 1946 Baylor's medical staff organized what is believed to have been the first hospital surgical tissue committee in the United States. It required that samples of tissue from each operation be thoroughly examined by the pathology department. The success of this committee caused the American College of Surgeons, the accrediting agency for hospitals at that time, to require that tissue committees be established in every hospital in the country. This requirement is still in effect.

Baylor's quality assurance has strengthened with time. The hospital routinely monitors a number of patient-care areas, including infection control rates, which is one of the reasons Baylor's surgical wound infection rate for clean and clean/contaminated procedures is 3 percent or under—compared with a national average of 5 percent. In April 1985 Baylor initiated a careful program of utilization review that precertifies the need to be admitted as an inpatient. This helps to ensure that only those patients who absolutely require hospitalization are admitted, cutting back on unnecessary hospital stays.

Patients at Baylor can expect the same attention to detail in their medical care, which encompasses a wide range of specialties and subspecialties.

Baylor's program of liver and kidney transplants, officially begun in April 1985, is already the second most active adult program in the United States, surpassed only by the program at Presbyterian-University Hospital in Pittsburgh (see page 269). More than 55 liver, 27 kidney, and three heart transplant procedures had been performed as of September 1986. The program will include pancreatic transplants in the near future.

Baylor's Sammons Cancer Center is home to one of only two bone marrow transplantation programs in Texas. The center offers a multidisciplinary approach that includes hematology, oncology, radiation oncology, surgery, and many other disciplines. In addition, patients learn to cope with their illness through special support groups. The families of cancer patients are also included in learning about the emotional and physical impact of the disease.

More than 25 disciplines in cardiology are combined at the H. L. and Ruth Ray Hunt Heart Center. Physicians here apply advanced techniques for the diagnosis, treatment, and rehabilitation of patients; they also conduct ongoing research in heart disease.

The Diagnostic Center for Digestive Diseases deals with chronic illnesses of the digestive tract, such as peptic ulcers or Crohn's disease. The center conducts extensive research and provides patient care for both children and adults.

Laser surgery is an important part of the work at Baylor. While there is no organized laser program or center, 75 members of the medical staff utilize lasers in their clinical practice. Five Ph.D.'s in the Baylor Research Foundation also use lasers in research activities.

Baylor was the first hospital in the Southwest to acquire a magnetic resonance imaging scanner for patient-care use.

The orthopedic service at Baylor is highly renowned in Dallas and throughout north Texas. Physicians here perform surgical reattachment of limbs and special hand surgery as well as other advanced orthopedic techniques.

Baylor's nationally known Psoriasis Center has been in operation for seven years. A comprehensive ambulatory center, the facility offers the latest treatments, including Goeckerman therapy, which utilizes crude coal tar and ultraviolet light; PUVA therapy, using psoralen and long-wave ultraviolet light A; and Ingram therapy.

At the Blanche Swanzy Lange Special Care Nursery, neonatologists help care for premature and high-risk babies.

Baylor also provides many services for the community. Anyone who is new to Dallas and seeking a physician can call the center's Helpline at 214-820-3312 and choose a doctor from an extensive list of qualified candidates. TelMed, a tape library of health information, is also available by phone (214-820-4000) and has received more than one million calls since its inception in 1980. Community programs in chemical and alcohol addiction, home health care, pregnancy and birth, stress management, and weight loss are also available.

Education is a major concern at the medical center. The A. Webb Roberts Center for Continuing Education in Health Sciences presents educational programs for physicians, nurses, and allied health professionals. Last year 50,000 people attended its programs. Nursing students at Baylor University in Waco receive two years of clinical training at the medical center. Baylor's medical education program trains 150 new doctors each year. Future hospital administrators also train at Baylor.

Founded as the Texas Baptist Sanitarium over eighty years ago, Baylor University Medical Center serves patients from Texas, the Southwest, and around the world. It is the second largest church-related hospital in the United States, acording to the *American Hospital Association Guide to the Health Care Field*, and it is the largest private hospital in Texas.

The medical center became the nucleus of a system that includes Baylor Medical Center, Ennis; Baylor Medical Center, Gilmer; Baylor Institute for Rehabilitation (formerly Swiss Avenue Hospital), Dallas; Baylor Medical Center, Grapevine; and Baylor Medical Center, Waxahachie. These community hospitals contribute primary and secondary acute care or long-term and specialized care and provide a referral base for the medical center in Dallas.

## Specialties

Baylor's medical staff represents every medical specialty. Some of its best-known specialties include cardiology; digestive diseases; heart, kidney, and liver transplants; intensive care; laser surgery; neonatology; ophthalmology; oncology; and orthopedics.

The medical center maintains centers of excellence in ambulatory surgery, arthritis, breast cancer, diabetes, drug/alcohol dependency, emergency medicine, medical imaging, physical medicine, psoriasis, and visual function testing.

---

**STATISTICAL PROFILE**

Number of Beds: 1,509 (licensed)
Bed Occupancy Rate: 73%
Average Number of Patients: 865
Average Patient Stay: 6 days
Annual Admissions: 43,630
Births: 4,393
Outpatient Clinic Visits: 97,800
Emergency Room/Trauma Center Visits: 38,840

Hospital Personnel:
  Physicians: 635
  Residents: 150
  Registered Nurses: 1,081
  Total Staff: 3,500

---

## Well-known Specialists

Dr. Reuben Adams, chief of obstetrics/gynecology.
Dr. Billie Aronoff, laser surgery.
Dr. Adrian Flatt, hand surgery; chief of orthopedics.
Dr. John Fordtran, gastroenterology; chief of medicine.
Dr. Patrick O'Leary, surgery.
Dr. George Race, M.D., Ph.D., chief of pathology.
Dr. Leonard Riggs, emergency medicine.
Dr. Marvin Stone, medical director of Sammons Cancer Center.
Dr. Jesse Thompson, chief of surgery.
Dr. Ralph Tompsett, internal medicine; specialist in infectious diseases.

# Research

The Baylor Research Foundation is a major component of the Baylor Medical Center Group. With approximately $4.5 million in funding, the foundation conducts active research in more than 100 diverse projects. Heart disease and cancer are two major research areas.

One of the current investigations is a study for NASA of bone loss in space. Other research projects involve lasers and their application to treating cancer. Researchers have been studying Photofrin II, an investigative drug that can be used in the treatment of certain infectious and parasitic diseases.

Research at Baylor is not restricted to the medical center campus. To extend its reach and share expertise in various research areas, Baylor entered into an agreement with the Pan American Health Organization in 1981. Baylor now has reciprocal working agreements with health institutions in Costa Rica, Brazil, and Venezuela.

# Admission Policy

Patients are not required to be referred to Baylor by a physician, although upon arrival all patients are admitted by a Baylor physician.

Baylor accepts assignment from insured patients. Noninsured patients are asked for a $1,000 deposit.

---

**ROOM CHARGES** (per diem)
Suite: $302–$480
Private: $223
Semiprivate: $215
ICU: $914

**AVERAGE COST PER PATIENT STAY:**   $3,737

**MAILING ADDRESS**       **TELEPHONE**
3500 Gaston Avenue    214-820-0111
Dallas, TX 75246

# The Texas Medical Center
# The Methodist Hospital

**HOUSTON, TEXAS**

In recent years the boom-to-bust economy of Houston has adversely affected many facets of life in this city. But there is still one boom town here, and it's The Texas Medical Center. Located just south of the downtown area on a 525-acre complex, it consists of 37 separate medical institutions housed in 50 permanent buildings. More than 50,000 people are employed at the center, and over 2 million outpatient visits and 180,000 inpatient admissions are recorded here every year.

Two of the nation's most highly regarded medical schools—Baylor College of Medicine and the University of Texas Medical School—are located at the center, as are the well-known Institute for Rehabilitation and Research and the New Age Hospice. There are a total of 6,000 beds in eight hospitals at the center. These include the 1,250-bed Veterans Administration Medical Center, a Shriners Hospital for Crippled Children, and two general acute-care hospitals (Ben Taub and Hermann Hospital), both of which contain designated Level I Trauma Centers. Four tertiary-care hospitals provide access to virtually every specialty and subspecialty of modern medicine, including oncology at M. D. Anderson Hospital (see page 297) and pediatrics at the world-renowned Texas Children's Hospital. The two flagship hospitals of the Texas Medical Center, the Methodist Hospital and St. Luke's Episcopal, provide acute care in many specialties; several departments in both hospitals are regarded as among the best in the world.

St. Luke's, a 930-bed facility staffed by some 1,300 physicians, offers excellent patient care in a variety of specialties, including general surgery, neurology, neurosurgery, ophthalmology, otolaryngology, plastic surgery, and urology. Widely regarded as one of the finest hospitals in the Southwest, St. Luke's is a well-known regional referral center for hand surgery, obstetrics (about 3,000 babies are born here every year), and high-risk pregnancy. Also located at St. Luke's is the world-famous Texas Heart Institute, the home of the legendary Dr. Denton Cooley and his staff of six cardiovascular surgeons, who annually perform about 2,000 open-heart operations and 20 heart transplants.

Cardiology and cardiovascular surgery are also well-known medical services at the Methodist Hospital, the primary teaching facility of Baylor Medical School. In addition to having its own legendary heart surgeon, Dr. Michael DeBakey, Methodist has an active heart transplant center, whose surgeons perform over 1,000 open-heart operations a year. Methodist's cardiovascular surgeons, led by Dr. E. Stanley Crawford, are also well known for their work with complex aneurysm procedures.

But there's much more here than cardiac surgery, as one would expect from the fourth largest nonprofit, nongovernmental, acute-care hospital in the United States. Staffed by over 700 physicians who also hold faculty appointments at Baylor medical school and a total medical staff of over 1,600, Methodist is an internationally known referral center serving about 40,000 inpatients a year. A little more than half the patients come from outside the Houston area; in 1985 they came from all 50 states and 62 foreign countries. Patient satisfaction is extremely high; 92 percent of the former patients who responded to a recent survey taken by the hospital claimed they would use the hospital again as well as recommend it to others.

Even a brief description of the programs offered at Methodist indicate why so many people are willing to travel long distances to obtain treatment here.

In concert with Baylor College of Medicine and under the direction of Drs. Michael DeBakey and Antonio Gotto, Jr., Methodist's comprehensive transplant center performs bone marrow, cornea, heart, heart-lung, kidney, and liver transplants. Through the multidisciplinary resources available here, patients receive comprehensive care before the transplant and long-term follow-up care.

Methodist is the home of the world's first center devoted to neurosensory disorders, which includes the following divisions. The Blue Bird Circle Clinic for Pediatric Neurology is the only center is the Southwest devoted to pediatric neurology and offers diagnosis and treatment for epilepsy and a variety of other neurological disorders in children. The Cullen Eye Institute offers cornea transplants, intraocular lens implants, radial keratotomy, and ultrasound treatment of glaucoma. The Institute for Otorhinolaryngology and Communicative Disorders encompasses ear, nose, and throat care and speech pathology and therapy. The Jerry Lewis Neuromuscular Disease Research Center investigates multiple sclerosis, ALS, and a variety of other disorders.

The hospital has the largest facility for outpatient surgery in the nation; 40 percent of all its surgical procedures in 1985 were performed on an outpatient basis.

The Sid W. Richardson Institute for Preventive Medicine of the Methodist Hospital was established in 1980 to reduce the risk of serious disease by providing individual and group programs of diet and exercise under constant scientific evaluation. The institute includes a health and fitness club, nutrition education, cardiac rehabilitation programs, corporate fitness programs, and Chez Eddy, an elegant gourmet restaurant serving cardiac-prudent meals.

Methodist's state-of-the-art technology includes a lithotriptor for nonsurgical treatment of kidney stones; complete imaging capabilities, including an in-house suite for magnetic resonance imaging; advanced anesthesia monitoring equipment; 13 lasers; extensive microsurgery capabilities; and large facilities for diagnostic cardiac procedures.

The quality of patient care at Methodist is enhanced by high nursing standards. For example, nurses who work in the operating rooms or critical-care units must have successfully completed a six-month training course. General-care nurses must come with previous experience or complete a three-month internship in medical/surgical nursing. Approximately 60 percent of all Methodist's registered nurses have bachelor's degrees.

## Specialties

Cardiology, Cardiovascular Surgery, Dermatology, General Surgery, Gynecology, Internal Medicine, Neurology, Neurosurgery, Obstetrics, Ophthalmology, Organ Transplantation, Orthopedics, Otorhinolaryngology, Plastic Surgery, Psychiatry, Radiology, and Urology.

---

**STATISTICAL PROFILE**

Number of Beds: 1,218
Bed Occupancy Rate: 70%
Average Number of Patients: 830
Average Patient Stay: 7.7 days
Annual Admissions: 39,028
Births: 2,236
Emergency Room/Trauma Center Visits: 16,227

Hospital Personnel:
    Physicians: 1,628
    Residents: 154
    Registered Nurses: 900
    Total Staff: 5,168

---

## Well-known Specialists

Dr. Bobby Alford, otorhinolaryngology; specialist in throat surgery.
Dr. Stanley H. Appel, neurology; specialist in ALS, Alzheimer's disease, neuromuscular disorders.
Dr. David S. Baskin, neurology; specialist in the treatment of stroke-caused paralysis and Alzheimer's disease.
Dr. Nick Bryan, radiology; specialist in magnetic resonance imaging.
Dr. C. Eugene Carlton, Jr., urology.
Dr. E. Stanley Crawford, general surgery; specialist in the treatment of aneurysms.
Dr. Michael DeBakey, surgery; specialist in cardiovascular and transplant surgery.
Dr. Alan J. Garber, internal medicine; specialist in diabetes.
Dr. Antonio Gotto, Jr., M.D., Ph.D., internal medicine; specialist in heart

disease and in lipid metabolism research, past president of the American Heart Association.

Dr. Donald P. Griffith, urology.

Dr. Robert Grossman, neurosurgery.

Dr. J. Alan Herd, internal medicine; specialist in preventive medicine.

Dr. Jimmy Howell, surgery; specialist in cardiovascular surgery.

Dr. David Huston, internal medicine; specialist in immunology.

Dr. Joseph Jankovic, neurology; specialist in Parkinson's disease.

Dr. Raymond H. Kaufman, gynecology; specialist in gynecologic oncology.

Dr. Gerald M. Lawrie, cardiovascular surgery; specialist in the surgical treatment of arrhythmia.

Dr. Larry Lipschultz, urology; specialist in male infertility.

Dr. Alice McPherson, ophthalmology; specialist in disorders of the retina.

Dr. George Noon, surgery; specialist in heart, heart-lung, and kidney transplants.

Dr. Peter Scardino, oncology.

Dr. Melvin Spira, plastic and reconstructive surgery.

Dr. Hugh S. Tullos, orthopedic surgery; specialist in hip surgery.

Dr. Hartwell H. Whisennand, surgery; specialist in liver transplants.

Dr. Christopher Wyndham, internal medicine; specialist in electrophysiological mapping of the heart.

## Research

In 1986 research funding for the Baylor College of Medicine amounted to over $35 million.

The Methodist Hospital, along with Baylor, is one of the nation's leading research centers in cardiology. Four of these major studies are the Cardiac Arrhythmia Pilot Study, Thrombolytic Intervention in Myocardial Infarction, Studies of the Left Ventricular Dysfunction, and Electrophysiology vs. Holter Monitoring in Malignant Ventricular Arrhythmia.

Dr. Antonio M. Gotto, Jr., is internationally recognized for his research on lipoproteins and their effect on the development of atherosclerosis. Methodist has one of three centers nationally that performs LDL (low-density lipoprotein) pheresis. This experimental treatment procedure, which filters cholesterol from the blood, is especially significant to patients whose conditions have not responded to diet modification or drug treatments.

Methodist is also the site of several pioneering treatments of cancer patients being developed under the guidance of Dr. Peter Scardino. One is the use of ultrasonography for imaging the prostate.

Neurological research performed by Dr. David S. Baskin includes investigation of the drug naloxone, which can in certain cases partially reverse paralysis caused by stroke. Within the next several years large-scale clinical trials of the drug will take place. Dr. Baskin is also involved in research in the treatment of Alzheimer's disease with Bethanechol.

Other areas of investigation at Methodist include a trial for the prevention of breast cancer that is part of a ten-year nationwide study involving more than 30,000 women, cardiovascular surgery, epilepsy, the development of hip prostheses, and hypertension drug treatment trials.

## Admission Policy

Patients can be admitted to Methodist without a physician's referral. The hospital has patient referral numbers by which anyone can make contact with a physician who practices here. The toll-free numbers are 800-222-6386 outside Texas and 800-222-6396 in Texas. (International inquiries: 713-790-5696.)

The hospital's financial requirements for routine admission are the same for all patients, regardless of income. As part of its preadmission procedure, the hospital provides patients with an estimate of the cost of the hospitalization so that appropriate financial arrangements can be made to cover expenses.

Methodist, a nonprofit, private health-care institution with no tax support or endowment, provides nearly $2 million in care annually for the needy. In addition, the hospital recorded more than $14 million in discounts and uncollectible accounts in 1985.

---

**ROOM CHARGES (per diem)**
Private: $167–$180
Semiprivate: $158
Ward: $152
ICU: $400

**AVERAGE COST PER PATIENT STAY:**   $5,699

**MAILING ADDRESS**       **TELEPHONE**
6565 Fannin                713-790-3311
Houston, TX 77030

---

# M. D. Anderson Hospital and Tumor Institute
# University of Texas System Cancer Center
# Texas Medical Center

**HOUSTON, TEXAS**

One of the foremost comprehensive cancer centers in the world, the University of Texas (UT) M. D. Anderson Hospital and Tumor Institute was developed in 1944 as a state cancer hospital offering care to all Texans, regardless of their ability to pay. Over 40 percent of the Texas residents treated here in 1985 obtained some portion of their health care free of charge. More specifically, the expense of medical care provided to medically indigent Texans exceeded $41 million.

Patients come to M. D. Anderson from every county in Texas, almost every state in the United States, and numerous foreign countries. (Approximately 76 percent of all patients treated over the years have been Texans.) In 1985 the 200,000th patient registered at the hospital: while it took almost thirty years for M. D. Anderson to record its first 100,000 patients, the second 100,000 were served in fewer than twelve years. These figures indicate both a rise in cancer incidence throughout the total population and rising demands from physicians who refer their patients here.

Activities in research, education, and prevention, along with patient care, have drawn leading scientific and medical talent to this institution. Even in the early years, M. D. Anderson physicians and scientists set new standards in innovative surgery, developed the Cobalt 60 unit to make radiotherapy a viable treatment alternative, and pioneered modern anticancer drugs. In more recent years staff members have embarked on studies of biological response modifiers and other immunologic processes to create a fourth arena for fighting cancer. M. D. Anderson currently has the largest clinical program of interferon studies in the world.

The majority of M. D. Anderson's patients are not hospitalized. Instead, they receive treatment as outpatients, either here or under the care of their hometown physicians, who are informed of the latest treatment methods through close collaboration with M. D. Anderson staff members and continuing education programs. M. D. Anderson operates the largest outpatient chemotherapy program in the country, with an average of 2,800 patients receiving such treatment each month. Additional hundreds of patients receive the latest anticancer drugs or radiotherapy in their hometowns, miles away from the hospital that makes such care possible.

Portable infuser pumps developed here allow some chemotherapy patients to receive treatment while continuing their usual daily activities. Other technological advances and special equipment at M. D. Anderson allow for more sophisticated treatment techniques. Lasers are used for delicate cancer surgery on an outpatient basis; in all some 200 outpatient surgeries are performed monthly. The nation's first hospital-based cyclotron was installed here to provide radiation treatment proven more effective for certain cancers than conventional radiation therapy and to offer short-lived radioisotopes for highly specialized diagnostic tests.

The hospital also operates five CAT scanners, new machinery to improve lung-scanning capabilities, and two diagnostic ultrasound units for use in localizing tumors during operative procedures. Interventional radiology techniques, largely developed and tested by UT System Cancer Center experts, block the blood supply to large tumors deep in the body and permit injections directly into cancers that otherwise might be impossible to treat.

Thousands of the patients treated at M. D. Anderson are children cared for in a program that has become a model. The Pediatric Star Community focuses on maintaining normal life-styles for young cancer patients. Emphasis is placed on the continuation of school lessons, both in the hospital classrooms and at home. Whenever possible clinical treatment is scheduled around classes. Shared mealtimes in the pediatric dining room are a normal part of the day for youngsters and their parents. Physical and social activities, including a summer camp program for patients and siblings, combine with expert medical care to prepare pediatric patients for life after cancer.

Although M. D. Anderson Hospital does not grant academic degrees, many students, including young researchers, receive a portion of their training here. Students in more than 30 categories participate in educational programs that vary in length from a few weeks to several years. The training offered ranges from intensive postgraduate work for physicians and scientists to special summer programs for high school and undergraduate students. During 1984–85 about 1,500 men and women received some portion of their education at the UT Cancer Center. An additional 4,000 health-care professionals from throughout the world participated in continuing education programs that year.

The general public is involved in another part of M. D. Anderson's education mission. A speaker's bureau and a toll-free telephone line provide detailed written and verbal information about cancer. Callers from anywhere in Texas can reach the Cancer Information Service through 800-4-CANCER (or in Houston, 792-3245). More than 100,000 Texans have contacted this bilingual service in the past decade, and the volume of calls has more than doubled in the last three years. Today nearly 75 percent of the callers request written materials on topics ranging from how to quit smoking and reduce dietary risks of malignant disease to the latest information about investigational therapies for specific cancers and resources for second medical opinions.

Public and professional education play a large role in the UT Cancer Center's mission of prevention. The center has implemented many programs in cancer screening, early detection, basic and epidemiological research, and education for groups at increased risk for certain cancers. Meanwhile, research here continues to investigate the causes of cancer in order to prevent these diseases from occurring. The Cancer Center's Science Park—Research Division is regarded as one of the world's foremost centers for carcinogenesis studies.

M. D. Anderson was designated one of the first three Comprehensive Cancer Centers in the United States. The UT System Cancer Center includes M. D. Anderson Hospital, the Rehabilitation Center, two research divisions of the UT Science Park, the R. E. "Bob" Smith Research Building, and the Anderson Mayfair, a patient-and-family hotel just across the street from the hospital.

## Specialties

Anesthesiology, Cancer Prevention, Chemotherapy Research, Clinical Immunology and Biological Therapy, Dental Oncology, Diagnostic Radiology, Experimental Radiotherapy, General Surgery, Gynecology, Head and Neck Surgery, Hematology, Internal Medicine, Laboratory Medicine, Medical Oncology, Neuro-Oncology, Neurosurgery, Nuclear Medicine, Pathology, Patient Studies, Pediatrics, Pharmacology, Clinical Radiotherapy, Thoracic Surgery, and Urology.

In addition, there are 27 outpatient clinics, including Immunology, Neurology, Orthopedics, Pain Control, and Radiotherapy.

---

**STATISTICAL PROFILE**

Number of Beds: 514
Bed Occupancy Rate: 86%
Average Number of Patients: 1,400
Average Patient Stay: 10.5 days
Annual Admissions: 14,365
Outpatient Clinic Visits: 348,548

Hospital Personnel:
  Physicians: 240
  Residents, Interns, and Fellows: 386
  Registered Nurses: 700
  Total Staff: 6,100
  Volunteers: 900

# Well-known Specialists

Dr. Charles M. Balch, authority on cancer immunology and the treatment of melanoma, head of the Division of Surgery.

Dr. Robert S. Benjamin, specialist in melanoma, professor of medicine.

Dr. Gerald D. Dodd, specialist in diagnostic radiology, head of the Division of Diagnostic Imaging.

Dr. Emil J Freireich, authority on adult leukemia and hematology, director of adult leukemia research.

Dr. W. K. Hong, head and neck medical oncology; specialist in leukoplakia.

Dr. Norman Jaffe, authority on pediatric oncology and solid tumors, chief of the Section of Pediatric Solid Tumors.

Dr. Bernard Levin, authority on cancers of the colon, pancreas, and stomach.

Dr. Eleanor Montague, radiotherapy; authority on conservative breast cancer treatment.

Dr. John A. Murray, orthopedic surgery; specialist in limb salvage surgery.

Dr. Donald Pinkel, chief of pediatric leukemia research.

Dr. Felix Rutledge, gynecology; authority on pelvic exenteration and gynecologic cancers.

Dr. Melvin Samuels, genitourinary oncology; authority on chemotherapeutic treatment of testicular cancers.

Dr. Jan van Eys, pediatrics; authority on pediatric oncology and psychosocial issues facing cancer patients.

# Research

Research expenditures at the UT System Cancer Center in 1985 exceeded $48 million, facilitating close to 500 research projects. These complex studies range from long-term investigations of subcellular components thought to have crucial roles in starting the cancer process to whether drugs, vitamins, or minerals may retard the development of cancer. Researchers also are learning how some naturally produced hormones help activate the body's immune system against cancer.

Among funding highlights was a $1-million grant from the American Cancer Society for accelerating studies to document how fat-rich diets contribute to the incidence of both breast and colorectal cancers.

Hundreds of research protocols continue work with investigational drugs and drug delivery systems to develop more effective chemotherapy treatments. In 1985 M. D. Anderson received a $3.1 million contract from the National Cancer Institute for research in new anticancer drugs; this was one of the largest contracts ever awarded for such a study. In 1986 M. D. Anderson received the largest grant ever awarded by National Cancer Institute for radiotherapy research—more than $9 million over five years.

Both basic and clinical research have been crucial to the UT System

Cancer Center's success. A major contributing factor has been the constant interaction of research team members—specialists from every related field who focus on a specific problem.

## Admission Policy

Patients are admitted to M. D. Anderson only upon referral by their physician. Referring physicians should call the New Patient Referral Office at 713-792-6161. While every patient is expected to pay for all medical services, Texas residents can make special arrangements for assistance after they have been admitted.

---

**ROOM CHARGES (per diem)**
Private: $190
Semiprivate: $175
Oncology ICU: $200
Medical ICU: $475
Surgical ICU: $500

**MAILING ADDRESS**         **TELEPHONE**
1515 Holcombe Boulevard     713-792-2121
Houston, TX 77030

---

# University Hospital and Clinics
# The University of Utah
# Health Sciences Center

**SALT LAKE CITY, UTAH**

Although the Salt Lake City area has only some 200,000 inhabitants, it is the most important urban center between Denver and northern California. For this reason two major referral centers are located here, the outstanding but little-known Latter-Day Saints Hospital and the internationally famous University Hospital and Clinics of the University of Utah Health Sciences Center.

The hospital and medical staff of the University of Utah gained national recognition in December 1982 when a dentist named Barney Clark received the world's first permanent artificial heart implant here. To the astonishment of many doctors and scientists, Clark lived for 112 days, a tribute to his determination and courage but also to the skill and dedication of the hospital staff, and, of course, to the Jarvik-7, the now world-famous mechanical heart developed at Utah.

Now known officially as The University Health Sciences Center, this complex consists of the Utah School of Medicine; colleges of pharmacy, nursing, and public health; a major library; laboratories; the University Hospital; and numerous outpatient clinics.

University Hospital is a major tertiary-care institution treating patients with all types of illness and injuries; it serves as a referral center for some 3.5 million residents of Utah, Idaho, Wyoming, eastern Nevada, western Colorado, and Montana—approximately 10 percent of the geographic area of the United States. University Hospital runs the largest patient air transport system in the United States, utilizing specially designed helicopters and fixed-wing aircraft. This system is particularly useful to five of the hospital's special units: the Burn and Trauma Center, the Newborn Intensive Care Center, the Poison Control Center, the Spinal Cord Injury Center, and the Transplant Center.

The Burn Center and the Transplant Center are among the best in the country. The Burn Center, one of seven founded by the NIH, has its own operating room, hydrotherapy facilities, and skin bank; it admits over 325 burn victims and has over 1,200 clinic visits a year. The Transplant Center performs approximately 50 kidney and 30 heart transplants a year. Only two heart recipients out of 58 have died here, a rate much lower than the national average.

Almost every kind of advanced medical practice is available here, including laser surgery, cornea transplants (there is an eye bank), and programs in specialized areas such as cystic fibrosis, high-risk obstetrics, and in vitro fertilization. The hospital is fully equipped with the most up-to-date medical machinery, including a lithotriptor and a magnetic resonance imaging scanner.

University Health Sciences Center is part of the University of Utah, a state institution. Less than 4 percent of the budget of University Hospital, however, comes from the state, and only 14 percent of the operating costs of the School of Medicine comes from state funds. The remainder comes from patient fees, faculty research grants, and gifts.

According to Dr. Don E. Detmer, University of Utah vice-president for health sciences, the university is actively involved in medical research. "Although many schools are de-emphasizing basic research and focusing on applied or clinical investigations, we have made a fixed, firm and formal decision to move forward in both areas."

The School of Medicine admits 100 students each year. In addition, every year nearly 1,000 health sciences students receive part of their training at the Health Sciences Center. This includes some 400 medical students as well as students of nursing, pharmacy, physical and respiratory therapy, and hospital social work—the full range of health-care professions.

In 1910 the two-year medical school at the university had 18 students and three faculty members with a budget of about $10,000. In 1986 the enrollment of the four-year school had soared to 400 students, and there were 613 faculty members with a budget of $79.5 million.

## Specialties

Adolescent Medicine, Anesthesiology, Arthritis, Burn Treatment, Cardiology, Clinical Pathology, Dermatology, Dialysis, Family Medicine, Family Planning, Gastroenterology, Genetics, Hematology, Hepatology, Immunology and Allergy, Internal Medicine, Laser Surgery, Neuromuscular Disease, Newborn Care, Nuclear Medicine, Neurosurgery, Obstetrics/ Gynecology, Oncology, Ophthalmology, Organ Acquisition and Transplantation, Orthopedic Surgery, the Pain Clinic, Pediatrics, Poison Control, Psychiatry, Radiology, Renal Disease, Spinal Cord Injury, Surgery, Trauma, Ultrasonography, and Urology.

Outpatient clinics serve more than 110,000 patients a year. Among the most important are the Pain Clinic and the Alcohol and Drug Abuse Clinic, but clinical services exist in almost every medical specialty, including Dentistry; Ear, Nose, and Throat; Orthopedic Surgery; and Plastic Surgery. The hospital has special rehabilitation programs for amputees and for victims of multiple sclerosis and stroke.

---

**STATISTICAL PROFILE (1986)**

Number of Beds: 370
Bed Occupancy Rate: 75%
Average Number of Patients: 277
Average Patient Stay: 8.9 days
Annual Admissions: 11,229
Births: 1,526
Outpatient Clinic Visits: 110,258
Emergency Room/Trauma Center Visits: 15,397

Hospital Personnel:
  Physicians: 378
  Interns and Residents: 411
  Registered Nurses: 495
  Total Staff: 1,870

---

## Well-known Specialists

Dr. William A. Gay, chairman of the Department of Surgery at the medical
  school, head of cardiothoracic surgery and of the heart transplant program.
Dr. Gerald Krueger, dermatology; specialist in psoriasis.
Dr. James L. Parkin, surgery; specialist in artificial ear implants, head of
  the Division of Otolaryngology.
Dr. John R. Ward, head of rheumatology.
Dr. Maxwell Wintrobe, author of the definitive text on hematology.

## Research

The medical education and patient-care programs of The University of Utah
Health Sciences Center are supported by more than 400 research projects
conducted by the faculty members of the School of Medicine. One of only
a few designated Clinical Research Centers sponsored by the NIH, the center
has researchers and physicians studying illnesses such as Huntington's disease, lupus, multiple sclerosis, and sudden infant death syndrome.

  Among the numerous research projects are studies in the removal of
bladder tumors, endometriosis, genetics, in vitro fertilization, radiology, and
retinal surgery. The Utah Cancer Registry, located at the university, conducts epidemiological studies in cancer and provides feedback for physicians
and hospitals. The registry operates under the sponsorship of the National
Cancer Institute, which recently agreed to fund several studies investigating
the possible links between diet and cancer.

  Researchers in the world-renowned Institute for Biomedical Engineering and Division of Artificial Organs refine developments in artificial hearing devices, hearts, kidneys, and limbs. The transplant program remains a vital part of the center's research and clinical activities.

## Admission Policy

Most patients at Utah are referred by their private physicians. Individuals may also make an appointment to be seen in any of the outpatient clinics and, in some cases, directly by hospital physicians. Patients requiring immediate care are admitted as soon as possible.

The hospital operates a toll-free referral and consultation hotline: 800-453-0122 (outside Utah), 800-662-0052 (in Utah). There is no financial requirement for admission.

---

**ROOM CHARGES (per diem)**
Private and semiprivate: $249.50
ICU: $659.50

**MAILING ADDRESS**          **TELEPHONE**
50 North Medical Drive       801-581-2121
Salt Lake City, UT 84132

# Medical College of Virginia Hospitals

**RICHMOND, VIRGINIA**

Unlike many of the academic medical centers described in this book, the state-supported 125-year-old Medical College of Virginia Hospitals (MCVH) is not highly publicized. Although MCVH is a major regional referral center and one of the largest and most active teaching hospitals in the nation, its proximity to Duke and Vanderbilt seems to have kept it from achieving the widespread recognition it deserves. In fact, what first brought MCVH to our attention were not recommendations from doctors but an analysis of the figures relating to complexity of patient care compiled by the people who administer Medicare. Over the last few years, MCVH has had one of the highest so-called case-mix indexes in the nation, higher than those of most of the prestigious Boston and New York hospitals. Since this means that MCVH is treating very sick people on a continuous basis, we decided to investigate further.

We discovered that virtually every form of contemporary medical service is available here, including one of the world's largest organ transplantation programs, a first-rate cardiac surgery department (about 800 bypass procedures are performed here annually), a major burn unit, and a regional head trauma center for special neurological and surgical services; there's also a Level I Trauma Center, a Comprehensive Cancer Center housed in its own four-story building, and a nationally famous neonatal intensive care unit, which is a vital regional resource for premature babies. In 1985 over 600 babies were born in this unit, and another 300 transferred from other hospitals.

Other special services include the Temporomandibular Joint and Facial Pain Clinic, which treats patients with facial injuries and those with severe chronic facial pain (such as that caused by stress-related tics), frequently women. The clinic has developed special heat treatment to relieve pain, but it uses medications as well. Research is also conducted here.

The first successful nontwin organ transplant was performed at MCVH in the early 1950s. Today this is the second oldest and one of the largest heart transplant centers in the United States; 240 heart transplants had been performed through the end of November 1986. Some 725 kidney transplants had been performed here through November 1986. And in 1984 MCVH added a liver transplantation program, which has since perfomed 34 transplants.

Another MCVH surgical specialty is artificial joint replacements; almost 3,000 such operations have been performed here since 1972, with more than 350 done in 1986 alone.

The Massey Cancer Center is a NIH-designated cancer center, one of only 20 or so in the country, and a regional referral center for the entire state. Dr. Walter Lawrence, the center's director, is a world-famous expert in head, neck, and stomach cancers. Virtually every form of cancer is treated here—on both inpatient and outpatient bases. The center is especially well known for its work in developing anticancer drugs. Massey is the only NCI-designated cancer center in Virginia.

The Children's Medical Center consolidates all programs related to pediatric patient care, education, and research. The center addresses major child health problems such as child and adolescent behavioral disorders, cancer, congenital heart defects, genetic problems, kidney and liver diseases, newborn respiratory distress, and trauma. The university operates the largest comprehensive hemophilia clinic for children in Virginia.

The Dementia Clinic is designed as a model for others nationwide. Its multidisciplinary team approach is expected to provide a prototype treatment plan for victims of Alzheimer's disease. The clinic offers resources and education to help the victim and the family. Currently more than 100 patients and their families are seen in the clinic, which is open one morning a week. A backlog of one and a half months indicates that many more people are in need of these services.

A consolidated inpatient and outpatient radiology department with over 30 procedure rooms, 24 operating rooms, two laser rooms, and an entire floor devoted to adult intensive care units, with 64 beds divided into specialty service areas, are all part of the new acute-bed facility at MCVH.

As an academic medical center, MCVH has a full-scale commitment to research and, as part of Virginia Commonwealth University, to the teaching of every health-related subject, including pharmacy, allied health professions, and health sciences, as well as nursing and medicine.

This hospital may not be very well known nationally but, according to a recent MCVH survey, the people of Richmond and the surrounding areas regard it as having the most qualified doctors and the best facilities. Among former patients of the hospital, opinions about the quality of care are consistently positive, especially regarding the nursing staff. In one recent MCVH survey, for example, almost 80 percent of those responding said the quality of nursing care exceeded their expectations. More than 60 percent of the registered nurses here have at least a bachelor's degree.

Still, when you are a patient of any large teaching hospital, it is not uncommon to feel lost or puzzled. To assist patients MCVH has two full-time patient representatives available to answer questions and act on behalf of any patients who need assistance with anything from a billing problem to an understanding of why they are being given certain tests. This is particularly impressive because hospitals need not offer this kind of service. So too is the fact that such an extraordinary medical facility is also the principal provider of charity care in the state.

## Specialties

Specialized inpatient and outpatient services include cardiac intensive care; dentistry; emergency medicine; heart, heart-lung, liver, and kidney transplants; newborn intensive care; neurology; obstetrics; oncology; open-heart surgery; psychiatry; radiation therapy; and trauma.

An outpatient department with 92 clinics covers a wide range of medical specialties, including allergies, burns, dermatology, genetics, glaucoma, head and neck tumors, infertility, nutrition, orthopedics, pediatrics, inpatient and outpatient renal dialysis, stroke, and urology.

---

**STATISTICAL PROFILE**

Number of Licensed Beds: 1,058
Average Number of Available Beds: 953
Bed Occupancy Rate: 80%
Average Number of Patients: 762
Average Patient Stay: 8.5 days
Annual Admissions: 32,389
Births: 3,884
Outpatient Clinic Visits: 161,333
Emergency Room/Trauma Center Visits: 101,050

Hospital Personnel:
  Physicians: 735
  Residents: 524
  Registered Nurses: 1,030
  Total Staff: 5,066

---

## Well-known Specialists

Dr. Joseph Boykin, plastic surgery; specialist in burn shock.

Dr. James W. Brooks, thoracic surgery.

Dr. Robert DeLorenzo, specialist in epilepsy, chairman of the Neurology Department.

Dr. I. David Goldman, oncology; specialist in anticancer drugs.

Dr. Stephen W. Harkins, experimental psychology; specialist in gerontology, research coordinator of the Dementia Clinic.

Dr. B. W. Haynes, Jr., specialist in surgery for burn victims, director of the burn unit, founder of the American Burn Association.

Dr. Walter Lawrence, surgical oncology; specialist in head, neck, and stomach cancers, director of the Massey Cancer Center.

Dr. H. M. Lee, director of the Clinical Transplant Program.

Dr. Richard R. Lower, cardiac transplant surgery.

Dr. Anthony Marmarou, neurosurgery.

Dr. Harold Maurer, pediatrics; specialist in childhood soft-tissue sarcomas.

Dr. Susan Mellette, specialist in cancer rehabilitation and continuing care.

Dr. Fay Redwine, one of the first obstetricians to perform fetal surgery, pioneer in methods for detecting fetal defects.

Dr. David Richardson, authority on cardiac arrhythmia, coronary artery disease, and hypertension.

Dr. Reno Vlahcevic, specialist in gallstones, chairman of the Division of Gastroenterology.

Dr. Robert S. Weinberg, ophthalmologic surgery.

Dr. Harold F. Young, researcher in using the body's immune system to fight certain kinds of brain tumors, chairman of the Division of Neurosurgery.

# Research

The Medical College of Virginia receives over $30 million in research grants and support programs annually. Projects cover a broad range of areas, including Alzheimer-type dementia, multiple sclerosis, and sudden infant death syndrome. Most of the clinical research reflects the hospital's strongest medical services; thus, cancer, neurology, obstetrics, organ transplantation, and trauma (especially head injuries and burns) are well-funded programs. Over the last decade, for example, Dr. Harold Maurer has developed a program for the diagnosis and treatment of childhood soft-tissue sarcomas that is now used throughout the world. In 1985 research scientists here identified a genetic abnormality as a major cause of Down's syndrome. Geneticist Dr. Barry Wolf developed a simple, inexpensive test to identify infants lacking an enzyme that controls the use of the vitamin biotin. Virginia now requires all newborns to be screened for biotinidase deficiency, which results in a form of mental retardation.

Other research is being conducted by Dr. Kenneth Kendler, well known for his work in the genetic/family studies of schizophrenia, and Dr. Philip Guzelian, a national leader in research on hazardous chemicals, who is pioneering methods for screening workers for potential cancer-causing chemicals.

Several key research grants have been awarded recently, including $1.5 million from the NIH for Dr. Anthony Marmarou and his staff to study brain swelling and increased intercranial pressure. Dr. Robert DeLorenzo has four major grants to study the causes of epilepsy, and Dr. I. David Goldman and his staff received $2.5 million from the National Cancer Institute for their work in developing anticancer drugs.

The hospital is also the site of an NIH-funded Clinical Research Center, where treatment for many disorders—including several forms of hepatitis, female infertility, and sleep disorders—is being investigated.

# Admission Policy

All patients must be admitted by an attending MCVH physician. While many patients are referred by outside physicians, many others come through the emergency room or through one of the specialty clinics on campus. For an appointment at one of these clinics call 804-786-0958.

Although MCVH offers an extraordinary amount of charity care ($78 million worth in 1985), it does require most patients to show they can pay. Only state residents are eligible for financial assistance, and charity care is provided only after financial screening and counseling. Even those with limited means are asked to pay something, and the hospital provides extensive help in financial planning so this can be achieved.

For most organ transplant procedures (except kidney), a deposit of $20,000 is required, and only very limited charity funds are available.

---

**ROOM CHARGES (per diem)**
Private: $231
Semiprivate: $220
ICU: $297–$722

**AVERAGE COST PER PATIENT STAY:**　$6,315.50

**AVERAGE COST OF ORGAN TRANSPLANTATION**
Heart Transplant: $78,300
Liver Transplant: $135,500
Kidney Transplant: Cost varies greatly and is covered by Medicare.

**MAILING ADDRESS**　　　**TELEPHONE**
401 North 12th Street　　804-786-4682
Richmond, VA 23298

---

# University of Virginia Hospitals

**CHARLOTTESVILLE, VIRGINIA**

---

In a recent survey taken by the University of Virginia (U of VA) Hospitals, 98 percent of the patients stated they would be willing to return for further treatment and 99 percent expressed satisfaction with the nursing care they received. These statistics represent one of the strongest expressions of patient satisfaction for any of the hospitals we have surveyed in this book.

The U of VA Hospitals are one of the nation's major acute-care referral institutions, serving central and western Virginia. Two units are located away from the main hospital: the 39-bed Children's Rehabilitation Center, which treats children with congenital or acquired handicaps, and the 120-bed Blue Ridge Hospital division, which houses programs in alcohol rehabilitation, diabetes, epilepsy, psychiatry, and tuberculosis.

Designated a Level I Trauma Center for the central Virginia region, U of VA is aided by the use of an emergency helicopter. The program developed here combines trauma-care expertise, an emergency room staffed by attending physicians, twenty-four-hour trauma care by a specially trained trauma team, trauma education programs, and a computerized trauma registry of injuries to measure patients' progress.

The Regional Burn Center here is one of three in the state that provides care to people suffering serious burns. It undertakes patient care, teaching, and research.

At Blue Ridge Hospital is the Diabetes Research and Training Center, one of eight similar centers in the United States funded by the NIH. The center offers programs in assessment, outpatient care, weight control, basic diabetes management, advanced management, and referral to other specialties of the U of VA Medical Center. A special obstetrics/gynecology clinic for diabetic women was recently opened.

Cancer patients are treated at the Surgical Oncology Clinic. Designed for the diagnosis and management of cancer, the clinic also provides follow-up for those whose cancer is treated primarily by surgery. All cases are entered into the Tumor Registry for careful tracking.

The Blue Ridge Poison Control Center intervenes in cases of poisoning, drug side effects, and suicide attempts. It receives about 10,000 calls a year concerning consumer protection, home treatment, or emergency referral.

The recently opened In Vitro Fertilization Clinic, the third such facility in Virginia, expects to treat 50 to 100 patients per year.

The Comprehensive Epilepsy Program encompasses teaching, research, and community service with a 15-bed unit in Blue Ridge Hospital. In a unique technique developed here, patients are videotaped while electroencephalograms are taken; this approach provides objective interpretations in testing patterns.

The state's first Stroke Hotline, established at the medical center, provides information to physicians and the public pertaining to cerebrovascular disease. Physicians can use the hotline to gain information, to facilitate referrals, or to assist with diagnoses. For the public the hotline provides information on the warning signs of stroke, emergency handling of stroke victims, and physician referrals.

The Lions of Virginia Hearing Foundation and Temporal Bone Bank, recently established at the medical center's Department of Otolaryngology, is the first in the state and one of about 50 in the nation, according to Dr. Robert Cantrell, chairman of the otolaryngology department and medical director of the temporal bone bank.

The Pain Management Center treats more than 2,000 patients every year and has served as a model for similar programs elsewhere. Says Dr. John Rowlingson, director, "Our goal is to help the patients develop methods for dealing with their pain themselves, so they can function normally with as little help as possible from doctors and medications."

The medical center provides its patients with all the latest equipment. It began operating one of the country's first six lithotriptors in August 1984. A magnetic resonance imaging device began operating here in August 1985. Since U of VA acquired the YAG laser in September 1984, it has been used in more than 100 operations, primarily for postcataract membranes.

The U of VA Hospital opened in 1901 as a 25-bed facility. Today a new 402-bed hospital is under construction at the university. Designed to ease

---

**STATISTICAL PROFILE**

Number of Beds: 762
Bed Occupancy Rate: 77%
Average Number of Patients: 550
Average Patient Stay: 7.8 days
Annual Admissions: 26,690
Births: 1,700
Outpatient Clinic Visits: 240,000
Emergency Department/Trauma Center Visits: 37,000

Hospital Personnel:
  Physicians: 310
  Residents: 420
  Registered Nurses: 750
  Total Staff: 3,700

overcrowding in the current medical center, the facility is to be completed by March 1988. In addition to the hospital, plans include renovation of the current medical center and other construction projected to cost $225 million.

## Specialties

Anesthesiology, Behavioral Medicine and Psychiatry, Cardiology, Cardiovascular Surgery, Dentistry and Oral Surgery, Dermatology, Endocrinology, Gastroenterology, Maternal and Fetal Medicine, Medicine, Neonatology, Neurology, Neurosurgery, Obstetrics/Gynecology, Oncology, Otolaryngology—Head and Neck Surgery, Orthopedic Surgery, Pediatric Surgery, Pediatrics, Plastic and Maxillofacial Surgery, Psychiatry, Radiology, Radiation Therapy, Rehabilitation, Surgery, Thoracic Surgery, and Urology.

## Well-known Specialists

Dr. Robert Blizzard, pediatric endocrinology.
Dr. Robert W. Cantrell, otolaryngology; medical director of the Temporal Bone Bank.
Dr. John Davis, rheumatology; specialist in lupus research.
Dr. Fritz E. Dreifuss, neurology; specialist in epilepsy.
Dr. Milton Edgerton, plastic surgery.
Dr. Robert M. Epstein, anesthesiology.
Dr. Jay Y. Gillenwater, urology.
Dr. Guy M. Harbert, obstetrics/gynecology; specialist in maternal-fetal medicine.
Dr. Edward W. Hook, specialist in infectious diseases.
Dr. Sharon L. Hostler, pediatrics.
Dr. John Jane, neurosurgery.
Dr. Thomas Richard Johns, neurology.
Dr. Rayford Scott Jones, surgery.
Dr. Neal F. Kassell, neurosurgery.
Dr. John Kattwinkel, neonatology.
Dr. Theodore Keats, radiology.
Dr. Frank McCue, sports medicine and hand surgery.
Dr. William H. Muller, Jr., cardiovascular surgery.
Dr. William O'Brien, internal medicine.
Dr. Warren G. Stamp, orthopedics and rehabilitation.
Dr. John Rowlingson, director of the Pain Management Center.
Dr. Michael O. Thorner, endocrinology.
Dr. Paul Underwood, obstetrics/gynecology.

# Research

In addition to several floors of laboratories, a seven-bed clinical research unit in the University Hospital is the site of a variety of studies under the rigid controls that this type of patient-care facility makes possible. Patients are admitted as volunteer participants in an intensive study of a disease problem, under a research plan or protocol developed by members of the faculty.

The Jerry Lewis Neuromuscular Center is one of ten such centers in the United States. It combines the fields of biochemistry, biology, chemistry, neurology, orthopedics, and physiology.

Basic research on wheelchair propulsion and efficiency is conducted at the Rehabilitation Engineering Center. Among many other mobility devices, computer-controlled chairs for quadriplegics and wheelchairs designed for air travel were developed here.

# Admission Policy

Patients may be admitted to U of VA only by a physician, either through the referral of an attending physician (on or off staff) or through a doctor on duty in one of the clinics or the emergency room.

The stated policy of the U of VA Hospital is to admit all patients requiring medical attention, regardless of their ability to pay. However, for other than emergency services patients are requested to pay the estimated amount of charges not covered by insurance either before or at the time of admission. Provisions are made to waive all or part of the deposit requirement if patients qualify under the established indigent care guidelines.

---

**ROOM CHARGES (per diem)**
Private: $285
Semiprivate: $270
ICU: $999

**MAILING ADDRESS**          **TELEPHONE**
Jefferson Park Avenue         804-924-0211
Charlottesville, VA 22908

---

# Fred Hutchinson
# Cancer Research Center

## SEATTLE, WASHINGTON

The Fred Hutchinson Cancer Research Center is devoted solely to cancer research. Its three divisions—Clinical Research, Basic Sciences, and Public Health Sciences—make up one of the best cancer research institutions in the world. The center, affectionately called the "Hutch" by the people who work here, is staffed by an extraordinary collection of biomedical research and clinical talent.

One of 20 or so Comprehensive Cancer Centers in the United States, the Hutchinson Center was established under the National Cancer Act of 1971. Opened in 1975, it is the only designated cancer center in the Northwest and as such serves Washington, Alaska, Montana, Idaho, and Oregon.

Although its primary function is research, the center accepts bone marrow transplant patients from around the world. In fact, more than 2,200 such transplants have been completed by Dr. E. Donnall Thomas, who pioneered the procedure, and his medical team. Dr. Thomas's team now performs approximately 350 of these transplants a year, making the Hutchinson Center the largest bone marrow transplant unit in the world. Bone marrow transplantation is used to treat patients with aplastic anemia, leukemia, other hematologic disorders, and selected solid tumors. Both children and adults are eligible for bone marrow transplants if they have donors and are physically able to undergo treatment.

Before receiving healthy marrow from a donor, the patient's own diseased or damaged marrow is destroyed with high-dose chemotherapy and/or total body irradiation. This intensive treatment usally takes seven to nine days. The actual transplant is relatively simple. The donor is given general or spinal anesthesia in the operating room. With a special needle, bone marrow is removed from the donor's hip bones, passed through screens, and placed in a blood bag. (The marrow may then be treated with monoclonal antibodies.) Usually within hours, the marrow is given intravenously to the patient, in much the same way as a blood transfusion, except the marrow is infused through a Hickman catheter, which has been implanted in the patient's chest before admission to the hospital.

While waiting for the new "graft" to begin to grow, approximately ten days to three weeks, the patient has no marrow function, leaving him or her susceptible to infection and bleeding problems. Some patients must be kept in laminar-airflow rooms, which provide a totally sterile environment for protection from infection.

There are many risks involved during the course of bone marrow transplantation. Bacterial, viral, and fungal infections, bleeding, and organ failure can all threaten the patient's well-being. Graft-Versus-Host disease occurs in approximately 50 percent of all transplant patients, and causes the patient's marrow to "reject" the patient by attacking major organs such as the skin, liver, and gut. There is also the risk of a nonsuccessful graft or graft failure and of a recurrence of the patient's disease.

Barring complications, the patient is usually discharged to outpatient care 30 to 40 days posttransplant and is treated in Seattle for another 60 to 70 days. It takes a minimum of six to nine months for the immune system to become fully normal.

Many transplant patients come to the Hutchinson Center as a last hope. Because the experience developed at the center has led to a steady increase in survival rates, patients come for this procedure from all across the United States and from 22 overseas nations.

Nearly 200 research projects are also in progress at the center, covering investigations into the fundamental causes of cancer, development of new treatment methods, and education and prevention programs.

The Hutchinson Center has affiliations with major health-care institutions in the Seattle area, including Children's Hospital and Medical Center, Pacific Medical Center, Swedish Hospital, University Hospital (see page 320), Veterans Administration Hospital, and Virginia Mason Medical Center (see page 325).

---

**STATISTICAL PROFILE**

Number of Beds: 60
Bed Occupancy Rate: 100%
Average Number of Patients: 60 (There are always at least 10–15
    patients on a waiting list.)
Average Patient Stay: The normal patient stay in the Seattle area is
    90–100 days; this includes approximately 45 days of inpatient
    care.
Annual Admissions: 350

Hospital Personnel:
    Physicians: There are approximately 50 physicians on the bone
        marrow transplant team; 15–20 of them are in clinical care.
    Total Staff: The transplant team consists of physicians, nurses,
        technicians, dietitians, and social workers, all of whom are
        specially trained in the care of the unique patient population
        here. The transplant program also serves as a training center for
        physicians and paramedical personnel from all over the world.

Most of the center's medical/research staff hold joint appointments in the Division of Oncology of the University of Washington School of Medicine. As a nationally recognized research institution, the Hutchinson Center has collaborative relationships with major research institutions across the United States.

The center was named for Seattle native Fred Hutchinson, a major-league baseball player who died of cancer in 1964 at the age of forty-five. Its funding comes from federal and private grants and contracts, contributions, third-party reimbursement for patient care, dividends, and interest.

## Specialties

Clinical Research, Basic Sciences, and Public Health Sciences.

Bone marrow transplantation is the best-known specialty of Clinical Research.

## Well-known Specialists

Dr. Fred Applebaum, bone marrow transplants.

Dr. Robert Hickman, developer of the Hickman catheter, which is used for access to the patient's circulation both for drawing blood and for administration of transplanted bone marrow, medications, blood products, and nutrition.

Dr. Paul Neiman, head of the Basic Sciences Division.

Dr. E. Donnall Thomas, pioneer in bone marrow transplants, associate director of the Clinical Research Division.

## Research

Clinical research at the Hutchinson Center is devoted primarily to developing effective means of curing a class of hematologic or blood-related cancers—leukemias and lymphoma (including Hodgkin's disease). Research studies within the Clinical Research Division are funded by the National Cancer Institute. Funds for specific projects are also provided by the American Cancer Society, the Leukemia Society of America, and private and civic contributions.

The Public Health Sciences Division studies the occurrence of cancer in human populations and the prevention of cancer. It operates a major registration of new cancer cases that serves as a resource for investigations into the causes of cancer. And it studies interventions that will prevent the recurrence of cancer and conducts public information programs about cancer prevention.

Basic Sciences is concerned with the study of fundamental life processes to help determine why cells transform from normal to malignant. Researchers in this division study cells and gene structures to find new ways of immunizing against cancer and other diseases.

## Admission Policy

A person cannot be admitted to the Hutchinson Center without a physician's referral. To be considered for a bone marrow transplant, a previous diagnosis is necessary; earlier test results must be submitted, along with information on procedures currently being followed. Next, information on the family must be provided to determine if there is a possible donor. The center prefers that the patient's physician call the center's consulting physician. However, if a prospective patient calls, the center's physician may answer some questions and then request that the patient have his or her physician call back.

Marrow transplantation is a complex and expensive procedure requiring intensive care for one to three months. Its costs must be borne by the patient. The hospital therefore requires a guarantee of funds to meet these expenses. For patients who are covered by medical insurance, there is usually no problem. Those who do not have adequate insurance must make a prepayment of $100,000. Billing is made against the prepayment, any unused portion is refunded, and fees in excess of the prepayment are charged to the payer.

When the consulting physicians determine that a patient is a candidate for a marrow transplant, an insurance representative from the center investigates the status of the patient's insurance coverage and obtains other information about the financial ability to provide coverage. If insurance coverage is not adequate, other means of providing the prepayment are discussed with the patient and family members.

Patients are hospitalized in either the Clinical Research Division of the Hutchinson Center or in the Swedish Hospital Medical Center. Swedish Hospital handles all billing.

---

**ROOM CHARGES** (per diem)
Private: $745

**AVERAGE COST OF A BONE MARROW TRANSPLANT**
Room: $35,000 ($745 per day for 45–53 days)
Ancillary: $24,500
Supplies: $10,500
Professional Fees (Staff and Consultants): $10,000

Puget Sound Blood Center (Processing Fees): $10,000
Outpatient Services (Pre- and Posthospital Stay): $7,000
Donor Charges: $3,000
  Total: $100,000

**MAILING ADDRESS**      **TELEPHONE**
1124 Columbia Street    206-467-5000
Seattle, WA 98104

# University Hospital
# University of Washington
**SEATTLE, WASHINGTON**

Although University Hospital is one of the smallest of all teaching hospitals in the United States, among some of the doctors consulted for this book, it is rated as one of the best. A major tertiary-care hospital serving residents of the Pacific Northwest and beyond, University Hospital is a teaching hospital staffed by faculty of the highly regarded University of Washington School of Medicine, who attract an enormous amount (over $70 million) of research funding.

In addition, the high caliber of the nursing staff at University Hospital accounts in large measure for the strength of patient services here. In 1982 the American Academy of Nursing named University Hospital as one of 41 magnet hospitals nationwide because of its success in recruiting and retaining nurses. University Hospital nurses must be registered nurses licensed by the state of Washington; 66 percent have bachelor's or more advanced degrees.

Yet the nursing staff is only one of the factors contributing to the quality of patient care here. The latest diagnostic and treatment equipment, such as a magnetic resonance imaging scanner, CAT scanner, and PET scanner, enhance patient-care services.

The hospital's interdisciplinary Cancer Center has a state-of-the-art cyclotron, for high-energy neutron therapy, funded by the National Cancer Institute. The center has also added four linear accelerators, an outpatient clinic for chemotherapy, equipment to provide external radio frequency therapy, and interstitial hyperthermia equipment. This expanded capability has meant a 300 percent increase in the number of cancer patients seeking treatment here in the past five years. With the opening of the cyclotron, University Hospital became a national referral center for cancer treatment.

The variety of services offered at University Hospital has increased dramatically since the hospital opened in 1959. Today the hospital offers complete medical, surgical, obstetric, psychiatric, and rehabilitation services. It has special units for critically ill adults, patients with kidney disease, and those suffering from heart disease requiring special treatment or surgery. A nationally recognized pain center is also based here. A wide range of specialty clinics provide initial evaluation, outpatient therapy, and follow-up care.

Special programs also include the Northwest Spinal Cord Injury Center (administered by the Department of Rehabilitation Medicine), which was ranked first in research in a 1985 survey.

Doctors at the hospital performed 28 kidney transplants in 1985 and launched a heart transplant program by performing three heart operations. Six more heart transplants were performed in the first half of 1986.

University Hospital's Regional Perinatal Care Center gives specialized care to high-risk pregnant women and premature and newborn ill infants. Many of these patients arrive on Airlift Northwest, an airborne intensive care unit sponsored by four Seattle hospitals, including University Hospital. The system affords everyone in the Pacific Northwest better access to the specialized medical services available in Seattle.

The Division of Reproductive Endocrinology in the Department of Obstetrics and Gynecology provides complete infertility and reproductive services, including in vitro fertilization and artificial insemination. Patients are usually referred by physicians in the Pacific Northwest region. Except for an occasional direct admission to the hospital, women are initially seen as outpatients in the Women's Care Center, one of the University Hospital clinics.

Cornea transplants for infants have been successfully performed at University Hospital, which houses the Lions Eye Bank and Eye Pathology Laboratory. Previously surgery was done on children no younger than three or four, but by that age the visual system's development can be severely retarded so that even a transplant of corneal tissue cannot restore optimal vision. Researchers here are also investigating the causes of diabetic eye disease, glaucoma, and a host of other visual problems.

The hospital's microbiology laboratories also serve as a regional referral center; a number of the tests performed here are not done in any other lab in the area. Technologists and technicians analyze samples for and act as consultants to critical-care medical centers in the Northwest.

In late 1986 University Hospital dedicated the East Wing addition, which provides 114 beds, bringing the hospital's total to 450. Even with these additional beds, University Hospital is still one of the smallest teaching hospitals in the country, which may only go to prove that size is not the only qualification for the best in medical care.

## Specialties

Allergies, Arthritis, Cardiology, Dermatology, Emergency Medicine, Gastroenterology, Genetics, Infectious Diseases, Internal Medicine, Medicine, Neurology and Neurosurgery, Obstetrics and Gynecology, Oncology, Ophthalmology, Oral and Maxillofacial Surgery, Orthopaedics, Otolaryngology/ Head and Neck Surgery, Pediatrics, Plastic Surgery, Psychiatry and Behavioral Medicine, Rehabilitation Medicine, Respiratory Diseases, Surgery, and Urology.

Some of the specialty clinics include the Family Medical Center, Family Service, Gastrointestinal Service, Geriatric Service, Hospital Dental Ser-

---

**STATISTICAL PROFILE (1985–86)**

Number of Beds: 450
Bed Occupancy Rate: 82%
Average Number of Patients: 369
Average Patient Stay: 8.2 days
Annual Admissions: 12,341
Births: 2,031
Outpatient Clinic Visits: 146,423
Emergency Room/Trauma Center Visits: 28,192

Hospital Personnel:
  Physicians: 300 active
  Residents: 500
  Registered Nurses: 545
  Total Staff: 3,064

---

vices, Hypertension, the Metabolic Clinic, Nutrition, the Pain Center, the Renal Clinic, the Thyroid Clinic, the Travel Clinic, Tropical and Infectious Diseases, and the Women's Care Center.

# Well-known Specialists

Dr. Herbert T. Abelson, pediatrics.
Dr. Marjorie E. Anderson, rehabilitation medicine.
Dr. Julian S. Ansell, urology.
Dr. C. James Carrico, surgery.
Dr. Charles W. Cummings, otolaryngology.
Dr. Philip J. Fialkow, medicine.
Dr. John P. Geyman, family medicine.
Dr. Thomas W. Griffin, radiation oncology.
Dr. Thomas F. Hornbein, anesthesiology.
Dr. Robert E. Kalina, ophthalmology; medical director of the Lions Eye Bank.
Dr. Frederick W. Matsen III, orthopedics.
Dr. Albert A. Moss, radiology.
Dr. Russell Ross, pathology.
Dr. Morton A. Stenchever, obstetrics and gynecology.
Dr. Paul E. Strandjord, laboratory medicine.
Dr. Gary J. Tucker, psychiatry and behavioral sciences.
Dr. H. Richard Winn, neurosurgery.

# Research

As of July 1986 research grants supporting University of Washington School of Medicine programs at University Hospital totaled more than $72 million. Primary research areas include AIDS, Alzheimer's disease, cancer, chronic pain, diagnostic imaging, fetal alcohol syndrome, organ transplantation, perinatal medicine, and rehabilitation medicine.

The Clinical Research Center, opened in 1960, was among the original 12 research centers established by the NIH. The first use of bone marrow transplants to treat leukemia, treatment of chronic kidney failure, new methods for the diagnosis and treatment of osteoporosis, and insights into the patterns of sleep and aging are among the research advances that have resulted from studies here.

The University of Washington was recently selected by the NIH to establish one of 14 AIDS Treatment Evaluation Units in the United States. A total of $100 million was awarded to these centers for five years, and the Seattle unit enrolled 50 to 60 patients in 1986.

The hospital's experience in infectious diseases research has led to its appointment as one of 90 hospitals in the United States to participate in an ongoing study conducted by the Centers for Disease Control. The centers and the hospitals are working together to keep track of infections in hospitals and patterns of resistance to antibiotics.

A three-year, $4.5-million grant from the National Cancer Institute has enabled the university to begin staffing the first full-scale imaging research center in the Pacific Northwest. The project, which involves researchers in many disciplines, will study some 20 patients in the first year of a long-term effort to improve cancer therapy by measuring tumor metabolism in response to therapy.

In other cancer research, university researchers have embarked on a new large-scale clinical trial using interleukin-2 and tumor killer cells called LAK cells to treat patients with melanoma and colon, ovarian, and renal cancer.

A newly established Alzheimer's Disease Research Center, one of about ten in the country funded by the National Institute of Aging, makes the University of Washington the only medical center in the United States to have two centers for Alzheimer's research. (An Alzheimer's Clinical Research Center was established a year ago with a grant from the National Institute of Mental Health.) The clinical center focuses on problems of patients with the disease, while the new research center will concentrate on its cause and development. The key project funded by the grant will attempt to show that a single major gene may be involved in families that appear to be hereditarily susceptible to Alzheimer's.

Extensive neonatal research makes University Hospital one of ten U.S. and Canadian clinical centers participating in the High Frequency Intervention Trial recently initiated by the National Heart, Lung, and Blood Institute. The purpose of this trial is to test a new form of mechanical ventilation used for low-birth-weight infants.

## Admission Policy

Patients may be directly admitted through the emergency room or any University Hospital clinic. Anyone may come to the hospital for care; if an individual does not have a personal physician, he or she may choose a primary-care physician or a specialist from the medical staff.

Patients may call the number for new clinic appointments (206-548-4333) to refer themselves, or physicians may call to refer their patients. Physicians may also call specific departments or University Hospital physicians to arrange referrals for inpatient or specialized tests, such as magnetic resonance imaging.

Patients who enter through the Emergency Department or because of medical necessity are admitted without consideration of their financial resources. Private pay patients scheduled for elective admission are asked to make a preadmission deposit. Charity care in fiscal year 1985 totaled close to $1.5 million, and the hospital absorbed another $3 million in bad debts that year.

---

**ROOM CHARGES (per diem)**
Room rates vary from $275 for acute medical/surgical to $780 for critical care. Unlike in most of the hospitals in this book, costs at University Hospital are based on intensity of care. There is no difference in cost between private and semiprivate rooms. (Charges also vary for neonatal intensive care, nursery, oncology, psychiatry, and rehabilitation units.)
ICU: $697

**AVERAGE COST PER PATIENT STAY:**   $4,549

**MAILING ADDRESS**              **TELEPHONE**
1959 Northeast Pacific Street    206-543-3300
Seattle, WA 98195

# Virginia Mason Medical Center

**SEATTLE, WASHINGTON**

While the city of Seattle has several first-rate teaching hospitals—Swedish, Harborview, and University Hospital (see page 320), for example—Virginia Mason Medical Center is decidedly among the best. About 1,000 people a day visit the clinic here, and each year over 280,000 receive some form of treatment. Several thousand come from outside Seattle, including many from Oregon, Idaho, and Montana; over 1,000 a year come from Alaska. Simply put, people come here because of Virginia Mason's excellent reputation in diagnostic medicine and because of the first-rate patient care the hospital offers in many areas, including cancer, diabetes, and heart disease.

Virgina Mason consists of a hospital, a clinic, six satellite clinics in and outside Seattle, and a research center. It offers acute-care services as well as routine treatment and is a major referral center for specialized care.

Founded in 1920 by eight doctors under the leadership of Dr. James Tate Mason (who named the facility after his daughter), the hospital was originally to be a place where people from all walks of life could obtain the care they needed. Patients would receive diagnosis and treatment in the clinic, additional care if needed in the hospital, and ultimate hope for cure from the research center. The concept was called "integrated care."

Since the hospital opened, it has undergone ten major building projects. The medical center has grown from a single five-story building to five separate buildings covering four city blocks.

Today the center functions in somewhat the same way as the Mayo and Cleveland clinics do. Almost 180 doctors representing 41 specialties pool their knowledge to diagnose and treat a wide variety of illnesses. Armed with the most up-to-date diagnostic medical machinery, including CAT scanners, nuclear magnetic resonance imaging, and ultrasound, the physicians here treat even the most complex disorders. Modern medical technology pervades the hospital and includes lasers for surgery and a lithotriptor for crushing kidney stones.

As vital as technology is today, it rarely counts for much when patients evaluate their hospital experience. In response to a recent hospital-sponsored survey, almost 95 percent of patients discharged from Virginia Mason indicated the highest possible recommendation. Predictably, most of the complaints were about the food, but on the most important items the responses were of the kind to instill confidence in all prospective patients. For example, 96 percent surveyed reported that they had received sufficient information about their illnesses and been given choices concerning treatment whenever possible. The nursing staff, too, received excellent marks; 96 percent said the nurses were "sensitive to the needs of families and visitors."

The nursing staff at Virginia Mason is exceptional. Over 40 percent have bachelor's degrees, and all have experience in specialty areas. A special program known as "collaborative practice" allows nurses to participate actively with doctors in planning and coordinating patient care. Nursing careers are given top priority by the Virginia Mason administration, and as a result the turnover rate for nurses is less that 10 percent a year. In 1982 the American Academy of Nursing recognized Virginia Mason as one of 41 magnet hospitals in the nation, that is, a hospital that attracts and retains a highly qualified nursing staff.

Staffed by nurses trained in cancer care, the N. Peter Canlis Cancer Care Unit has 26 beds. Virginia Mason is one of the largest cancer treatment and diagnostic centers in the region, treating more than 70 patients a day and 1,600 new cancer patients a year.

Approximately 300 patients receive operations for heart disease here annually. Coronary bypass surgery mortality risk is under 1 percent at Virginia Mason, and the hospital has a high success rate for kidney transplants and open-heart surgery. In 1985 doctors at Virginia Mason completed 34 kidney transplants, the highest number of transplants in the area.

The hospital has its own private hotel—the Mason House—with seven floors of rooms for out-of-town patients and their families. Short Stay Surgery is designed for patients requiring procedures that do not necessitate an overnight hospital stay. This was the first such program in the region. Seattle's first hospital-based midwifery program was initiated here. Virginia Mason was also one of the first hospitals to permit fathers to be present during deliveries.

Other special facilities include the largest hyperbaric chamber and facility in the Northwest; The Buse Diabetes Teaching Center, where diabetic patients learn to live with greater independence (over 10,000 diabetics are treated annually at Virginia Mason); and the Sports Medicine Center, which provides care for athletes with sports injuries as well as conditioning facilities and educational programs for all athletes. A health promotion service called SENSE provides consulting services to local businesses and offers a range of programs.

In the 1920s Virginia Mason instituted the region's first postgraduate program for doctors. In 1985, 75 physicians (chosen from over 600 applicants) received postgraduate training here; 27 of them completed residency specialties.

Since the hospital's first intern came in 1925, more than 1,000 medical school graduates have received their internship, residency, or fellowship training here—and the physician training program is still growing. Through Virginia Mason's clerkship program, more than 100 students from around the United States have come to the hospital for brief periods to train in special areas.

Virginia Mason was one of the first medical centers in the Seattle area to offer continuing education programs to doctors and is a regional provider of accredited continuing medical education. Twelve workshops, symposiums, lectures, and practical demonstrations are offered each year.

## Specialties

Treatment at Virginia Mason encompasses everything from primary practice in the satellite clinics to subspecialties in all aspects of medicine. Major specialties include Anesthesiology, Cancer, Cardiology, Critical Care, Diabetes, Diagnostic Medicine, Infectious Diseases, Intensive Care, Kidney Dialysis and Transplantation, Obstetrics and Midwifery, Oncology, Physical Medicine, and Surgery.

---

**STATISTICAL PROFILE**

Number of Beds: 309
Bed Occupancy Rate: 72.5%
Average Number of Patients: 224
Average Patient Stay: 6.3 days
Annual Admissions: 13,002
Births: 1,177
Outpatient Clinic Visits: 315,280 (including satellite clinics)
Emergency Room/Trauma Center Visits: 16,048

Hospital Personnel:
   Physicians: 175
   Residents: 75
   Registered Nurses: 423
   Total Staff: 1,892

---

## Well-known Specialists

Dr. Richard P. Anderson, cardiothoracic surgery.
Dr. L. Frederick Fenster, liver and biliary tract disorders.
Dr. Patrick L. Freeny, radiology.
Dr. Robert P. Gibbons, urology.
Dr. Lucius D. Hill, general, thoracic, and vascular surgery; developer of the Hill procedure for hernias.
Dr. Robert J. Metz, endocrinology; specialist in diabetes.

Dr. Willis J. Taylor, radiation oncology; former president of the American Cancer Society.

Dr. Gale Thompson, anesthesiology.

Dr. Kenneth R. Wilske, immunology, allergy, and rheumatic diseases; author of several books on arthritis.

Dr. Richard H. Winterbauer, chest and infectious diseases.

# Research

The Virginia Mason Research Center is not as large or well known as many of the research groups described in this book, but the scientists here have made contributions in many fields, especially arthritis, asthma, cancer, and diabetes. The 100 ongoing research projects are usually linked to the hospital's concerns. For example, bone marrow transplant patients can receive care at Virginia Mason while participating in the studies of the Fred Hutchinson Cancer Research Center (see page 315). The research center also conducts national studies on bladder, lung, and prostate cancer, leukemia, and lymphoma.

Other fields of research include implantable prosthetics for the deaf, decompression, diagnostic equipment such as arterial dopplers, eye surgery, heart problems, high blood pressure, synthetic hip replacements, immunology, infection, the insulin pump, pain relief, patient treatment studies, and the use of carbon fibers in wrist surgery.

The research center receives funding from a variety of sources, including many donations by area residents, physicians, and corporations. Grants have also been made by the NIH, the American Cancer Society, Battelle Northwest, the Cancer Research Institute, the Seattle Foundation, and the Washington Lung Association. In 1984 the center received over $2.3 million in grants and $700,000 in donations.

# Admission Policy

Patients are seen at Virginia Mason twenty-four hours a day, with or without a physician referral. Although patients have to be formally admitted to the hospital by a physician with privileges, anyone can come to the clinic or to one of the satellites for treatment and then be admitted. In fact, 95 percent of all hospital admissions are through the clinic.

The hospital does not have a financial requirement except for certain kinds of elective surgery. While no one in need of medical treatment is turned away, Virginia Mason and several other area hospitals share the burden of indigent care, so the hospital may arrange to send an incoming patient without resources somewhere else.

**ROOM CHARGES** (per diem)
Private: $265
Semiprivate: $265
ICU: $865
Room Charges at Mason House:
  Single: $36
  Double: $41
  Suite: $52

**AVERAGE COST PER PATIENT STAY:**   $4,434

**MAILING ADDRESS**          **TELEPHONE**
Hospital:                    Hospital: 206-624-1114
  Box 1920                   Clinic: 206-223-6600
  925 Seneca Street
  Seattle, WA 98111
Clinic:
  Box 900
  1100 Ninth Avenue
  Seattle, WA 98111

# University of Wisconsin Hospital and Clinics

**MADISON, WISCONSIN**

The University of Wisconsin Hospital and Clinics (UWHC) is a major tertiary-care referral center servicing all of Wisconsin and parts of Illinois, Iowa, upper Michigan, and Minnesota. Almost 20 percent of patients here are from out of state, and about 70 percent of those from Wisconsin are from out of the county. Attending physicians at UWHC are members of the UW Medical School faculty. As a major teaching institution, UWHC is a leading center for patient care, biomedical research, education of health professionals, and public service. Its range of medical specialties and services is among the most complete we've come across.

According to the National Transplant Registry, UWHC has the nation's third largest renal transplant center (after the University of California at San Francisco and The University of Alabama [see page 15]) and the second largest pancreas transplant center (after the University of Minnesota [see page 185]), a distinction of special note given the small size of the surrounding community. The hospital significantly advanced its role as a regional transplant center by incorporating active heart and liver transplantation programs in 1984–85. The state of Wisconsin has the highest per capita rate of organ donation in the nation, and the UW procurement team is on twenty-four-hour alert to take calls from any donor hospital or clinic. Since 1966, 1,589 kidney transplants have been performed here. The hospital's program offers both living-related and cadaveric renal transplants. It is also a leader in nonrelated living donor transplants, specializing in spousal transplants.

Success rates in transplantation of UWHC have exceeded the national average. For example, since July 1984, 39 liver transplants have been performed by Dr. Munci Kalayoglu with a patient survival rate of 91 percent, compared with the national rate of just over 65 percent. (Dr. Kalayoglu's patients include nine children, with a 100 percent success rate.) Worldwide, pancreatic transplant patients have a 25 percent success rate after one year. The 66 pancreatic transplants performed by Dr. Hans Sollinger at UWHC between 1982 and 1985 have had a 50 percent success rate. University of Wisconsin Hospital and Clinics is also a leading innovator in transplanting bone marrow between mismatched donors and recipients.

The University of Wisconsin Clinical Cancer Center is one of 20 or so Comprehensive Cancer Centers in the United States funded by the NIH. The center offers a broad range of standard and specialized treatments for cancer and is pioneering new therapies such as hyperthermia, immune modulators such as interferon and interleukin-2, and radiobiology. The center made headlines in 1985 as the second site nationwide for clinical tests of interleukin-2.

Each year the center treats more than 300 children with cancer. The first formal protocol in the world for marrow transplantation in children with brain tumors was developed here. The center is internationlly known for its work in areas such as breast and bladder cancers and medical oncology. The Chemosurgery Clinic for the treatment of skin cancer offers a technique developed and refined at UWHC. Cancerous growths are removed under plane-by-plane microscopic control, assuring complete excision of the cancer without removing extra skin. The center's Cancer Prevention Clinic offers cancer risk assessment, preventive health care counseling and education, and special medical examinations and tests.

The cardiology department at UWHC is one of the largest in the Midwest, with 15 full-time cardiologists on staff. They have teamed with a cardiac surgery department that specializes in all aspects of adult and pediatric cardiac surgery and transplantation. This is among the few facilities in the country to have developed expertise in the repair of complex thoracoab-dominal aneurysms and was among the first institutions to introduce a promising clot-dissolving drug, TPA (tissue plasminogen activator), in 1986.

The University of Wisconsin Hospital and Clinics is also a major center for the study and treatment of children's lung disease and was recently designated a federal Pediatric Pulmonary Center through a $1.5-million training grant from the U.S. Department of Health and Human Services. The UW Pediatric Center is a major center for the study and treatment of cystic fibrosis.

Ophthalmologists here have played leading roles in the National Eye Institute trials demonstrating the effectiveness of lasers in treating diabetic retinopathy and macular degeneration. The department is also known for its program in ophthalmologic plastic and reconstructive surgery and main-tains clinics in all other subspecialty areas of ophthalmology, such as cornea transplants, glaucoma, hereditary retinal disease, and low vision. Lasers are being successfully used here to halt disease, and the Ophthalmology De-partment was a key participant in national studies demonstrating the effec-tiveness of laser treatment for various eye disorders.

Special programs in the department of psychiatry include its nationally renowned Center for Affective Disorders, which treats mood swings, par-ticularly depression and manic depression; the Lithium Information Center; Child and Adolescent Psychiatric Services; the Couples/Family Therapy Clinic; and the Anxiety Disorders Clinic, which provides care for patients who suffer from anxiety, panic attacks, phobias, and other related disorders.

The UW Sports Medicine and Fitness Center offers comprehensive care to improve health fitness and well-being. Diagnosis, treatment, and reha-bilitation of sports-related injuries, as well as specialized care for acute and chronic medical problems, are among the services provided by the center's team of sports medicine physicians, athletic trainers, exercise physiologists, and physician therapists.

The department of plastic and reconstructive surgery offers expert care in all aspects of plastic surgery. Major specialty areas include cancer surgery, cleft lip and palate anomalies, cosmetic surgery, craniofacial and maxillofacial surgery, hand surgery, microsurgery and replantation, and reconstructive surgery.

The Rehabilitation Center provides a comprehensive program for patients with chronic pain, head injuries, neuromuscular disabilities and related disabling conditions, and spinal cord injuries.

The Neuromuscular Retraining Clinic, part of the center's Brain Injury Program, is the only program of its kind in the nation, offering intensive outpatient rehabilitation therapy for patients with debilitating brain injuries leading to paralysis, muscular spasms, or tremors. The innovative therapy involves "retraining" portions of the brain to assume functions once controlled by the damaged area. Notable successes have been observed, some in patients chronically disabled for years. Unfortunately, the waiting list for the clinic can be as long as two years.

The University of Wisconsin Hospital and Clinics is rapidly expanding services to the community. For instance, it has opened the Women's Health Center. The new Immunology Clinic will continue to probe the causes and treatment of immunologic diseases, including AIDS. A state-of-the-art image processing laboratory enables physicians to combine findings from the catheterization lab with results from nuclear scanning, echocardiography, and electrophysiological tests.

Recognizing the need to share resources, UWHC has recently expanded affiliation agreements with other health-care providers. Cooperative arrangements with Southwest Health Center, Beloit Memorial Hospital, Neillsville Memorial Hospital, and Freeport Memorial Hospital permit UWHC to provide educational, clinical, and administrative support in a wide range of professional disciplines.

The hospital also offers a critical-care helicopter service and a mobile unit that functions as an intensive care unit on wheels.

The quality of health care at a hospital can often best be described by its former patients. "I'm kind of a 'regular patient' at your hospital because of my condition. I live 230 miles away from your hospital but still drive that far just for checkups at the clinic. I've been to several other hospitals years ago but after coming to the UW Hospital, Madison, I'll never go anywhere else. In my opinion, it's the best hospital in the country."

This comment is fairly typical of the glowing testimonials given to this hospital by its former patients. In 1984, 95 percent of the people who responded to the hospital's questionnaire reported they were very satisfied or satisfied with their stay at the hospital according to 16 variables. Nearly 97 percent were very satisfied with the care provided by their physicians and nurses.

Part of this high measure of patient satisfaction is attributable to the hospital's new facility on a forty-five-acre site on the University of Wisconsin, Madison, campus. Here, patient rooms were specifically designed for maximum privacy; all hospital rooms have their own bathrooms and large windows with views.

## Specialties

Anesthesiology, Family Medicine and Practice, Internal Medicine (including Cardiology and Emergency Medicine), Neurology, Obstetrics/Gynecology, Oncology, Ophthalmology, Pathology, Pediatric Intensive Care, Pediatrics, Psychiatry, Radiology, Rehabilitation Medicine, and Surgery.

Special areas of expertise include bone marrow transplantation, burn treatment, cancer, cardiac intensive care, cardiovascular surgical care, children's lung disease, critical care, eating disorders, eye care, in vitro fertilization, organ transplantation, poison control, sleep disorders, sports medicine, and trauma.

All the major departments at UWHC run specialty clinics. Among the more than 70 clinics, several are particularly well known: Affective Disorders, Cardiac Rehabilitation, the Eye Clinic, Neuromuscular Retraining, Oncology, and the Sports Medicine and Fitness Center. In addition, five outpatient clinics are located around Madison and surrounding communities. Home programs exist for patients needing intravenous care or respiratory treatments.

---

**STATISTICAL PROFILE**

Number of Beds: 503
Bed Occupancy Rate: 70%
Average Number of Patients: 350 per day
Average Patient Stay: 8.3 days
Annual Admissions: 15,618
Outpatient Clinic Visits: 299,084
Emergency Room/Trauma Center Visits: 15,000

Hospital Personnel:
  Physicians: 575 (402 active; 173 courtesy)
  Residents: 434 (356 house staff; 73 fellows)
  Registered Nurses: 812
  Total Staff: 3,510

# Well known Specialists

Dr. Folkert O. Belzer, surgery; transplant surgeon and researcher, developer of the Belzer perfusion pump used to preserve donor kidneys.

Dr. Paul P. Carbone, oncology; specialist in breast cancer.

Dr. John W. Chandler, ophthalmology; specialist in corneal disease and transplantation.

Dr. William G. Clancy, orthopedic surgery; specialist in sports medicine.

Dr. David G. Dibbell, plastic and reconstructive surgery; specialist in cleft lip and palate surgery.

Dr. Philip M. Farrell, pediatrics; authority on children's lung diseases.

Dr. Richard Hong, pediatrics and medical microbiology; specialist in pediatric immunology, leader in new immunologic techniques.

Dr. Manucher Javid, neurosurgery; pioneer of the chymopapain injection procedure for slipped discs.

Dr. James Jefferson, psychiatry; specialist in manic depression and the use of lithium.

Dr. Dennis G. Maki, infectious diseases.

# Research

With over $40 million in public and private grants coming to the medical school each year, UW is one of the leading research institutions in the country. Almost half of this money is given for clinical research, so the hospital and clinics have extensive ongoing programs.

The largest single research area is oncology, which receives about $15 million in funding a year. Clinical work includes use of drug therapies, such as interferon and interleukin-2, as well as new treatments including whole body hyperthermia and localized hyperthermia in conjunction with radiotherapy.

Other major research programs exist in pediatrics, where important work in immunology and cystic fibrosis are under way, and ophthalmology, especially in diabetic retinopathy. Another diabetes project still in the experimental stage is seeking a way to inject diabetics with material bearing the islets of Langerhans.

Doctors at UW are also researching techniques to prevent rejection of transplanted organs. In the 1970s physicians found that blood transfusions from a living related donor prevented early rejection. This procedure has been undergoing continued research at UW and has been adopted for use in non-living-related transplants.

Organ preservation techniques are being investigated to increase preservation time for hearts, livers, and pancreases. One goal is to be able to perform these operations on a nonemergency basis, as is now possible with kidneys. Preliminary laboratory work at UW indicates that liver perfusion may extend liver storage time from ten to as many as seventy-two hours.

Research into a new cold storage solution may increase pancreas storage time to forty-eight hours or more.

Physicians in the UW Cardiology Department are investigating TPA as well as other new drugs for heart arrhythmias and cardiomyopathy. A variety of basic research projects are also under way, from study of the heart's microcirculation to investigation of how disease impairs heart muscle function and metabolism.

Physicians in UW's Radiology Department are working to improve diagnostic techniques. Using magnetic resonance imaging technology, researchers are investigating the chemistry of the body, detection of substances in diseased tissue, and new ways to image the heart and blood flow. Digital subtraction angiography, a process allowing more accurate X-ray examination of blood vessels, was developed in part through research conducted at UW.

## Admission Policy

A doctor's referral is not necessary for admission to UWHC unless it is required by the patient's health insurance plan. Patients can be admitted without referral through the emergency room or one of the clinics. Any patient may make an appointment at one of UWHC's clinics by calling the hospital. The phone number for general information about the clinics is 608-263-8580.

The hospital does not have a financial requirement for admission, except for certain elective procedures, such as cosmetic surgery and in vitro fertilization. In 1985 charity care totaled $1.5 million, and another $2.5 million in uncollectible debts was absorbed.

---

**ROOM CHARGES (per diem)**
Private: $199
Semiprivate: $199
ICU: $708

**AVERAGE COST PER PATIENT STAY:**   $5,923.20

**MAILING ADDRESS**      **TELEPHONE**
600 Highland Avenue   608-263-6400
Madison, WI 53792

---

# Index to Names
## of Medical Professionals

# General Index

Absorptive disorders, treatment, 117
Accreditation, of hospitals, 5
*Accreditation Manual for Hospitals*, 5
Acne, treatment, 232
Acoustic neuromas, 65
Acquired immune deficiency syndrome. *See* AIDS
Acupuncture, 47
Addiction, 61. *See also* Alcohol and drug dependency
Admission policy, 11
Adolescent disorders, specialists in, 152
Adolescent gynecology, hospitals/clinics specializing in, 156
Adolescent health. *See* Adolescent medicine
Adolescent medicine
  hospitals/clinics specializing in, 17, 33, 39, 52, 76, 91, 103, 123, 146, 151, 211, 226, 303
  specialists in, 43
Adolescent pregnancy, 122
  hospitals/clinics specializing in, 123
Adolescent psychiatry, 75, 117, 226. *See also* Child psychiatry
  hospitals/clinics specializing in, 84, 175, 181, 229
  specialists in, 113
Adoptive immunotherapy, 127
Adrenal disease, specialists in, 103
Adult respiratory distress syndrome, specialists in, 91
Affective disorders. *See also* Bipolar disorder; Depression; Mania; Manic depression
  hospitals/clinics specializing in, 123, 152, 228, 333
  specialists in, 91
  treatment, 259, 331
Aging, 17. *See also* Geriatrics and gerontology
  hospitals/clinics specializing in, 241
  research, 35, 54, 63, 92, 127, 225, 239–40, 247, 323
    specialists in, 134
  specialists in, 76, 129
AIDS
  hospitals/clinics specializing in, 52, 129
  research, 35, 49, 54, 77, 119, 125, 129, 134, 158, 229, 236, 268, 323

  specialists in, 267
  specialists in, 133, 163, 167, 235
  treatment, 332
Air embolism, treatment, 260
Alcohol, research, 92, 213, 247
Alcohol abuse. *See* Alcohol and drug dependency
Alcohol addiction. *See* Alcohol and drug dependency
Alcohol and drug abuse. *See* Alcohol and drug dependency
Alcohol and drug dependency
  adolescent, hospitals/clinics specializing in, 181
  hospitals/clinics specializing in, 91, 112, 151, 171, 181, 188, 228, 290, 303
  research, 40, 127, 152, 286
  specialists in, 113, 129
  treatment, 28, 37, 84, 167, 227, 289
Alcohol dependency. *See* Alcohol and drug dependency
Alcoholism
  children at risk for, research on, 177
  hospitals/clinics specializing in, 224
  research, 40, 127, 213
  specialists in, 113, 129, 152, 224
  treatment, 121, 122, 167, 227, 283
Alcohol rehabilitation, 311
Allergy
  hospitals/clinics specializing in, 17, 34, 39, 52, 57, 76, 86, 96, 102, 107, 118, 123, 132, 138, 146, 156, 162, 171, 177, 181, 187, 211, 217, 234, 240, 260, 266, 303, 308, 321
  pediatric, hospitals/clinics specializing in, 181
  research, 127
  specialists in, 40, 44, 58, 129, 183, 229, 328
  treatment, 18, 21, 38, 56, 57, 61, 75, 95, 210
ALS. *See* Amyotrophic lateral sclerosis
Alzheimer's disease, 2
  hospitals/clinics specializing in, 34, 52, 107, 129
  research, 54, 98, 109, 125, 129, 134, 138, 152, 189, 213, 219, 229, 236, 262, 295, 323
  specialists in, 53, 76, 108, 125, 138, 188, 212, 235, 242, 294

Joint motion, research, 202
Joint repair, 84
Joint replacement, 22, 23, 89, 137, 155, 180, 190, 200, 248. *See also* Artificial joints
specialists in, 23, 91, 218
Joint scans, 16
Joint surgery, reconstructive, 16
Joint transplantation, 259
Juvenile diabetes
hospitals/clinics specializing in, 76, 103
research, 30, 63, 98, 139
specialists in, 77, 212
treatment, 95, 210, 217
Juvenile rheumatoid arthritis, 18, 57

Karposi's sarcoma, research, 236
Kidney cancer, research, 163, 178, 323
Kidney disease
hospitals/clinics specializing in, 187, 303, 322
research, 40, 63, 127, 134, 286
specialists in, 63
treatment, 15, 27, 101, 144, 170, 307, 320
Kidney failure
in children, specialists in, 188
research, 323
treatment, 15, 101
Kidney function, research, 285
Kidney stones
hospitals/clinics specializing in, 91, 172, 217
specialists in, 71, 97
treatment, 32, 38, 80, 101, 155, 170, 187, 192, 227, 258, 293, 325
Kidney transplantation, 15, 16, 27, 32, 33, 46, 51, 53, 60, 69, 70, 80, 89, 95, 101, 102, 106, 116, 121, 136, 138, 155, 170, 174, 180, 185, 190, 211, 216, 228, 239, 248, 250, 258, 269, 283, 284, 288, 290, 293, 302, 306, 308, 321, 326, 327, 330
pediatric, hospitals/clinics specializing in, 103
pretransplant blood transfusion, specialists in, 193
specialists in, 18, 34, 43, 72, 81, 97, 138, 193, 212, 241, 246, 295
Knee, artificial, 22
Knee disorders, specialists in, 103
Knee injury, research, 202
Knee replacement
research, 92
specialists in, 202

Laboratory medicine
hospitals/clinics specializing in, 28, 123, 187, 250, 260, 299
specialists in, 322
LAK cell therapy, research, 323
Language disorders, research, 54
Laryngeal cancer, treatment, 192, 205
Laser bronchoscopy, 27
Laser catheterization, research, 251
Laser linear accelerators, 106, 107
Lasers, 106, 169, 185, 190, 293
dermatologic applications, 174
in lung cancer treatment, 169
in neurosurgery, 183
for ocular disorders. *See* Lasers, ophthalmologic applications
in oncological surgery, 298
research, 242, 291
ophthalmologic applications, 75, 122, 191, 275, 331
research, 278
specialists in, 124
in port wine stain treatment, specialists in, 133
research on, 35, 77–78, 158
specialists in, 147, 162, 290
surgery, 32, 51, 52, 79, 80, 84, 144, 161, 283, 289, 303, 325
hospitals/clinics specializing in, 53, 290, 303
in treatment of dermatologic birth defects, 155
in treatment of precancerous conditions, specialists in, 188
in vasectomy reversal, 166
Lead poisoning, hospitals/clinics specializing in, 217
Learning disorders, 17
hospitals/clinics specializing in, 118, 157, 181
research, 54
treatment, 66, 75, 111, 187, 265
Left ventricular dysfunction, research, 295
Leg reattachment, 166
Leprosy, specialists in, 147
Lesch-Nyhan syndrome, specialists in, 53
Leukemia
acute lymphocytic, treatment, 279
adult, treatment, 204
childhood, 140
psychological treatment, 280
research, 143
specialists in, 300
treatment, 101, 161, 205
lymphatic, hospitals/clinics specializing in, 224

Orthotics, 240
Osteoarthritis
  research, 202
  treatment, 102
Osteogenesis imperfecta, research, 202
Osteogenic sarcoma, 140
  treatment, 280
Osteomalacia
  research, 202
  treatment, 102
Osteomyelitis, treatment, 260
Osteoporosis
  hospitals/clinics specializing in, 91, 177,
    197, 200
  rehabilitation, 22
  research, 139, 158, 172, 183, 202, 323
  specialists in, 104, 172, 202
  treatment, 61, 84, 102, 170, 175, 211
Osteoradionecrosis, treatment, 260
Otolaryngology/Otorhinolaryngology
  hospitals/clinics specializing in, 33, 62,
    71, 80, 86, 96, 102, 107, 118, 123,
    146, 155, 167, 171, 176, 181, 192,
    212, 217, 231, 234, 240, 256, 260,
    292–94, 312, 313, 321
  research, 213
  specialists in, 43, 44, 86, 162, 218, 251,
    285, 294, 313, 322
Otology, 39, 234
Otorhinolaryngology. See Otolaryngology
Outpatient surgery, 181
Ovarian cancer
  research, 235, 268, 323
  specialists in, 103
  treatment, 22, 51, 123, 140, 232
Ovulation induction, 161

Pacemaker, 134, 217
Paget's disease
  research, 158
  treatment, 47
Paget's disease of bone, treatment, 102
Pain
  with cancer (oncologic)
    specialists in, 207
    treatment, 74, 92, 205
  in children, treatment, 66
  hospitals/clinics specializing in, 197, 267,
    299, 303
  intractable
    research on, 38
    treatment, 74
  research, 198, 323
  in rheumatoid arthritis, research, 139
  specialists in, 241
  treatment, 16–17, 28, 38, 47, 61, 91, 108,

122, 123, 138, 157, 161, 162, 167,
  175, 177, 206, 217, 226, 238, 240,
  254, 259, 265, 270, 283, 306, 312,
  320, 322, 332
  research, 328
  specialists in, 177, 313
Pancreas cancer, specialists in, 300
Pancreas surgery, 144
  specialists in, 147
Pancreas transplantation, 16, 46, 80, 106,
  121, 155, 174, 185, 248, 254, 258,
  269, 283, 330
  research, 262
  specialists in, 188
Pancreatic autotransplants, 144
Pancreatic disease
  research, 72
  specialists in, 124
  treatment, 144
Panic attacks, treatment, 331
Paralysis, stroke-caused, specialists in, 294
Parasitic disease, research, 35
Parathyroid gland, treatment, 170
Parent Care Unit, 103
Parenteral nutrition, research, 177
PAR Image Analyzer, 275
Parkinsonism. See Parkinson's disease
Parkinson's disease
  research, 98, 213, 220, 229, 236, 286
  specialists in, 91, 235, 295
  treatment, 74, 183, 211, 215, 283
Patent ductus arteriosus, indocin treat-
  ment, research, 49
Pathology, 74
  hospitals/clinics specializing in, 17, 28,
    33, 39, 48, 52, 62, 67, 71, 74, 80,
    86, 96, 107, 118, 123, 156, 167, 176,
    187, 192, 197, 206, 212, 217, 234,
    240, 245, 256, 260, 272, 277, 281,
    303, 333
  specialists in, 40, 86, 108, 285, 290,
    322
Patient satisfaction, 9
Patient studies, hospitals/clinics specializing in, 299
Pediatric critical care, 89
Pediatric intensive care, 28, 70, 117, 186,
  226, 250, 333
  specialists in, 30, 158
Pediatric metabolism, specialists in, 242
Pediatrics
  hospitals/clinics specializing in, 17, 21,
    22, 26–28, 33, 34, 39, 42, 43, 48, 52,
    62, 67, 71, 76, 80, 86, 95, 96, 107,
    121, 123, 146, 156, 171, 175, 176,
    181, 185, 187, 206, 212, 217, 228,